W9-BVS-075

Supercharge Your Health,
Strip Away Pounds, and
Eliminate the Toxins Within

the detox
prescription

Woodson Merrell, MD,
with Mary Beth Augustine, MS, RDN,
and Hillari Dowdle

With a foreword by **DEAN ORNISH, MD**

RODALE.

This book is intended as a reference volume only, not as a medical manual. The information given here is designed to help you make informed decisions about your health. It is not intended as a medical prescription or a substitute for any treatment that may have been prescribed by your doctor. If you suspect that you have a medical problem, we urge you to seek competent medical help.

Mention of specific companies, organizations, or authorities in this book does not imply endorsement by the author or publisher, nor does mention of specific companies, organizations, or authorities imply that they endorse this book, its author, or the publisher.

Internet addresses and telephone numbers given in this book were accurate at the time it went to press.

© 2013 by Woodson Merrell, MD

All rights reserved. No part of this publication may be reproduced or transmitted in any form or by any means, electronic or mechanical, including photocopying, recording, or any other information storage and retrieval system, without the written permission of the publisher.

Rodale books may be purchased for business or promotional use or for special sales. For information, please write to: Special Markets Department, Rodale Inc., 733 Third Avenue, New York, NY 10017.

Printed in the United States of America

Rodale Inc. makes every effort to use acid-free ∞, recycled paper ♲.

Book design by Chris Rhoads

Medical Symptom Questionnaire © 2013 by the Institute for Functional Medicine. Used with permission.

Dirty Dozen Plus and Clean Fifteen © 2013 by Environmental Working Group, www.ewg.org. Reprinted with permission.

Library of Congress Cataloging-in-Publication Data is on file with the publisher.

ISBN-13: 978–1–60961–535–2 hardcover

Distributed to the trade by Macmillan

4   6   8   10   9   7   5   3   hardcover

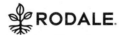

We inspire and enable people to improve their lives and the world around them.

rodalebooks.com

For my brilliant and beautiful wife, Kathy, and my bundles
of joy and inspiration, Caitlin and Isabel. —W.M.

To my superduper amazing daughters, Brynne and Rhiannon; to my husband
and best friend, Tim; to my wonderfully supportive parents, siblings, family, and friends;
to cancer survivors everywhere; and to all the individuals who have allowed me
the great honor of using food as medicine to share in their care. —M.B.A.

To the brilliant writers Martha Hume and Chet Flippo, my newly minted
guardian angels. And to the Turczyn boys, Truman and Coury, who remind me that
health and happiness are life's biggest priorities. —H.D.

Contents

Foreword by Dean Ornish, MD vii • Introduction x

CHAPTER **ONE**

What's the Problem?   1

A thorough explanation of what toxins are, where they come from, and how they're
wrecking your life. Plus: case studies of real people—and real results.

CHAPTER **TWO**

How Toxic Are You?   29

Two self-administered tests help you determine how toxins are affecting your health and
your home, and let you decide how serious the problem really is.

CHAPTER **THREE**

The Detox Continuum   48

Whether you need a little tune-up or a major overhaul, the Detox Prescription can meet
your needs with a 3-, 7-, or 21-day plan based on the best in current nutrition science.

CHAPTER **FOUR**

Get Ready, Get Set . . . Go!   71

Once you decide which plan is for you, we'll help you prepare your kitchen, body, mind,
and spirit for success.

CHAPTER **FIVE**

The 3-Day Turbo Cleanse   98

Three days' worth of juices, smoothies, and nut milks will yield quick results and kick-start
your energy! Plus: a guide to the best possible smoothie boosters.

CHAPTER **SIX**

The 7-Day In-Depth Detox 134

A weeklong juices-and-foods plan that will deepen your detox results and reset your health. Plus: detoxifying teas and grab-and-go snacks.

CHAPTER **SEVEN**

The 21-Day Clean and Lean Diet 177

Three weeks to cleanse your mind and body, gain great new eating habits, and lose weight in a sustainable way. Plus: sensationally sweet desserts that offer detoxifying side benefits.

CHAPTER **EIGHT**

Beyond the Detox Prescription 289

What to do if you've tried everything and still need help: our guide to meditation, elimination diets, integrative therapies, saunas, probiotics, enzymes, medical foods, smart supplements, and more.

CHAPTER **NINE**

The Science of Detox 319

Every cell in the body can go through the phases of detoxification. We'll explain how that happens, why nutrition is so critical to the process, and what measures you can take to support the detox process at the cellular level through smart use of targeted foods and nutraceuticals.

Acknowledgments 338 • Index 340

Foreword

This book can transform your life. Here's why:

Our bodies often have a remarkable capacity to begin healing if we allow them to do so—to a much greater degree and more quickly than had previously been realized—if we simply stop doing what's causing the problem.

So much of Western medicine is based on the supposition that we need to get our health from outside ourselves. The internist says, "Take this pill, you'll feel better." The surgeon says, "To cut is to cure."

But we now know better. For most people, health is not something we *get*; it's something that we already have until we damage it.

The concept of detoxification is to identify what is harmful to your health and to stop doing it. This simple idea allows your body to maximize its potential for healing.

In this context, the most useful question can be, "What am I doing that is disturbing my inner health?" For a surprising number of chronic diseases, the answers are:

• what we eat;

• how we respond to stress;

• how much we exercise;

• whether or not we smoke cigarettes;

• how much we sleep;

• how much love and support we have in our lives.

In this wonderful new book, Dr. Woodson "Woody" Merrell broadens the concept of detoxification beyond food to include these other aspects of our lives that so profoundly affect our health.

When we realize what's causing the problem, we can make different choices that allow our bodies to begin healing. Dr. Merrell shows how, and why. He can help you tailor a program that's just right for you, one that is based on good science and extensive clinical experience. You've come to the right place.

I've known and admired Dr. Merrell for many years. He is a renowned leader and pioneering clinician helping to create a new paradigm of true health care, rather than just sick care—one that is more caring and compassionate as well as more cost effective and competent. He is an extraordinary healer and educator. His patients love him, and so do I. You're in good hands.

We often think of advances in medicine as something high-tech and expensive: a new drug, a powerful laser, an innovative surgical technique. It may seem hard to believe that such simple aspects of our lifestyles can have such a powerful impact on our health and well-being, but they often do.

For the past 36 years, my colleagues and I at the nonprofit Preventive Medicine Research Institute have conducted a series of clinical research studies showing what a potent difference changes in diet and lifestyle can make and how quickly they can occur. These lifestyle changes include stress management techniques such as yoga and meditation; a mostly plant-based diet; moderate exercise; and increased social support, community, and love.

We used high-tech, state-of-the-art scientific measures to prove the power and efficacy of these simple, low-tech, and low-cost interventions.

We showed that these lifestyle changes alone may reverse even severe heart disease. At any age. We also found that these lifestyle changes may reverse type 2 diabetes and may slow, stop, or even reverse the progression of early-stage prostate cancer.

Because of these findings, Medicare and many insurance companies are now covering our program of comprehensive lifestyle changes for reversing heart disease for those with type 2 diabetes and early-stage prostate cancer. Dr. Merrell and his colleagues at the Continuum Center for Health and Healing at Beth Israel Medical Center in New York are now offering this program.

The major determinant of our health and well-being is not our genes but primarily the lifestyle choices we make each day. When we change our lifestyle, it actually changes our genes. In our research, we found that more than 500 genes were beneficially affected in only three months—upregulating (turning on) disease-preventing genes and downregulating (turning off) disease-promoting genes, especially those controlling inflammation, oxidative stress, and the RAS oncogenes that promote prostate cancer, breast cancer, and colon cancer.

Also, these lifestyle changes may even begin to reverse aging by lengthening your telomeres, the ends of your DNA that control aging. Telomeres are like the plastic tips at the ends of shoelaces that keep them from unraveling. They keep your DNA from unraveling. As your telomeres get longer, your life gets longer.

But living longer isn't the only goal. The detox prescription that Dr. Merrell eloquently describes in this book is designed to help you live better as well as live longer.

I'm continually amazed by how dynamic the biological mechanisms are that affect our health and well-being—for better and for worse. When you follow Dr. Merrell's recommendations, you're likely to feel so much better, so quickly, it reframes the reason for making and maintaining these changes from fear of dying (which is not sustainable) to joy of living (which is).

If it's pleasurable, it's sustainable.

Dean Ornish, MD
Founder and President, Preventive Medicine Research Institute; Clinical Professor of Medicine, University of California, San Francisco; author, The Spectrum *and* Dr. Dean Ornish's Program for Reversing Heart Disease
www.ornish.com

Introduction

You may have heard about the detox process before. You may have read one of the dozens of books on the market about the subject. You may have followed some sort of cleanse you found on the Internet. You may have fasted, or purged, or abstained for the sake of your health. You may be sick, you may be tired, you may be wracked with problems that result from being overweight, overworked, and overstressed. You may have tried everything—and still be seeking "the" answer.

Here it is.

I have dedicated my entire 35-year career as a medical doctor to helping patients heal themselves. For the last 10, I've focused on detoxification as one of the most powerful proactive steps that any modern human can take in evolving toward better health. Sleep, relaxation, social connection, and exercise are also key to an overall sense of well-being. But detox, done my way, naturally includes a healthy diet and yields results you can really feel within only a day or two. It is the quickest way I know to jump-start a healthy new life.

I know that much of what is out there in terms of advice is questionable, if not outright quackery. A lot of it is a thinly disguised way to sell you pricey supplements, powders, and other such fairy dust. "Detox" has become the new Wild West, full of shoot-from-the-hip healers and modern snake-oil salesmen, looking to profit from the desperate and debilitated, who are willing to embrace magical thinking in their search for a real cure.

I have to tell you that there is no magic involved. Indeed, the answer is not ethereal but completely down-to-earth. You just need a knowledgeable guide. And you can trust me to be that. I've spent 15 years reviewing the science and applying medically proven techniques in my role as director of the Continuum Center for Health and Healing at Beth Israel Medical Center in New York City, as a medical professor at Columbia University's

College of Physicians and Surgeons, and in my own private practice on Manhattan's Upper East Side. I have seen real results in literally hundreds of patients, and I can tell you with authority that the Detox Prescription has nothing to do with abnegation and everything to do with embracing and eating food. Real food. Healing, healthful, detoxifying food.

This is the work I was born to do. I have always been interested in helping others support their own health: I was raised by parents who took me to see the pediatrician when I was sick but also understood that homeopathy and other self-healing therapies could work just as well in some situations. As I moved through high school and college, I took up yoga and meditation and began to see for myself how the mind, breath, and body are completely interconnected.

I had planned to enter medical school but loved these metaphysical practices so much that I was hesitant to leave them behind in pursuit of what was thought at the time to be "harder science." So I didn't—I vowed to combine Eastern wisdom with Western medical understanding, aiming to create a new kind of medicine focused on supporting the body's incredible power to heal itself.

Don't misunderstand: My training in Western medicine is unimpeachable. Like most doctors, I was taught in depth how the body functions and how it is susceptible to disease. At Columbia—where I teach to this day—I was trained to put my trust in the findings of gold-standard medical studies and to make calls based on the field's cumulative body of experience. Yes, my instructors told me, I should always listen to my patients and examine them carefully, but I should also weigh their complaints carefully against the canon of knowledge held by the medical establishment. I was trained to sort patients into relatively fixed categories based on their symptoms, the standard practice in 20th-century American medicine, fundamentally laid out in the game-changing Flexner Report published in 1910. They taught me to use pharmaceuticals for frontline treatment of just about everything.

All this I accepted readily and learned fully—it's what we know today as evidence-based medicine, and it is a great guide for many problems. But I think of it now as just a starting point.

As my experience and knowledge in medicine matured, I began to realize that no two patients with similar symptoms, or even the same diagnosis, ever have the same exact problems. That is to say, each is the product of a unique set of genetic factors, environmental influences, and lifestyle habits. They don't fit easily into the neat boxes that medical school had so exquisitely equipped me to use. Some patients who came to see me were really, truly sick and in need of medical intervention—for them, drugs and/or surgery were lifesavers. Too many, however, were basically healthy by every medical measure but often felt horrible. They were living in a gray area: tired, foggy, flabby, irritable, achy, depressed, and, in some cases, despondent. They were just beginning to slip into illness and wanted nondrug ways to reverse it.

These patients helped me realize that each one of us is longing only for health and happiness, in search of a way of living in the world that will let us appreciate our bodies, make good use of our minds, and fulfill our spirits. To treat my patients well, I needed to treat them as souls rather than symptoms. I needed to help them learn how to live, and live well.

This was not a set of tools I'd been given in the course of my medical training. For most of my career, lifestyle recommendations regarding diet, exercise, and relaxation had been dismissed by the medical establishment as "soft science." Any additional outside-the-box approaches to healing—including acupuncture, massage, herbal medicine, meditation, breath work, and therapeutic use of vitamins and minerals—were considered at best to be a form of benign neglect, and at worst viewed as outright quackery.

But these were exactly the approaches I used with my gray-area patients to help them regain the balance in their lives. And they often were working far better than most any drug ever could or would have!

Now, of course, medical practice has come around to my way of thinking. Over the past 10 or 15 years, we've seen an explosion of studies in peer-reviewed medical journals showing that lifestyle interventions and complementary practices really do work. (In fact, the most recent wave of evidence shows that even most complementary practices are rendered unnecessary if proper changes to diet, exercise, and lifestyle are made.) Researchers at the Stanford Prevention Research Center found that of the $2.5 trillion we Americans spend annually on health care, 78 percent goes toward treating chronic diseases such as diabetes, high blood pressure, and heart disease. At least 50 percent of these chronic diseases are preventable or even reversible with lifestyle changes: This means a potential savings of about $1 trillion a year in health care spending, while improving patient lives.

So why doesn't this happen? Medical schools *are* beginning to tiptoe into these waters now, but many doctors simply don't learn much about lifestyle medicine or complementary practices in their training. If they don't seek out the information, they don't know how diet changes, or meditation, or yoga, or social support, or supplements, or a daily walk can change your life; they don't know how to prescribe this new kind of medicine. In some cases, you the patient might have to tell them about it!

Pharmaceuticals are still the favored recourse among the American medical elite. God knows that drugs can work wonders, in so many cases greatly improving and even saving lives. But just as often (dare I say *more* often?), they are unnecessary! Rather than treat discomfort and disease with chemicals, I think it better to work with food and lifestyle measures that support the body's own internal healing processes whenever possible.

I like the taxonomy of disease recently proposed by the brilliant physician and health researcher Stephen Genuis. He tells us that all disease and discomfort in the body can be traced to one of only five root causes:

Infectious agents
Inherited tendencies (that is to say, what's bred into our DNA)
Psychological dysfunction
Nutritional deficiency
Toxicity

Modern medical practice is largely focused on the first three of these, all of which can sometimes respond marvelously to our pharmaceutical arsenal. Still, the psychological bases of disease (and many of our "functional" problems) are primarily practiced and reimbursed on the pharmaceutical model, rather than engaged on more fully realigning our minds with more productive thought processes. The last two—nutritional deficiency and toxicity— are rarely addressed at all, and when they are, it is only in the most severe cases—anemia, say, or ingestion of rat poison.

That is a shame, since nutritional deficiency and toxicity, along with psychological dysfunction, offer our greatest opportunity to intervene in disease before it manifests in chronic symptoms and before our patients need to step on the treadmill of Western medical care. They are a kind of medical "sweet spot," the areas in which I believe we doctors have our greatest opportunity to do good in the world. We can help our patients make simple changes in their lives that can not only really, truly make them feel and operate better but actually circumvent the kinds of serious diseases—heart disease, diabetes, cancer—that are eating away at their bodies and bank accounts and even our social structure.

Today we've mapped the human genome and logged the potential to treat many inherited diseases right at the source. Though the technology for direct intervention in the disease process is still nascent, we know now—through the work of such pioneers as my brilliant, groundbreaking colleague Dean Ornish, MD, and Nobel Prize–winning geneticist Elizabeth Blackburn, PhD—that heredity is not destiny. Our lifestyle choices, our sleep and stress levels, our bad habits, and our diets dictate whether or not many disease-producing genes get "turned on" or "turned off" and literally how quickly our chromosomes age. This exciting new field of epigenetics—meaning literally "around" the gene—allows us to see how environmental factors alter our gene expression in a specific place within each cell. As a result, we now know that when we take active control of these factors, we can literally help control our health and genetic destiny—no doctors or drugs necessary!

I keep a prescription pad handy for those cases where drugs really can provide a solution. I keep an entire medical center, and a good one, behind me for the patients who need advanced screening or surgical interventions. But by and large, the work I mainly do is to educate and empower my patients to take charge of their own body-mind-spirit health and to enable their own bodies to be their best healer. Ironically in some ways, I have dedicated my career and my life to making myself absolutely redundant.

Still, the work of balance can be a struggle for many of us, as it is for my patients. I see people from all walks of life—from schoolteachers to corporate accountants to movie stars. As I mentioned above, they don't always show up sick. In fact, because some of them make their living based on their looks (actors and actresses, models) or physical performance (musicians, athletes, dancers, etc.), they take great care to take care of themselves. But across the board, most are not living up to what they feel is their true potential in terms of capability, resilience, and energy.

I love to help people with all of it: I teach people how to breathe deeply and reduce their stress with meditation. I educate them about the importance of rest and show them how to get a good night's sleep. I help them devise exercise plans that are both efficient and effective. I tell them how to use the power of their thoughts to create more of what it is they want. And I help them understand the importance of making meaningful interpersonal connections. It's *all* important.

But truthfully? It can be a struggle to eat in a way that is truly optimal;

there are so many different diet plans, trendy superfoods, and strong opinions out there that people get confused, if not completely overwhelmed. It's worth the effort to sort through the dross, because when you discover the way to eat right and eat well, results are profound. That's because food allows us to directly address the last two of Genuis's disease factors, the most overlooked in our society: toxicity and nutritional deficiency.

In my opinion, the scariest thing happening today is the typical American diet, and its truly monumental environmental and health consequences. Our culture has become focused on quantity over quality and given birth to a food industry that cranks out ever more of what we most like to eat: meats and sweets. We do that by bullying nature into producing more, too—with chemical pesticides and herbicides and fertilizers that can be nearly as damaging as industrial waste. As a result, most of us are overfed but undernourished, toxic, chronically inflamed, and well on our way toward the whole range of symptoms that comprise metabolic syndrome, characterized by high blood pressure and serum cholesterol levels, obesity, and prediabetic insulin resistance—the chronic conditions that increasingly rule over our health care mess.

We all know this, if only subconsciously. And yet we are surrounded by an onslaught of messages encouraging us to eat highly processed foods. They're quick! They're easy! They're cheap! Never mind that they're also potentially harmful, or even deadly.

> You *can* get off the crazy train. In fact, you have the chance to turn things around pretty quickly by combining the arts of detoxification and optimal nutrition.

The situation sounds dire because it *is* dire, but don't get too depressed. You *can* get off the crazy train. In fact, you have the chance to turn things around pretty quickly by combining the arts of detoxification and optimal nutrition. That's what this book is about.

You can build a better new you every time you pick up a spoon, a fork, or a straw. You've heard it before, but I'll say it again: Food is medicine. Every bite you eat (of unprocessed real food, that is) or sip you take (of juice or tea) is composed of hundreds of thousands of tiny molecules that make your cells what they are and tell them what to do. That's right. Food components are literally genetic signaling molecules that tell those disease tendencies bred in our bones to stay dormant by providing the nutrition your body needs to keep on functioning optimally. When you eat well, you have a chance to create energy, forestall disease, remove toxins from your system, and improve every aspect of your health.

Because you replace every molecule of every cell in your body within the course of only 1 year, I am not being flip when I refer to the "new you." It is quite literally possible, no matter how bad you're feeling or eating today, to be utterly transformed in just 365 days. But it won't take you that long. You can be feeling significantly better in just a couple of days and make lasting changes to your health within a month. It's amazing, really, the potential you have for health and healing—if you only can recognize it and can learn to work with it, rather than against it.

You can, and I am here to tell you how to do it!

Consider *The Detox Prescription* a giant leap from where you are right now toward where you want to be. As the name suggests, this program is a cleanse plan, carefully designed to help you undo whatever damage has already been done, prevent further damage, and release toxins that have accumulated in the body's tissues. But beyond that, it's also a crash course in optimal nutrition, teaching you how to nourish your own body with all the phytonutrients and antioxidants it needs to support the processes of detoxification and health. Eating a diet based on fruits and vegetables, preferably organic, you can become maximally healthy, cleaning out toxins, putting out free-radical fires, improving metabolism, and supporting your own disease-fighting capacity.

The evolution of my career has led to developing the 7- and 21-day detox cleanses offered in this book, based on all the solid science I've seen supporting a plant-based diet, modified with limited amounts of fish, as the absolute healthiest on Earth. The anecdotal evidence is just as strong. Hundreds of my patients have done this most gentle cleanse to rave results. They have lost weight. They have found more energy. They experience less headache, indigestion, and achiness. Most important, they feel empowered to take control of their health.

I started using the 3-day cleanse a little later, emboldened by a series of medical studies published in Scandinavian medical journals in the 1990s. These followed a group of patients suffering from the notoriously debilitating autoimmune disease rheumatoid arthritis. Researchers found that what worked best for these difficult patients was a weeklong juice cleanse, followed by 3 weeks on a vegan diet (free from dairy, eggs, and meat), after which symptoms were dramatically reduced and the need for medication mediated or even eliminated. Better yet, the positive changes accrued in only 28 days lasted for a full *2 years*—even after many returned to their normal diet. Incredible! As these studies were also published in prestigious American arthritis journals, I couldn't see why rheumatologists weren't using this dietary technique. I didn't understand why every doctor in America wasn't looking into it for patients experiencing any kind of chronic pain, fatigue, or discomfort.

I felt that I'd found the Holy Grail of nutrition. These studies provided me with proof positive that my own ideas and experiences in the field of detoxification were valid and showed me precisely how to kick my own cleansing plan up a notch. By adding only 3 days of juicing, which virtually anyone can do without risk or discomfort, I could let my patients rest their digestion, powerfully nourish their bodies, and kick-start a new state of health. The 3-day juice cleanse is the best way I know to unwind damage from past behavior and rapidly begin to reduce systemic inflammation. When I started introducing it to my patients, I, too, began to observe amazing results in them. Having seen and felt the changes in their own bodies, these patients were thrilled with their new selves (and with me). Eager to keep up the good work, they found it both easy and unintimidating to move on to the 7- or 21-day plant-based cleanses.

> The 3-day juice cleanse is the best way I know to unwind damage from past behavior and rapidly begin to reduce systemic inflammation.

What you will see in this book is the sum total of all that I have learned, taught, practiced, and studied over the last 35-plus years—and carefully refined over the last 10—about how to change your health by removing toxins from your life and eating optimally healthy foods. Read this book and you'll understand how food can be used every day to detoxify the body, flood the system with beneficial nutrients, and keep health gremlins at bay.

With the help of Mary Beth Augustine, MS, RDN, an incredibly experienced and knowledgeable colleague I've worked with for 15 years, I've made it easy for you, providing a detailed plan along with recipes, convenience options, and even little healthy "cheats" to keep it absolutely real . . . and completely doable. Moreover, this plan is not about subtraction, as so many Western diet plans are. Rather than harping on what you can't or shouldn't eat, it keeps its focus squarely on the delicious foods you *can* enjoy. That's addition—a net positive for you and your body.

You will not be starved. You will not feel horrible. You won't have to radically change your life. You won't need thousands of dollars' worth of herbs or colonic therapy sessions to do it. I'm not selling any special vitamin formulas or protein shakes or any product at all; I'm simply telling you how to do what you already do three times a day (at the minimum) in a way that can transform your health.

In fact, the entire 21-day cleanse is delicious, nutritious, and ultimately life enhancing. It will not only stop the madness but leave your body in better shape than it was before toxins and bad choices began to take their toll in the first place. It can begin to reverse many of the disease processes you might be experiencing and put you in a better place to start healing. It can lower blood pressure and blood sugar, quell systemic inflammation, and eliminate nagging problems like headaches and indigestion. It may even allow you, with your own physician's permission, to cut out (or cut back on) medications. You won't even need to replace them with a fistful of over-the-counter supplements.

Try it, and you will experience all the benefits my patients do: weight loss, glowing skin, abundant energy, clear mind, and solid health. You don't even have to take my word for it. Try any one of the three plans offered here (or combine them, as I suggest, for maximum effect). *You* be your own doctor: Prescribe it for yourself! Study it carefully in the laboratory of your own body. Log your own progress. With a little effort, and a willingness to change a few things around, you will at the very least really see how it feels to eat well and eat clean.

I've accomplished a lot in my career but feel especially proud to have the information and experience at my disposal now to offer the first detox book in the marketplace to be fully grounded in good science. (To learn more about the studies underpinning the program, visit www.woodsonmerrell.com.) Read it, do it, and you will find yourself transformed and better educated about how to be clean and clear for the rest of your life. I hope it will be only a first step on *your* journey toward true health . . . truly, a life's work.

what's the problem?

I see them every day: the walking wounded. They drag themselves into my office looking pasty, bloated, and wan. They are tired—often bone tired, with barely enough energy to make it through the day. At the same time, they are working harder than ever, running 100 miles an hour on scant fumes, stepping on the stress accelerator all day until it's time to pass out. But then they don't. Then they lie awake, fraught with worry, trying to sleep, knowing they need to recharge. As with big tired-wired toddlers, much-needed rest is out of their reach.

They're overweight (maybe just a little, maybe a lot). They're achy. They complain of arthritis, or back pain, or stiff neck, or one of the millions of other painful little messages that their bodies are sending, trying to prompt them to slow it all down. To take care of themselves.

There's no time, though, so they've got a few other complaints, too. Heartburn, irritable bowel, constipation, and reflux are common—their digestion just isn't what it used to be. Blood pressure may be going up; blood sugar levels might be teetering right on the edge of what's normal. Cholesterol has become an issue. They're flirting with metabolic syndrome (a combination of the preceding three problems—blood pressure, cholesterol, and blood sugar)—and they know just enough about it to get worried. Enough to come to me for help, seeking a diagnosis that will make sense of their symptoms, and perhaps a prescription that will allay all their ills.

These patients are each unique, of course, with their own personal blend of hereditary challenges, life stressors, and health histories. But even so, they are all suffering from the same pervasive, insidious disease: modern American life.

The majority of my patients have the best of intentions. They try to eat well, but they're more likely to eat easy—relying on what's fast and available to fill their stomachs. That means too many processed foods, high in sugars, fats, and preservatives. They try to get a few fruits and veggies each day, but it's hard. Do potato chips count?

When sleep won't come, they stay up late into the night, watching the news on television, surfing the Internet, keeping up with their friends on Facebook. They wake up exhausted, grab some coffee, get the day going. Maybe there are kids to wrangle, maybe not. But there *is* work, whether it's at home or in the office, and lots of it. More coffee. Perhaps a doughnut or two; a 4 p.m. candy bar reward.

There's a commute, a trip to the grocery store, then it's back home. The house is a mess, but they do what they can, relying on chemical-filled cleaning products to do for them what elbow grease could and would do (if only they had the time). They're thankful for the miraculous plastics that make life easy for them, letting them take their coffee or cola to go, cordoning off single servings of salads, soup, sandwiches. What did we ever do before such convenience items existed? How did we live?

They're thankful, too, for the handful of pills they take every day to keep going—high-tech supplements, antidepressants, statins, blood pressure medication, antacids, etc. Modern medicine's pharmaceutical arsenal really is a miracle, they'll tell me. They want to believe it.

The only thing is, why do they feel like they're lurching through life like the undead—functioning in their lives, but not really living. Why do so many of them feel so *bad*?

Toxic Avengers

Although, as I said earlier, all of my patients are unique, they are also alike in one key way: They are all toxic to some degree, simply as a result of living in our chemically dependent society. This toxicity may or may not manifest itself. But nearly every pathological diagnosis is accompanied by an underlying systemic toxicity, which (especially if accompanied by nutritional deficiencies) can undermine the body's inborn genius for healing itself.

Toxins are a fact of modern life—and there is really no escaping them. (By *toxin*, we mean a substance that is in some way essentially poisonous to the body.) They are in the air and the water and the food; they're in nearly everything we touch. They're in our bodies, created within as we struggle to keep up the pace. They're in our media and minds. And yes, they're even in our medicine.

More than 80,000 different chemicals are produced and used in the United States—in everything from cosmetics and cleaning products to food and furniture; most of them are new to us, at least in terms of evolutionary history. Nobody really knows the full story of how they work on us or what they can do to us, as the Environmental Protection Agency has required testing on only about 200 of them. Science is showing that some big offenders, like bisphenol A, dioxins, or DDT (see "The Usual Suspects," page 8), can act like hormones in the body, disrupting its natural function and tinkering under the hood of our natural metabolic machinery. We know that many of them even have the ability to interact with our genes themselves, effectively "turning on" innate tendencies to develop disease. It's compelling and scary stuff. But the truth is, I think we're barely scratching the surface.

Chemical agents are everywhere, and messing with every bodily function. In fact, a very recent study out of Tufts University, published in the journal *Endocrine Review*, suggests that we are more sensitive than we ever knew to more substances than we could possibly suspect. It revealed that our bodies are sensitive to a very minute amount of chemicals—equal to one-twentieth of one drop of water in an Olympic-size pool.

In the vast majority of cases I see, there is no "smoking gun" toxin to point at, no one trigger of the discomfort and dysfunction of mind and body that motivates the person to get help.

The real problem, as I see in my practice every day, is a chronic onslaught of multiple chemical exposures. The Centers for Disease Control and Prevention (CDC) has confirmed that the average person's body contains 153 chemical agents known to be toxic or probably toxic to the human body. And that's just what is known; many other chemicals are so new that we just don't understand their long-term effects.

The body was designed to deal with many toxic substances, both outside the body (exogenous) and inside it (endogenous)—think about our ancestors eating an occasional poisonous mushroom or flooding their systems with cortisol so that they could outrun a saber-toothed tiger. Such an occasional physical insult could easily be addressed by the body's system of detoxification, ever ready to wage all-out war. But it was not meant to be in contact with so very many toxins 24/7. The body is simply not equipped to deal with the daily load of hundreds or even thousands of chemicals, many at or just below the level of what's acceptable.

The liver, kidneys, and the bowels—our main organs of detoxification and elimination and our body's natural defense against the dark arts of modern chemistry—are overloaded; our natural detoxification mechanisms don't work as well as they should because they just can't keep up with the burden. A truly effective detox means not only flushing out unwanted chemicals absorbed from air, food, water, and the body's own internal metabolic and stress-related processes, but also binding them efficiently with nutrition drawn from a healthy diet, then eliminating them from our bodies effectively and efficiently. It can be hard to keep up.

Because we are overloaded, our bodies have no choice but to store unprocessed toxins in bodily tissues—especially fat cells, since most toxins are fat-soluble. We accumulate toxins over time. No wonder we feel so bad.

No wonder we all need a little help!

The Phases of Detox

The help you need—that we all need—is a detox cleanse.

But not just any detox will do. Despite what a cursory Internet search will tell you, there are no magic formulas for detox, including the so-called "Master Cleanse," which involves drinking a mixture of water, lemon juice, maple syrup, cayenne pepper, and salt. There is no way to bully your body into doing a better job through deprivation, fasting, or purgation.

Detox isn't something that requires extreme measures—in fact, radical plans can cause much more harm than good, flooding and overwhelming the system with too many toxins without supporting their elimination.

In the simplest terms, here's why: The body's detoxification system operates in two phases. In phase I, the body identifies toxins and transforms them into unstable molecules, or free radicals, to be excreted. In a sense, phase I makes the toxins *more* toxic, so that the body can't help but notice them and try to get rid of them. Most detox plans focus solely on phase I, which offers incomplete support and can be downright dangerous.

During a healthy and normal phase II, these hypertoxic free radicals are then bound up with specific dietary nutrients to render them water soluble so that they can be eliminated from the body via the urinary or digestive tract. Here is where most detox plans come up short—phase II requires maximal (not minimal) nutrition, meaning that vitamins, minerals, and phytonutrients needed for the successful binding of phase II must be readily available. If they are not, you are only releasing, reprocessing, and restoring toxins. (For a complete explanation of this process, see Chapter 9.)

> Your body simply cannot process toxins without adequate nutrition.

In other words, for phase II to work optimally, the body must be well nourished with the dietary nutrients (or "substrates") needed for this crucial binding process. The body has six primary pathways for successful detoxification (the most important being sulfation, glucuronidation, glutathione, methylation, acetylation, and amino acids). All of these require the nutrients found in a plant-based diet, as well as adequate fiber and hydration. By definition, these come from food.

If you are doing a detox that focuses on phase I at the expense of phase II, you are allowing free radicals to roam about like a crazy man with a loaded gun, doing damage anywhere and anyhow they can. Fruits and vegetables are nature's phase II SWAT team—there to neutralize the threat before things get lethal! If you're overweight, sick, and toxic, 2 weeks of an imbalanced diet such as the Master Cleanse can make you look and feel worse than ever. *Any plan that requires fasting or reliance on one, two, or three foods will be a net loss.* Your body simply cannot process toxins without adequate nutrition. Without it, you may never even get to phase I!

Where Do Toxins Come From?

Everywhere, is the short answer. But for the purposes of understanding the scope of toxicity, here's a brief list of the primary sources of our cumulative exposure:

Fruits and vegetables: Conventional produce is routinely exposed to pesticides and herbicides, which can contain neurotoxins or carcinogens. Organics are a far better bet, though they, too, can be exposed to chemicals that have persisted in the soil or water. One good example is DDT, which has been illegal since 1972 but will take thousands of years to break down in nature. It is ubiquitous and was found by scientists at Consumers Union to be present in nearly 25 percent of organic produce.

Meat and dairy: Beyond the health-depleting burden of animal fats, which have been linked to heart disease, obesity, and even cancers, conventionally raised meat and dairy are exposed to chemical pesticides (in the feed) and, in many cases, hormones and antibiotics used to promote growth and fend off disease. Dairy is especially toxic if you are among the 60 percent of Caucasians, 75 percent of African Americans, or 90 percent of Asians who are lactose intolerant (in which case lactose acts as a toxin to your system).

Sugar: Sugar is a sneaky subverter of health, but in excess (which isn't a lot) it's nearly as toxic as any man-made substance. Because sugar, or glucose, raises blood insulin levels and promotes inflammation, constant exposure leads inexorably to diabetes, high blood pressure, and heart disease—not to mention any of numerous cancers that have been linked to elevated insulin levels. Fructose, another kind of sugar that does not raise insulin, has been shown to perhaps be even worse for health.

Plastics: Chances are you've heard about the problems associated with the use of bisphenol A (BPA) in plastic bottles, food storage containers, can liners, and packaging materials. Guess what? It's even worse than you know, as cash register receipts can deposit literally a thousand times more of the substance than containers can. Worse, literally hundreds of chemical compounds are used to create plastic products, which have been proven to leach chemicals into air, water, and food when under pressure from heat or routine wear and tear. Perfluorooctanoic acid (PFOA), a chemical used in creating nonstick plastic coatings in cookware and some clothing, was recently associated with heart disease in a study published in the *Archives of Internal Medicine*. Researchers found what appears to be a direct relationship: The more PFOA you have in your body, the more likely you are to experience cardiovascular disease. Hundreds of good published studies chronicle the adverse health effects of dozens of common man-made chemicals to which we are exposed daily.

Air: Particulate matter (smog), containing toxic organic compounds and heavy metals, is mostly the result of cars or power plants. Chemical fragrances, cleaners, synthetic furniture, and building materials add to the chemical burden indoors.

Water: Municipally treated water is likely to be free of microorganisms. But it likely contains chemicals, excreted pharmaceuticals (including birth control pills), or lead leached from old pipes, unless you are purifying it yourself through reverse osmosis. Treatment plants were not designed to filter out most chemicals (including environmental toxins and medications).

Household and personal care products: Take a close look at the labels on the products under your kitchen sink (surface, floor, and tile cleaners) and in your bathroom (shampoos, lotions, sunscreen, and deodorants). You'll likely see a long list of chemical agents, which you're exposed to through the air or, in the case of personal care products, the skin. "Fragrance" is a tip-off that toxic chemicals such as endocrine-disrupting phthalates and benzophenones, which can interfere with thyroid function, are present. How susceptible you will be to them is a matter of genetics—and diet, because these toxins compete strongly with others for control of detox pathways.

Drugs: Not many docs will tell you this, but I will: Drugs, even the prescription kind, can be toxic to the body. We use chemicals to cause a reaction in the body, and the huge list of side effects you will see on the package insert demonstrates that one man's medicine is another man's poison. With Western pharmaceuticals, we can only hope that more good is done than harm.

Excess weight: Obesity takes a toll on every human system. Once thought of as inert, fat is now understood as a systemic stressor, and is itself a creator of inflammatory chemicals that add to your own body burden. If you're overweight, you need to lose weight to feel your best. But one word of caution: Fat is the body's favorite storehouse for unprocessed toxins, which are released when pounds are dropped. Keep weight loss low and slow to avoid making things precipitously worse.

Smoking: Are you smoking? Quit now—and for good. Evidence that smoke of all and any burning inhalants is toxic is overwhelming.

Stress: Stress is a catch-all term for the cascade of human hormones, neurotransmitters, and other biochemical events that occur when we respond to our environments and life situations with anxiety. The two major "stress hormones"—cortisol and adrenaline—are useful in short bursts but toxic in the long term. These endogenous toxins can disrupt sleep, lead to weight gain, and undermine brain function.

Let me say that again, a little bit louder: Your body cannot process toxins without adequate nutrition.

In my opinion, the *only* medically sound way to detoxify your system,
create better health, and lose weight sustainably is to support your body
with a clean, nutritious diet. No disastrous deprivations or superexpensive
supplements or consultations with elite doctors or dietitians are necessary.
Food, as ever, is the very best medicine—and with a little education and
detox savvy, you can prescribe it for yourself every time you pick up a fork.

In fact, consider this book your prescription pad. This is the best detox

The Usual Suspects

Here are a few of the biggest chemical offenders in our modern environment. Many
of these are known to have hormone-disrupting effects; others are carcinogenic.
Each of these has studies to prove it is deleterious to human health. Yet this is just a
small sampling of what is out there!

BPA: *What is it?* Shatterproofer. *Where is it?* Plastic bottles, plates, containers,
packaging; also can linings. *What's it do?* Mimics the effects of estrogen and has
been associated with obesity.

Atrazine: *What is it?* A pesticide. *Where is it?* Corn. *What's it do?* Causes
reproductive dysfunction.

Dioxin: *What is it?* Good old industrial waste. *Where is it?* In soil and food, particularly animal products. *What's it do?* Associated with lower sperm counts, breast
cancer, and reproductive and mental disorders.

PCB: *What is it?* Insulating material. *Where is it?* In household items, wiring,
paints, foams. *What's it do?* Linked directly to cancer and to problems with the
immune, reproductive, nervous, and endocrine systems.

PFOA: *What is it?* Plastic coating. *Where is it?* Coated pans, Gore-Tex clothing, drinking water. *What's it do?* Associated with increased cardiovascular disease.

Phthalate: *What is it?* Plasticizer and fixative. *Where's it found?* Perfumes,
cosmetics, toys, adhesives. *What's it do?* Carcinogenic and disrupts hormones—
interferes with male reproductive system.

plan available, period, one I've dedicated 35 years of practice to developing. I use it to treat nearly every category of patient I see—whether they're healthy and looking to get healthier, basically well but in need of more energy, or seriously sick and seeking to heal themselves in the most holistic way possible.

The Detox Prescription plan can change your life in as little as 3 days. Because it starts with an intensive focus on whole-food juices, teas, and nut milks, it works to give digestion a break, unwind inflammation, and flood the system with the vital phytonutrients it needs to do the entire job of detoxification (not just phase I). From there, it adds back whole foods

DDT: *What is it?* Pesticide. *Where's it found?* Outlawed in 1972 but persists in soil and water for thousands of years. (It's still being used legally in high-mosquito-risk countries.) *What's it do?* Toxic to the liver and nervous system, disrupts reproduction.

PBDE: *What is it?* Flame retardant. *Where's it found?* Couches, pillows, carpets, children's clothing. *What's it do?* Linked to problems with brain development as well as thyroid and reproductive function.

Paraben: *What is it?* Preservative. *Where's it found?* Cosmetics, lotions, personal care items. *What's it do?* Mimics estrogen; linked to breast cancer.

Perchlorate: *What is it?* Rocket fuel. *Where's it found?* The water supply. *What's it do?* Disrupts thryoid hormone, interferes with energy production in the mitochondria of cells.

Triclosan: *What is it?* Antibacterial agent. *Where's it found?* Personal care and housekeeping supplies. *What's it do?* Depresses production of testosterone and thyroid hormones in humans. Contributes, via infiltration of the water system, to the infertility of frogs and other species.

EMF: *What is it?* By-product of electrical gadgets and appliances. *Where's it found?* Computers, phones, televisions, power lines. *What's it do?* Depresses production of testosterone and thyroid hormones, with long-term effects on brain function (in studies, hyperactivity of the brain cells has been demonstrated near where the cell phone is pressed to the ear).

judiciously, allowing the body to recover and reset itself over the course of a week. And finally, it introduces a 21-day plan to make a low-toxin, high-energy diet and lifestyle a way of life, rather than an emergency measure.

The 3-day juice cleanse can require a bit of self-discipline, at least for the first 24 hours. But this is not a plan for die-hards or ascetics. I'm not preaching any particular dietary gospel. Despite my appreciation for the healthy benefits of a plant-based diet, I'm no vegangelist. Rather, I simply want to help you come to grips with a way of eating that enhances, rather than undermines, your life. I know that the senses of taste and smell are primary to an enjoyable life—they make us feel good. So this plan is designed to have you looking forward to every meal, every snack.

I could go on and on about the science behind it, the outcomes I've seen. But rather than *tell* you what the Detox Prescription can do, let me show you. The following case studies are real people in real life (though names have been fudged a bit to protect privacy). Each represents a real struggle and reflects real results. I'll let those results speak for themselves, beyond which I'll only say this: If they can do it, you can, too!

CASE HISTORY

The Headachy Thinker

Celeste had always dreamed of being an editor, of working with brilliant writers and helping them to create the kind of literature that could change lives. She pictured herself at the top someday, calling the shots, promoting pure excellence in the publishing industry. At age 32, she was on her way, situated as an associate editor with a prestigious publishing house.

She was, she told me, what her industry called a workhorse (as opposed to a show pony—those editors who do nothing but look good and schmooze). She spent long hours in the office poring through manuscripts, volunteered for weekend duty, and frequently took work home at night in an effort to catch the eye of her talented, demanding boss. She drank copious amounts of coffee to keep her going. She was willing to work longer, harder, and faster to make her dreams come true. Trouble was, her body seemed to be balking at the workload.

Celeste is the perfect example of someone who lives in her head—bright, intellectual, curious, driven, and all about ideas. And ironically (or not?), her big problem was headaches. Specifically migraine headaches—whopping pounders that would put her in bed for at least a day, then lead to another day or two of functioning at half speed. She'd had them for several years, but now they were happening more frequently—once a week, sometimes more. "And they happen at inconvenient times," she said, clearly frustrated. "They don't care about my deadlines."

Luckily, she had decent health insurance and could afford to keep a triptan drug (like Imitrex or Zomig) with her at all times. These, if taken soon enough in the process, can stop a migraine in its tracks. But Celeste felt she was missing that mark too often, and once the pain came—accompanied in her case by nausea and blurred vision—nothing would ease it.

When her boss made a note of her increasing absences at work, Celeste was motivated to call me. She'd talked to her doctor about this and had been referred to a neurologist, who promptly suggested Topamax, an anti-seizure medication often used as a migraine preventive. She tried it for a while, but the side effects were simply not tolerable: slowed speech, muddled thinking, and difficulty finding the right word. Clearly, not acceptable for someone who thinks, speaks, edits, and writes for a living!

She was aware that in certain cases migraines could be triggered by foods but had never been able to detect a pattern in her own diet—red wine, hard cheese, processed meats . . . they all seemed to be okay. Based on her medication use, as well as her dependence on caffeine (which can both hurt and help migraines), I also knew that Celeste was likely to be toxic. So I recommended that she spend a week weaning herself off of coffee and onto green tea and then undertake the 7-day cleanse, kicked off with 3 days of juices. By doing this, I explained, she could start to clean up her system and make it easier to identify her triggers and maybe even stop migraines for good. So she did it happily and reported the usual results: better thinking, clearer head, more energy. No migraines.

Still, it was hard to tell what was going on—her body responded well to a cleaner, plant-based diet, but adding foods back in might prove tricky. Dietary irritants specific to Celeste were likely to be setting off her migraines. With input from our senior nutritionist, Mary Beth Augustine, I devised a special 21-day elimination/challenge designed to identify Celeste's problem foods. (If you'd like to try an elimination diet for yourself, you'll find a general version on page 292.)

Finally, through trial and error, the culprit was identified: She was sensitive to histamine-containing foods, which include eggplants and spinach (both of which she adored), avocado, mushrooms, and dried fruits, as well as many commonly used condiments and fermented foods such as sauerkraut, vinegar, or yogurt. That's a list of very healthy and nutritious foods—for most people. But it goes to show the truth behind the axiom "One person's medicine is another's poison." Celeste's highly reactive nervous system was easily triggered by these comparatively mild food irritants. She needed to cut them out to experience relief.

Diet had a major positive impact, but it wasn't the whole story. As long as Celeste continued to work around the clock and turn over her whole body and mind to stress and worry, migraines would be there. She needed an "off switch" for these to restore order in her life, whether she liked it or not. She dismissed yoga as "too time-consuming" and meditation as "too hard." But she was willing to sit quietly and learn a simple breathing technique, which she perceived she could take on the road of her fast-paced life. It was a perfect choice for a patient I had observed to be breathing shallowly and likely to hold her breath when concentrating.

Moreover, I recommended that she combine her dietary changes with a couple of nutritional supplements that would serve as natural migraine prevention: magnesium and butterbur. And I had her undergo a course of acupuncture to treat both her headaches and the associated body imbalances that come from overwork and overworry.

Four months later, Celeste had all but eliminated her migraines—though she gets them occasionally, they happen no more than once every few months and are much less intensive and shorter in duration than they had been. Having gone through the process with me, she felt more confident that she could predict risk factors—foods, stress, lack of sleep, her menstrual cycle—and know when to take her triptans to abort the headache cycle. She knew she could use the 3-day juice cleanse anytime she needed to "reset" her mind and body.

Despite her initial resistance, Celeste had signed up for a meditation course at a local community center—and was even enjoying it. It calmed her nerves and gave her perspective, she reported. Better yet, her boss had noticed and appreciated her consistency and new steadiness on the job, enough to suggest her for a new job within their company—one that would lead to a promotion, the next logical step along Celeste's career path.

TOXIC TRIGGER: **OVERWORK**

Because she was both ambitious and driven, Celeste worked in overdrive nearly all the time. That meant she was stuck in sympathetic nervous system mode—that classic fight-or-flight state that taxes the adrenal system and pumps cortisol and adrenaline into the body. This leads, as we've seen, to weight gain over time—though Celeste was not quite there yet. It also leads to shallow breathing, anxiety, higher pulse rate, and an increase in vascular tone . . . all migraine stage setters, if not outright triggers. She needed to get active in stimulating her body's natural antidote: the calming parasympathetic nervous system. We have learned to measure real and lasting health in terms of heart rate variability—meaning that our heart rate goes up and down as our nervous system dominance switches from sympathetic to parasympathetic. The more variability, the better. If you are stuck, as Celeste was, in sympathetic overdrive, do all you can to cultivate a better relationship with your parasympathetic system—the more the better.

MY ADVICE

Meditation is the gold-standard practice for relaxation and perspective. The health benefits are innumerable and are being borne out by study after study showing that it promotes very real and beneficial changes in body and brain. It doesn't have to be hard; in fact, my favorite technique is one used by the Vietnamese Zen monk Thich Nhat Hanh. Simply sit, breathe, and connect your breath to this mantra: "Breathing in, I feel calm. Breathing out, I smile." Even four or five rounds of this simple meditation can change your mood, improve your health, and create balance between your sympathetic and parasympathetic system dominance.

CASE HISTORY

Type-A Wonder Woman

Mara had been my patient for years, and she was a real go-getter. A high-powered attorney with a keen intellect and nerves of steel, she was ruthless in her negotiations. She was also ruthless with herself. She woke at 5 a.m. every morning to squeeze in a 2-hour, cardio-focused workout. She worked intensely and late into the night, allowing herself a meager 4 hours of sleep per day. She carefully tracked her calories to keep her weight under control, but emphasized protein (meat) at the expense of complex carbohydrates (fruits and vegetables). She drove her kids nearly as hard, running them through the typical "tiger mom" demands that they study hard; participate in sports, music, and arts; and set themselves up neatly for a life as successful as she perceived her own to be. To say she was a control freak would be vastly understating the case. She was a hard taskmaster, for herself and everyone around her.

My advice at the outset was pretty simple: Sleep more, exercise less, and pay as much attention to the quality of the food you are eating as you do to the quantity. I explained the benefits of eating organic food to eliminate exposure to pesticides and herbicides and encouraged her to reduce her meat consumption. She initially scoffed at this idea, unable to imagine living any other way. When I suggested putting her on a 7-day cleanse, she flatly refused. There was nothing she couldn't cure with her own mighty willpower, she thought, and would keep doing what she was doing, ever harder and faster.

Then the unthinkable happened. Despite doing "everything right," Mara gained 10 pounds. She had reached her midforties, with years of hard-driving self-discipline under her belt, and yet here she was, busting through the seams of her immaculately tailored designer suits—not technically overweight, but not where she wanted to be. She amped up her efforts to diet and exercise her way down to her ideal weight, but nothing worked.

Feeling frustrated and desperate, she came back to me. I knew that what she needed most was sleep—she just wasn't getting enough to allow her body the respite it needed to complete the processes of healing, assimilation, and detoxification. I told her so, but she still couldn't hear it.

She wouldn't change her lifestyle around—she was unwilling to even consider that every single thing she was doing wasn't the best, most perfect thing—but she finally agreed to do the 3-day juice cleanse, and no more. The plan dovetailed nicely with her controlling nature, after all.

Imagine Mara's surprise when she found that she didn't need to gather all her inner strength just to make it through 3 days. In fact, she enjoyed the structure and strictures of the juice cleanse. She felt energized, yes, but also lighter. There was something here, Mara realized, something powerful.

So she kept it up, moving on through the 7-day cleanse and learning to focus on an organic, plant-centric diet. She began to embrace the idea that food wasn't just about calories; she could change her diet in ways that would make her feel and look better. The needle on the scale began to move for her, and she was sold.

Mara began to eat clean and to return to the 3-day juice cleanse whenever she felt she needed a boost. As she went on, she developed a new kind of clarity: She realized, and told me, that though she had always felt that she was in control of her life, her life had gotten out of control. Aha!

She was only willing to make so many changes, but they were important ones. Rather than exercising full-bore 7 days a week, she agreed to dedicate at least 2 days to a mellower routine. She agreed to sleep more, and went to 6 hours a night—a huge improvement, and, in Mara's case, just as important as the food in helping weight loss and creating a lifestyle of wellness.

As the weight came off, the lightbulb went on: Mara was living in a toxic environment of her own making. She began to relax—just a little!—with herself and her kids. She rearranged her caseload to ease—just a little!—the pressure. She was still a master of the universe, but now her universe was a less toxic, more benevolent place to be living.

TOXIC TRIGGER: **LACK OF SLEEP**

For the body's innate processes of detoxification to work at their best, you need plenty of rest. In Mara's case, she was working out too much, flooding her body with the free radicals naturally created by exercise, and resting far too little. Add the random bad food choice or cocktail, and you get a system overloaded with toxins from both internal and external sources.

MY ADVICE

To be your healthiest, aim to get 8 hours a night. Go to bed a little bit earlier; sleep in when you can. If you wake in the night, practice dream remembrance—that is, as soon as you start to feel that you are going to wake, instead reject conscious thinking and keep your attention on the dream as tenaciously as you can. If that doesn't do the trick, try some meditative breath work: Inhale for a count of four, hold for a count of one, then exhale for a count of five. Repeat as necessary to induce sleep—or at least reduce your anxiety about being awake.

Overweight Couch Potato

Brett wasn't a lazy sort of fellow; in fact, he had climbed the corporate ladder into a very respectable management position in the insurance business by the time he came to see me in his mid-thirties. He considered himself a self-made man, willing to work hard to get ahead. Which he did, to the tune of 10 to 12 hours a day sitting in front of a computer.

At home, he did what he thought he needed to do to relax, what he thought everyone did. He watched the game, drank a few beers. He ordered Chinese food for dinner and later had a few snacks, too. He was a single man, so his diet consisted mostly of what was easy to get and close by or what satisfied his cravings.

Problem was, he was getting fat—and his cholesterol and blood pressure started creeping up. He wasn't too worried about it, but just enough to come and see me. Heart disease figured prominently in his family health history. Better safe than sorry.

It's a good thing he did, as he was on the same path that has led millions of Americans to develop heart disease, diabetes, obesity (he was right on the borderline), and/or hypertension. He was the poster boy for the problems engendered by our sedentary lifestyle and by eating what's known as the Standard American Diet, or—appropriately—SAD: high in refined sugars, low in fiber, based largely on wheat and corn, and featuring plenty of factory-farmed, high-cholesterol meats. But he wasn't too late to change his destiny—far from it. He was glad to hear that.

As we talked about his life, Brett revealed that he'd been feeling sluggish and foggy. He felt a little achy on most days, too. His sex drive was down. He was enjoying the fruits of his labors, but felt that his head wasn't really "in the game." But that was typical, right? Didn't everyone feel that way?

No, I assured him, they did not. I explained that though these were problematic symptoms of toxicity, they were easily addressed. He had no compounding medical issues other than weight. He could do the 3-day juice cleanse and see marvelous results.

Brett—a get-along guy to the core—agreed to do it, though he worried mightily that he'd be hungry, that he might not be able to "stick it out." He thought of it in terms of "fasting" and considered himself to be a poor candidate for self-denial. Still, I encouraged him to try and made it easy for him by referring him to one of New York's many excellent juice-delivery services.

After a bit of procrastination, which I pointed out wasn't making him feel any better, he finally did it. As I had predicted, he was very surprised. It wasn't so hard; he wasn't so hungry. In fact, for the first time in years, he felt that he was in control of his cravings. By day 2, in fact, he felt invigorated, he told me later. "It was like a slap in the face," he said. "I felt so much better that I was able to see how my life is just floating by me."

That slap literally snapped him out of the ennui that had become his default emotional temperature. Now, he was more than willing to make other lifestyle changes. He cut back on the meat and the carryout. He learned to cook a few simple things at home and started shopping with an eye toward his health.

Moreover, he started to use a breath-work technique I gave him to keep himself present in the moment—which is where every decision happens. He began to engage more in his job, to "feel lit up" in meetings. He started exercising a little, then more. He started dating again.

Best of all, his health got better. He's got a bit more weight to lose, but all of his critical numbers—cholesterol, blood sugar, blood pressure—improved in only a few weeks. I am proud to use Brett as an example. He is the poster boy for how little steps toward a less toxic lifestyle can lead to dramatic positive changes.

TOXIC TRIGGER: **CONVENIENCE FOODS**

Convenience foods aren't inherently evil; in fact, they can be quite helpful to busy Americans . . . if you take care to limit them and balance your intake with healthier choices. Brett was relying on restaurants or fast-food joints for most of his meals or grabbing quick microwave entrées—and not the organic, healthy kind. He didn't really know what was in his food in the way of additives and preservatives, not to mention pesticides in the produce or plasticizers in the containers.

MY ADVICE

Try not to eat out more than a couple of times a week, particularly from purveyors of cheap processed foods; the rest of the time, cook your own simple, organic fare. Never microwave in plastic containers or plastic-lined cardboard ones, which may leach chemicals into food. Use glass or lead-free ceramic instead.

The Aging Model

The minute Eloise walked into my office, I could see why she'd been a top model for so long. Of course, I knew of her and had seen her in a million advertisements; she was the face for a major beauty brand, an elite even among supermodels, and a real household name. Her career had taken off in her teens and skyrocketed throughout her twenties.

But now, at 37, she was fraught with anxiety about what the future might hold for her. The modeling industry is not kind to aging women, in general; Eloise was lucky to still be on the job at all at her age. Genetics had obviously been kind to her, but she found it harder and harder to keep up with the glamorous lifestyle she'd been living, with all its drinks, and smokes, and occasional forays into drug abuse. She'd cleaned up her act by the time I saw her but felt she was still suffering consequences.

Most notably, she reported, she gained weight more easily. Her strategy had always been to eat nothing—or as close to it as she could manage. (Think one-lettuce-leaf lunches.) Now she couldn't operate that way. She would feel terrible physically if she skipped out on meals. But if she ate well, she felt terrible emotionally, worried that the food would run straight to fat. She'd tried several diets and cleanses—including the Beverly Hills Diet and the Master Cleanse—but hated them all, finding them onerous or impossible. Her decisions around food were becoming increasingly stressful; each bite she took felt like a little step toward her demise in her business.

Eloise wasn't overweight. Far from it. But she told me, "I find myself having to suck in my stomach more and more often." Examination revealed very little body fat but a good deal of bloating—a sign of weak digestion and a not-uncommon problem for models. Her love-hate relationship with food wasn't helping, nor was her intensive and erratic travel schedule. She needed to get on a diet that could support her from the inside out.

I put her on the 21-day cleanse to begin flushing out the toxins she'd accumulated during her party-girl days, reset her digestive system, support her body without adding to (or subtracting from) it, and introduce her to a way of eating that was sustainable. Eloise needed to have the weight of decision making lifted from her shoulders long enough to cultivate a friendlier relationship with her food choices.

The 3-day juice cleanse was—as it so often is—a real eye-opener. Eloise felt great, calling me to tell me how much more radiant she was feeling. "I feel like I'm glowing," she told me. "Like I'm incandescent." And that's a good feeling for a model.

I took the opportunity to talk to her about the phytonutrients—plant-based chemicals that protect and promote health—that were creating her inner glow and about how she could begin to look at food as so much more than carbs and calories. Though she'd started with a delivery service cleanse, Eloise felt committed to keeping wholesome green juice in her diet, and so she invested in a juicer. She began to take it with her when she traveled, to add in to her contracts that she needed an assortment of fresh, organic, whole foods on every set. The bloat had dissipated, taking many of her fears with it.

Six months later, she was more optimistic about her future. She had a diet she could finally feel good about and a healthful secret weapon (juice) in the fight on weight gain. Better, she was able to feel that she really was doing everything she should (and eliminating what she shouldn't) do to protect her most valuable business asset: her good looks. But more important, the improvement that came from knowing how to take charge of being maximally healthy had her feeling wonderful.

I see a lot of models and celebrity clients who have similar stories. For them, even though it may seem shallow, looking good is good business. The secret to their long-term success is that they invest in their health because they intuitively know (or find out the hard way) that the outward beauty that the world gets to see is a reflection of what's going on inside. To look radiantly healthy, you have to *be* radiantly healthy!

TOXIC TRIGGER: **A CHECKERED PAST**

Ah, youth . . . that magical time when we think we are invincible, able to do, eat, or consume anything without consequence. Experimenting with drugs, alcohol, and cigarettes is so common in our youth culture that we nearly consider it a rite of passage. Though we grow out of those habits, our bodies hold on to the memories—literally. When the system is overloaded with toxins, it is forced to find a home for them. Mostly it tucks them away neatly in a nest of body fat, to be dealt with later. Problem is, most of us are carrying on in lifestyles that create ongoing toxic stressors—the body is so busy processing our daily exposures that it never has a chance to go back and clean up the past. (One of my patients, a 50-something member of a prominent rock-and-roll band, told me that if he had known he would live so long, he'd have taken better care of himself during his youthful heyday.) A detox creates space for it to do just that—and you need to do one, even if your transgressions occurred in the distant past. If they're more immediate, take steps to curtail bad habits now.

MY ADVICE

Stop smoking immediately, limit your alcohol intake to one or two drinks 5 days per week, and avoid recreational drugs. You might also want to look askance at some of your prescriptions. Talk to your doctor about potential for toxicity and—if risk is high—about other options.

CASE HISTORY

Midlife [Health] Crisis Couple

By any measure, Jon and Emily Ehrlich had had a successful life. They'd worked together for years in the entertainment industry, helping to stage some of the most successful concerts in history. They'd hopped from coast to coast, keeping up an exhausting, toxic travel schedule by anyone's standards. But by the time they reached their early sixties, they were able to retire comfortably and travel at leisure. Which they did, exploring the far corners of the world together: this time for pleasure rather than work.

But 2 years into their "golden years," the Ehrlichs realized that instead of feeling invigorated by the attainment of their lifelong dreams, they felt run down. At loose ends. Like they didn't have the energy to do much of anything. They were slowing down. Moreover, they were feeling very old . . . before their time.

Still, they *were* mortal, and a bit of caution was in order for them both. Both were overweight, to the tune of about 40 pounds apiece. With aging had come the usual creeping up of blood pressure levels. Both were on statins to keep cholesterol under control. Cardiovascular health was especially important to Jon, whose father had died of a heart attack at age 50.

I was in heaven; the Ehrlichs were my favorite kinds of patients. Just motivated enough to make changes, at a time when they can really be critical in determining how well you live your life, and for how long.

Target one was the weight. My prescription? Detox.

I explained that weight loss would improve the quality of life for both of them and move those problematic health measurements back to where they could optimally. No, they wouldn't have to adopt a severe liquid diet, or go in for laparoscopic surgery, or do any other extreme measures. Rather, they could try the 3-day juice cleanse to help them break some bad eating habits and introduce a few new healthy ones.

For patients like the Ehrlichs, low and slow is the ideal weight loss plan. Because the body stores up pesticides, PCBs, and other potentially hormone-disrupting chemicals it encounters in fat tissue, they are released into the bloodstream as the pounds melt away, adding further toxic burden to the body. Extreme diets can flood and even overwhelm the system with these chemicals, undermining the benefits of the weight loss. Also, extreme dieting measures are likely to yield a weight loss of up to 50 percent muscle mass. If weight is regained, chances are it will comprise only 20 percent muscle mass—meaning every time you yo-yo, you end up with more fat at the same weight. Not only are you much worse off health-wise, but it is also much harder to lose weight the next time.

The philosophy made sense to them, and they decided to embrace the 3-day juice cleanse as a team, with Emily saying, "Let's bite the bullet together." And together they did, sharing their thoughts and insights throughout the process.

The results were dramatic. Not only did they feel energized by the 3-day plan, they "got" the low-toxin lifestyle. Because they could really *feel* the difference and *see* the results quickly, they were able to transition seamlessly into a healthier, happier life and lifestyle.

With all this new energy, they not only got back on the road, they got back in business—cherry-picking their projects, enjoying their newfound creativity with unloaded bodies and hearts. Best of all, they realized the true joy of retirement: the prospect of living into their nineties together, healthy and happy and whole.

TOXIC TRIGGER: **TRAVEL**

Travel can be life enriching; it can also be quite draining, especially if you're a frequent business traveler. Airlines routinely spray insecticides throughout the cabin before international flights, fouling the air quality on board—and that's to say nothing of the ambient germs or air fresheners or flame retardants that build up in recirculated air. Furthermore, during long, high-altitude flights, such as those the Ehrlichs frequently took to Asia and Australia, passengers are literally exposed to cosmic radiation, which can be a stress to the human system. (Unfortunately, there's not much you can do to avoid it if you're going long distances.)

MY ADVICE

Do what you can to limit the number of trips you take in a year, break your flight into smaller segments, and support your body by drinking plenty of water and choosing the healthiest foods that detoxify naturally—organic fruits, vegetables, and whole grains.

CASE HISTORY

Two Exhausted Caregivers

On the face of it, Annie and Britney had little in common beyond geography. Annie was a 70-year-old retired business executive who'd successfully raised three kids on the Upper East Side of Manhattan, having lived a life of jet-setting glamour. Britney was a late-twenties stay-at-home mom in Brooklyn with two little boys. But they both came to me completely depressed and utterly depleted, and for the same reason: They were caregivers.

Annie's husband, Max, had developed Alzheimer's, cutting short their happy retirement. His decline was swift and brutal. The three adult children were happy to help Annie when they could—which wasn't much, since they all lived at least one plane ride away. Max needed around-the-clock care, and Annie felt it was her job to give it to him. Because his dementia was so severe, Max could not be left alone safely. Ever. And so Annie stayed with him, 24/7, afraid to leave the house, unable to even take a short walk or meet a friend for coffee. She loved Max, but she hated what he had become—and the life she now felt trapped in.

Britney's younger son, Jackson, was severely autistic. Though she and her husband, Chase, reached out into the community and availed themselves of every resource they could, they felt overwhelmed by their child's special needs. Determined to beat the disease, they'd tried everything to help Jackson, at considerable expense of time and money. They'd see little breakthrough moments, a glimmer of hope, then Jackson would backslide and Britney would return to her normal state of mind: despair. Chase did everything he could to help her, but he also had to hold down his job in order to keep the family's health insurance and pay for Jackson's treatments. Meanwhile, their older child, Spencer, was just coming into his own as a 10-year-old—he wanted to play sports, he wanted to take art lessons. Britney very much wanted his childhood to be normal and tried to accommodate Spencer's requests, but it was all too much.

Both women were eating spottily, serving the healthy stuff to their charges as best they could, though perhaps too often settling for whatever those charges would eat, which was often high-carb comfort food (the crutch of every caregiver). Both were running on stress, feeling that they could not escape it. Because they were dealing with anxiety all day long, they were fueled by adrenaline—becoming toxic from the inside out. I prescribed a 3-day juice cleanse for both of them and emphasized how important it would be for them to find some kind of stress relief. I emphasized the need to make time for social connection *outside* the realm of the caregiving. Though it's an old analogy, it works: You put the oxygen mask on yourself first, so that you stay alive to help the others you care for.

Annie, at my urging, availed herself of one of New York's juice delivery services. She loved it—here was one less thing to think about! Even more, she loved the resulting revelation, which came for her on day 3. "It was like something lifted," she told me. "I could see that life could go on."

With this new perspective, Annie made other changes. She didn't go vegan, exactly, but she ate a lot less meat. She also eliminated all the cake and cookie comforts she kept around the house to soothe herself. She felt great about these changes, in part because Max's diet improved, too. It wasn't always easy, but with some creative thinking, Annie was able to cre-ate for him delicious, real, nutrient-dense foods and serve them to him with genuine love.

Though she resisted my suggestion that she see a therapist, she did find a support group for Alzheimer's caregivers at her neighborhood community center and hired help so that she could go out. Finally, a circle of friends who could really understand what she was going through! It was a huge relief, and with their help Annie committed to extending to herself the same excellent care she was offering to Max.

Britney decided to juice for herself, thinking that she could share the nutritional benefits with Jackson (which she did). She had never done anything like this before, but she embraced the idea wholeheartedly, knowing she needed to make exactly this kind of healthy change. For her, making the choice to do it was one small step toward taking care of her-self again. It was empowering for her and made her feel like a better wife and mother. Determined to eliminate toxins from her family life, she delved into her research and overhauled not only her diet but her house-hold routines as well. Because Jackson was always sick, she was a fanati-cal cleaner and never hesitated to use antibacterial soaps and industrial surface cleaners—all of which were introducing even more toxins to her home environment.

For Britney, as for Annie, clarity was the biggest side benefit. Britney saw how limited her life had become. She had been a runner but gave it up com-pletely to be with Jackson around the clock. While on the cleanse, she sim-ply *knew* (or maybe remembered) that she needed to run to keep her sanity. So she found a cooperative parenting group that traded hours of care for their autistic children and suddenly had time to go on three runs a week.

When, on a return visit, she told me, "I feel like the person I was 10 years ago," I had to laugh. She'd just been a kid! But I was tickled to see her calm and centered and feeling she had enough energy to live her life fully.

TOXIC TRIGGER: **SOCIAL ISOLATION**

Loneliness is one of those ubiquitous toxins that fly under the radar, but its effects can nonetheless be devastating. Every day new studies are confirm-ing that social isolation leads to degenerative health conditions, most nota-bly depression and heart disease. Annie's stress over the condition of her husband was only compounded by her determination to stay with him around the clock, to the exclusion of anything or anyone else. Social support can be the key to relieving stress.

MY ADVICE

Make time for friends weekly (and, no, Facebook updates will not do). If you're facing a crisis, try to find a support group with whom to share your feelings.

TOXIC TRIGGER: **HOUSEHOLD CLEANING PRODUCTS**

Any parent with a sick child will take pains to create a home that is free from bacteria and viruses. Often the parents will choose antibiotic soaps and surface sprays, as Britney did. In her quest for clean, Britney loaded up on antibacterial cleansers and power cleaners of all stripes. She was also fastidious in making sure the air in the house smelled fresh and frequently used chemical air fresheners and scented candles. When we made a list of all her industrial cleansers, we counted 15—all of them toxic.

MY ADVICE

Soap and water has been proven just as effective in keeping bacteria and viruses at bay, so switch to natural cleansers, powered by essential oils. Ditto for air fresheners and candles, if you must use them, though a better investment would be in a houseplant or two, which are proven to clear the air pollution.

CASE HISTORY

The Sensitive Superstar

Leila seemed to have it all: She was a famous movie actress with a loyal husband and a couple of healthy, loving children. She was catered to and pampered by nearly everyone who ever came into contact with her. She had a slew of agents, assistants, personal trainers, stylists, makeup artists, and dietitians at the ready to help her keep getting work and looking good. She had looks, she had money, and she had enough box-office power to pick and choose her projects. What she didn't have was something no one in her world seemed to know (or care) much about: her health.

Despite appearances, Leila didn't feel well much of the time. Since her early teens, she had suffered an array of bothersome, if oblique, digestive complaints: gas and bloating, diarrhea alternating with constipation, indigestion, and heartburn. By the time she found her way to my office at age 40, Leila had been through the medical wringer. She had seen every specialist in the book and endured many times over a full battery of testing, colonoscopies, endoscopies, sonograms, and blood work, but the doctors had failed to find anything definitive. She had already tried eliminating dairy, as one doc suggested, to no avail. So they slapped her with the label irritable bowel syndrome (IBS), a grab-bag "diagnosis" that doctors use to cover digestive troubles that come and go. (It is medical speak for "we really don't know what's happening.")

Because she was a respected and powerful Hollywood star, they catered to Leila, of course, prescribing an array of medications aimed to allay her symptoms. Mostly Leila found the side effects either scary (as with the gastroesophageal reflux disease [GERD] meds, which she'd heard could cause bone loss) or onerous (as with the antianxiety and antispasmodic drugs commonly prescribed for IBS patients). The antianxiety medication was the only thing that really eased the symptoms, but it left her feeling drowsy and dopey and dependent. In her career, she said, she couldn't afford to lose her edge. She needed a different approach. Moreover, she wanted to know why this was happening and address the problem at its source.

She'd been tested several times for celiac, an autoimmune disease caused by gluten, but had always been negative. Still, I suspected wheat sensitivity (less an allergic condition like celiac than a chemical sensitivity to other ingredients within wheat besides gluten), which is usually overlooked by a medical establishment that's always viewed things in black (celiac) or white (no celiac, therefore, A-OK). A diet journal revealed that, indeed, she was eating tons of the stuff—making what she thought were healthy choices, opting for whole wheat breads and pastas. But gluten is only one of many potentially problematic compounds found in modern American wheat, many of which can create chemical reactions that the human digestive tract is ill equipped to deal with. Trouble is, even small reactions, over time, will begin to sabotage the digestion and result in all kinds of tummy troubles . . . just as Leila was experiencing.

The wheat was toxic to her system. She needed to quit consuming the stuff, overhaul her diet, release accumulated toxins, and heal her gut. This made a big difference quickly—as it does for nearly half of my over-40 patients. So I prescribed the best medicine at my disposal: the 21-day cleanse.

The 3-day cleanse did for Leila exactly what I knew it would: It gave her digestion a rest and infused her system with phytonutrients, which gave her energy and confidence in our plan. As she worked through the entire 21 days, she felt better and better and watched her symptoms slowly disappear. When she started to eat "normally" again, she stuck with most of the principles of the Detox Prescription and vowed to stay wheat free for life. Within 3 months, she said, she felt like a whole new person.

TOXIC TRIGGER: **WHEAT**

The modern wheat we eat today is in fact a highly hybridized, genetically modified foodstuff that contains dozens of carbohydrate and protein molecules that are new to the human body and likely to create a chemical sensitivity. For more on this, read the fantastic book *Wheat Belly* by William Davis, MD. In it, he argues that modern wheat bears little resemblance to the grain our caveman forebears ate; it's so new in our relative evolution that the body hasn't had time to create coping mechanisms to deal with it! Celiac disease and gluten sensitivity are only a small part of an overall epidemic of wheat-related woes . . . ongoing exposure can result in symptoms like Leila's and eventually in obesity, heart disease, and even diabetes. Don't get me wrong: Whole grain foods can be a healthy choice if you're among those who can tolerate them. If you are sensitive to them, however, they can wreck your health.

MY ADVICE

Cut the wheat entirely if you're experiencing IBS or GERD; even if you're not, cut back on the stuff significantly to see if your condition improves. Consider looking at other problematic foods, too, especially dairy, soy, eggs, nuts, and seafood. Together with wheat, these five foods are thought to account for 90 percent of all food allergies and sensitivities. Talk to your doctor about a simple panel test for IgG or whole blood allergic reactions—which are not as severe as the classic IgE reaction associated with anaphylactic shock but can contribute to chronic problems such as headaches and IBS. Definitely experiment with quinoa, a rarely allergenic grain that's also a great source of protein.

You might have seen a little of yourself in one of these case studies. Maybe you have a little overworker or couch potato in you; maybe you tend to isolate yourself in times of stress or fret about growing old. Maybe you eat anything and everything; maybe you eat practically nothing. I chose these case studies not because they are extraordinary (though in some cases the people behind them certainly are) but because they are so very common. Each and every one encapsulates the human condition in the early 21st century, fighting to thrive in an increasingly toxic world.

But it may well be that your story is completely different. Every one of us has a different tale to tell, a different set of circumstances and symptoms and exposures. If you are feeling bad and can get to an integrative physician who specializes in functional medicine to help you work through your individual set of problems, by all means make an appointment today (for local references go to functionalmedicine.org). If not, turn to the next chapter and let me help you help yourself. The journey starts with a simple question: *How toxic am I?*

how
toxic
are you?

W hen I tell my patients that they're likely to be "toxic," many of them are very surprised. They want to know how it could have happened, the most likely culprits in their food and environment, and just what level of toxicity I'm talking about. If they're new to the model of integrative medicine, they might demand some testing to see "proof positive" that they have a problem.

Proof can be had, of course, if you are willing to pay for it. We can test the human body for thousands of chemical stressors. We can test blood serum levels, we can test hair and urine and feces for traces of chemicals and metals. We can test for specific dysfunctions known to be a direct result of toxic exposure, such as high levels of lipid peroxides. We can do stress testing to check the overload factor of specific detox pathways. With the latest technologies, we can even look at the genome itself for evidence of weaknesses—in the form of single-nucleotide polymorphisms, or SNPs (pronounced "snips"). SNPs are defects in the DNA that make us more susceptible to diseases like breast cancer or Alzheimer's—and though they are not the direct result of toxins, they are more likely to assert themselves in a negative way when exposed to environmental stressors.

The thing is, most insurance companies won't cover such testing, which can easily tally in the thousands—if not tens of thousands—of dollars. If you have the money and want to spend it, I'm happy to help. But aside from testing for heavy metals (which I often suggest under certain circumstances, see "Don't Be a Metal Head," page 34), proper evaluation and treatment can be done with a few of the tests. As I said in Chapter 1, for most of us there is no single bullet (as in aha, it's PFOA!). Battling toxins is more like handling a dirty bomb. If it's a financial stress, you can save your money on diagnostics and mostly skip right to the treatment, especially if you feel chronically unwell and are working with a doctor who is looking at the whole picture with you. In all but a very few instances, such as when you're doing chemotherapy, have Crohn's disease, or are pregnant (see "Proceed with Caution," page 96, for more details), a simple food-based detox improves symptoms—often dramatically—and is incredibly safe.

> The evidence that we are all toxic, to varying degrees, is now overwhelming.

The evidence that we are all toxic, to varying degrees, is now overwhelming. We are all exposed to toxins in the air, water, and soil. Tens of thousands of chemicals are in use in modern industry and agriculture, and it's hard to know exactly how many of them are problematic for us—our government and industry leaders don't exactly have the best track record in being proactive about protecting human health at the expense of economic expansion.

Worse, most of us are exposed to toxic chemicals even before we are born. Thanks to an excellent—though shocking—study conducted by the watchdog organization Environmental Working Group, we know that not only BPA is present in the cord blood of babies, but 232 other synthetic chemicals are, too. The list includes all of the chemicals listed on pages 8 and 9, as well as heavy metals, which are known to interfere with neurological development.

I hesitate to share the full picture with every patient—it's scary stuff and can be overwhelming. But I do urge them to make the connections between their own lifestyle exposures and health stressors. To that end, I encourage nearly everyone who walks through my clinic door to take the two quizzes on the following pages. The first is a Medical Symptom Questionnaire developed by the Institute of Functional Medicine. It is a proven, reliable way to link niggling health concerns we've accepted as part of our "okay, not great" health picture—or as a natural by-product of aging. It shows us how an accumulation of little annoyances can lead to chronic, often debilitating problems—such as undermining energy, detracting from performance, deflating happiness, and eventually snowballing into serious health crises. My patients are often surprised that these "little issues," so small that they didn't even think to mention them, add up—and how each one can be linked to toxin overload.

The second is the Environmental Factors Questionnaire, which I've developed myself to assess a broad range of lifestyle exposures. It asks you to consider chemical exposure in your food and in your environment, but also habits and patterns that create toxins from within. Unchecked stress, sleeplessness, lack of exercise, excess weight, and social isolation can be nearly as toxic on the system as any of the chemicals dreamed up by the maddest of scientists. Even if you are feeling well, the effects of living a toxic lifestyle will catch up with you over time. Why wait to do something about it?

Each test can stand alone; you don't have to do both. However, I recommend that you consider both sets of results. Chances are, if you're reading this book, you are curious about whether you are toxic and understand (or at least hold out hope) that you could be feeling much better. If your score on one or the other of these tests is very high, I recommend that you seek professional help and the individual attention required to cope with your situation and to right your sinking health ship. Try to find yourself an integrative/functional medicine practitioner, who is trained to combine Western medicine with nutrition and integrative approaches, to assess your situation and design an intervention plan that can help you in more depth than this book can provide. The Institute for Functional Medicine offers an incredible directory; find it at functionalmedicine.org.

If you're in the middle range—which most of us are—you can take charge of your health right now by eliminating toxins from your diet and your household, by embracing positive health habits, and by kick-starting your new, healthy life. Even if you're on the low end of the scale, you'll benefit from the nutritious and delicious recipes and irresistible mind-body practices you'll find in *The Detox Prescription*.

Do You Need Further Testing?

Although I don't usually submit my patients to a battery of tests to learn which toxins might be causing their problems (with the exception of heavy metals—there are too many to count, and it's very expensive), I do use both general and specialized testing when I suspect an underlying condition. This allows me to rule out specific nutritional deficiencies, infections, and degenerative diseases that might be yielding symptoms similar to those experienced by healthy patients who are in need of a simple detox.

Because your physician may not be aware of the importance of looking into toxins as a cause of problems—and even if he is, he may be constrained by cost—you might need to be proactive about requesting the tests required to rule out any of the following conditions—especially if you have a family history:

- Infections (such as chronic viral, amoebas, gingivitis, or Lyme disease)
- Hormone imbalance (thyroid, adrenal, or female or male sex hormones)
- Autoimmune disease (rheumatoid arthritis, lupus, Sjögren's)
- Heart disease (arrhythmia, high blood pressure, angina)
- Neurodegenerative disease (multiple sclerosis, early Alzheimer's)
- Liver or kidney dysfunction
- Malabsorption (especially from leaky gut syndrome)
- Inflammatory bowel disease (Crohn's and colitis)
- Celiac disease
- Silent reflux
- Small intestinal bacterial overgrowth ("SIBO")
- COPD (poor respiratory function)

How Toxic Are You Feeling?

This is the gold-standard questionnaire for gauging toxicity based on physical symptoms, developed by the Institute for Functional Medicine.

Because I am a member of this group, and because I know that it represents the best science available, I use this questionnaire to get a quick

- Chronic sinusitis

- Migraine

- Allergies (either inhaled or food)

- Heavy metal accumulation

- Nutritional deficiencies (such as B_{12}, iron, vitamin D, calcium, iodine, magnesium)

- Genetic predispositions (SNPs)

The best practitioner to consult is one who is trained in functional medicine, since he or she is trained to look past symptoms to the underlying causes. You can find a functional medicine practitioner in your area through the Web site of the Institute for Functional Medicine (functionalmedicine.org). Additionally, integrative practitioners use the best of allopathic medicine as well as botanical medicine, Eastern practices, mind-body therapies, and cutting-edge nutrition and are trained to take a personalized lifestyle medicine approach.

If you and/or your doctor do decide to pursue more in-depth toxin testing, it will benefit you to seek out an environmental medicine expert. You can find a list of practitioners trained in this area from the American Academy of Environmental Medicine (AAEMonline.org). But be aware that such testing can run you way north of $1,000 (and is typically not covered by insurance). And most conventional physicians won't know how to interpret abnormal toxin findings—much less what to do about them. Again, functional and environmental medicine experts are typically most knowledgeable about toxicity and can guide you through this process if needed (including which are the most reliable labs to use for testing).

Find more information on these and other tests at www.woodsonmerrell.com.

Don't Be a Metal Head

The heavy metals arsenic, lead, and mercury are number one, two, and three on the priority list of hazardous substances tallied by the Agency for Toxic Substances and Disease Registry (ATSDR). Testing for them is wise, especially if you're having serious cognitive difficulties (see the lists of symptoms below) or feeling agitated all the time. These may not be entirely eliminated from the body through normal detox processes; you may need to undergo chelation therapy to bind the metals and safely eliminate them from the body. Your doctor can administer blood, urine, or hair-analysis tests, most of which are covered by insurance.

Lead is commonly found in old houses—particularly in lead-based paints, which may flake or chip over time, even if they are covered up—and in outmoded plumbing. Many city water systems may feature some lead pipes—or lead welding—that can leach into the water even in new homes. Though lead paint has been banned for use on toys in the United States, it is still used in those manufactured overseas. Also, a recent study conducted at the University of Florida found lead in 8 of 22 commonly used brands of calcium supplements. *Symptoms may include memory loss, high blood pressure, and mood disorders.*

Mercury exposure comes mainly from fish in the diet—those caught in polluted waters are risky, as are large, predatory species like tuna or swordfish. As a rule of thumb, the bigger the fish, the more likely it is to be contaminated (salmon is an exception), because these larger fish feed on smaller fish and the mercury accumulates in their fatty tissue. Mercury is also found in the particulate matter emitted into the air by coal-burning power plants and in old silver mercury–based fillings, especially if they are damaged. *Symptoms may include tremors, vision disturbances, muscle weakness, and lack of coordination.*

Arsenic is classified by the FDA as a carcinogen. It's both ubiquitous in the environment and insidious in its effects. Human exposure comes via produce, which absorbs arsenic from water, soil, and fish. One recent *Consumer Reports* study showed that arsenic, which was previously used as an insecticide in cotton fields, is present in nearly all rice—a troubling development. *Symptoms include headaches, abdominal pain, and confusion.*

baseline for nearly every one of my patients. But as much as it helps me to see exactly how toxins and other toxic influences are interfering with their health and vitality, it helps *them* to get a sense of the subtle web toxic exposure can weave throughout the entire body.

Nothing here is a smoking gun signifying danger; indeed, we all suffer from headaches, fatigue, stuffy heads, food cravings, and/or anxiety from time to time. But as you weigh your answers, you may begin to see patterns—ways in which you've been undermined by *poor lifestyle choices*. Maybe you'll realize that you've been feeling bad for a while, but simply soldiering forth—figuring that everybody must feel this way, that it's normal. It's not.

Good health should feel that way—good. And while it's true that age does slow things down and bring on natural aches and pains, *toxic lifestyle factors* introduce a kind of unpleasant background noise—maybe not overt sensations or even namable complaints, but a constant grating drag. It's the "ugh" zone.

The questionnaire is organized into categories associated with body systems. Your own symptoms may cluster around one, two, or more of these—or be spread pretty evenly throughout. In some cases, answers might seem contradictory or impossible. Can you be sluggish *and* hyperactive? Have diarrhea *and* constipation? But toxins are not normal—and neither are the array of symptoms they cause.

Take this quiz at the outset of your detox, but don't set it aside—you can use it throughout the plan to see how you are doing. Take it again on days 3, 7, 14, and 21 of the Detox Prescription plan—or whenever you need a little inspiration to keep on going. Chances are you'll be pleasantly surprised how quickly, thoroughly, and measurably better you feel.

SELF-TEST #1: MEDICAL SYMPTOM QUESTIONNAIRE

Answer each question on a scale of 0 to 4:

    0 = I never experience this symptom.

    1 = I occasionally experience this symptom, but it's not severe.

    2 = I occasionally experience this symptom, and it *is* severe.

    3 = I often experience this symptom, but it's not severe.

    4 = I often experience this symptom, and it *is* severe.

(continued)

Head

Do you have headaches? ___

Do you feel faint? ___

Do you feel dizzy? ___

Do you suffer from insomnia? ___

Subtotal ___

Digestion

Do you feel nauseous or have
bouts of vomiting? ___

Do you have diarrhea? ___

Do you have constipation? ___

Do you feel bloated? ___

Do you frequently burp or pass gas? ___

Do you have heartburn? ___

Do you have stomach or intestinal pain? ___

Subtotal ___

Muscles and Joints

Do you have pain or aches in your
joints? ___

Do you have arthritis? ___

Do you feel stiff or feel limited in your
movements? ___

Are your muscles stiff, painful, or achy? ___

Do you feel physically weak? ___

Subtotal ___

Eating and Weight

Do you indulge in binge eating
or drinking? ___

Do you crave particular foods? ___

Are you overweight? ___

Are you underweight? ___

Do you retain water? ___

Do you eat compulsively or mindlessly? ___

Subtotal ___

Energy Level

Do you feel fatigued or sluggish? ___

Do you feel apathetic or lethargic? ___

Do you feel hyperactive? ___

Do you feel restless? ___

Subtotal ___

Mind

Is your memory short or faulty? ___

Do you have trouble comprehending
information? ___

Do you have trouble concentrating? ___

Are you uncoordinated? ___

Do you find it difficult to make decisions? ___

Do you stutter or stammer? ___

Do you slur your speech? ___

Do you suffer from any
learning disabilities? ___

Subtotal ___

Emotions

Do you have mood swings? ___

Are you anxious, fearful, or nervous? ___

Are you angry, aggressive,
or irritable? ___

Are you depressed? ___

Subtotal ___

Eyes

Are your eyes itchy or watery? ___

Are your eyelids swollen, sticky,
or reddened? ___

Do you have bags or dark circles
under your eyes? —
Do you ever have blurry or tunnel
vision? —
Subtotal —

Ears

Do your ears feel itchy on the inside? —
Do you suffer from earaches
or infections? —
Do you have drainage from your ears? —
Do you experience ringing
in your ears? —
Subtotal —

Nose

Do you have a stuffy nose? —
Do you have sinus problems? —
Do you suffer from hay fever? —
Do you have sneezing attacks? —
Do you have excessive mucus
formation? —
Subtotal —

Mouth and Throat

Do you have a chronic cough? —
Do you frequently feel the need
to clear your throat? —
Do you have a sore throat, hoarseness,
or loss of voice? —
Are your lips, tongue, or gums
swollen or discolored? —
Do you have canker sores? —
Subtotal —

Skin

Do you have acne? —
Do you get hives, rashes,
or patches of dry skin? —
Do you have hair loss? —
Do you suffer from flushing or hot
flashes? —
Are you excessively sweaty? —
Subtotal —

Heart Health

Do you ever experience
an irregular or skipped heartbeat? —
Do you ever experience a rapid or
pounding heartbeat? —
Do you ever experience chest pain? —
Subtotal —

Respiratory System

Do you have chest congestion? —
Do you suffer from asthma
or bronchitis? —
Do you have shortness of breath? —
Do you have difficulty breathing? —
Subtotal —

General Health

Do you get sick frequently? —
Do you feel the need to urinate
urgently or frequently? —
Do you suffer from any genital itch
or discharge? —
Subtotal —

GRAND TOTAL —

Test courtesy of the Institute for Functional Medicine

Scoring the Medical Symptom Questionnaire

0 to 50: Keep It Clean

In short: Everything is fine. A detox diet plan is not urgently needed. How-ever, the Detox Prescription will enhance your life by flooding your body with nutrition, lending vitality and energy. Keeping your organs of diges-tion, assimilation, and detoxification strong and healthy is the best way to ensure that your numbers stay in this range permanently.

50 to 70: Toxins on Board

You are just starting to see the effects of accumulated toxins—and may be witnessing the beginnings of disease processes. Undertaking the Detox Pre-scription will be a real lifesaver for you—the sooner you start, the sooner you will see improvement. Better, you'll also stand a real chance of avoiding long-term health problems through lifestyle changes alone. At this stage, you truly can be your own best physician.

70 to 100: Take Action Now

If you haven't already received a significant diagnosis—high blood pres-sure, sugar, or cholesterol—you are working on one. The Detox Prescrip-tion diet is absolutely essential for you. In addition, you'll need to clean up your home environment (see Chapter 4). If your symptoms tend to cluster around one particular area—digestion, say, or emotions—you may benefit from taking nutritional supplements related to your particular health chal-lenge (see Chapter 8).

100 and above: 911!

There's no doubt: You are sick and in need of serious medical attention. Find an expert in the field of functional medicine (consult the directory at functionalmedicine.org if you don't already have one) and make an appointment today. You can do days 4 through 21 of the Detox Prescrip-tion diet, but you will benefit the most from doing it under medical supervision. Don't do the 3-day juice cleanse until you have your doc-tor's okay.

How Toxic Are You Living?

What follows is a tool I've developed myself for helping patients assess their toxic exposure risks based on environmental factors. It looks first at the externals—mostly what's in your air, water, and food. And a lot of the usual suspects are accounted for here—pesticide-laden produce, chemical-heavy home cleaners, hormone-disrupting plastics. If you've given the previous chapter a careful read, not much on this list should surprise you.

But this questionnaire also considers the *internal* environment you create for yourself with your own lifestyle choices. Burning the candle at both ends, indulging your anxieties, keeping yourself isolated, or nursing grudges and other negative thoughts—all these habits create intrinsic toxins, the by-products of the body's stress mechanisms. Whereas they are "completely natural," these can weigh as heavily on the body as anything cooked up in an industrial laboratory.

Patients are often surprised to see how these toxic stressors are weighted against one another. In particular, this questionnaire lets them see that little lifestyle habits they've been holding on to, maybe thinking to themselves, "it's not so bad," can add up. Maybe you like to snack on microwave popcorn, spritz on perfume, satisfy your sweet tooth, wash your hands frequently with antibacterial soap, or even sneak a smoke every now and then. These choices come with consequences. I don't want you to feel that you should deny yourself every pleasure—indeed, an occasional indulgence won't hurt much, even if it's less than healthy. But little "cheats" and "crutches" do add up. And when you see the toll they can exact, you may choose to choose differently.

We cannot control many toxic factors—in the face of increasingly polluted water, air, and earth, we may feel like walking around in a hazmat suit. But the truth is, by controlling our habits of mind, body, and spirit, we do control many more harmful factors than we might previously have known. We can choose what we drink, eat, take, say, and do; most of us have a lot of leverage about what we spray into the air, slather onto our bodies, and scrub onto our homes' surfaces.

The science on this subject is absolutely clear: Lifestyle changes are powerful medicine. When we make good choices, we literally have the power to write most of our own health destiny—to decide not only how well we will

The Medication Equation

Do you take a number of prescription and over-the-counter medications every day to keep health problems in check, to feel better, or to stave back symptoms of stress? Most Americans do. Medications compete with each other in the body's detox pathways for a limited supply of phase I cytochrome enzymes and phase II conjugators—and also compete in those same pathways with pesticides, herbicides, and other incidental toxins we run into every day. When we turn to drugs as easy answers for every little annoyance, we could be unwittingly boosting our body's toxin burden.

I do not advocate stopping or reducing any medication suddenly, and certainly not without the consent and guidance of the prescribing physician. Some pharmaceuticals are real lifesavers and must be continued. But if you're on an arsenal of self-prescribed over-the-counter medicines, or lean too regularly on prescriptions that are meant only for occasional usage (such as sleep aids or painkillers), consider weaning yourself off them.

Even drugs that might have once seemed essential—blood pressure or cholesterol medicine—might be eliminated (or significantly reduced) once proper lifestyle changes are firmly in place. Consider talking with your doctor about reducing your use of these pharmaceuticals:

Acetaminophen: This drug (also known by the brand names Tylenol and Panadol) is often recommended for aches, pain, and fever for those with sensitive stomachs. However, in large doses or taken frequently, it can be toxic to the liver. An occasional NSAID (such as ibuprofen, taken with food/antacids for those with stomach issues) can sometimes be a better choice for pain and fever. And for inflammation (something acetaminophen doesn't help with anyway) consider an enzyme, herbal, or homeopathic formula (more on this in Chapter 8). And do *not* take Tylenol if you drink alcohol regularly, as it increases the burden on your liver.

Acid-suppressing medications: Antacids (like Tums or Alka-Seltzer) are okay to take occasionally—as are drugs that inhibit the production of acid in the stomach, such as H2

feel today and tomorrow, but even how our genetic tendencies will play out over the long haul.

When we educate ourselves about toxins in the environment—both internal and external—we can begin to get out of protection mode and

blockers (Tagamet, Pepcid, Zantac, and Axid) and proton-pump inhibitors (Prilosec, Zegerid, and Prevacid). But taken long term—over a period of months, or even years as some people do—they can interfere with bone health, the digestive process, and even with nutrient uptake: The longer you take them, the more pronounced these deficits can be (including osteonecrosis of the jaw and femur fractures). Instead of taking these drugs, you can talk to a knowledgeable integrative doctor about reducing acidic foods with natural substances that help the stomach lining heal (such as special forms of licorice [DGL], mastic gum, zinc carnosine, and enzymes). I will review all of these options in Chapter 8.

Corticosteroids: Though these drugs can be lifesaving for acute, severe problems such as asthma or allergy attacks—and even long term for certain autoimmune conditions—they also create many deleterious effects on mind, mood, and emotion. When steroid drugs are taken chronically, their side effects can manifest quickly, causing weight gain, ulcers, high blood pressure, and immune system suppression. When they are inhaled, however, it's harder to feel the effects—though this doesn't necessarily mean they're safer (they have been shown to be absorbed over time). Avoid these long term when you can—and always question if you really have to use them instead of other choices with less-far-reaching consequences for reducing inflammation such as herbs and food-based nutrients (e.g., turmeric, omega-3 oils, and enzymes).

Chemotherapy (and radiation): If you are undergoing radiation and/or chemotherapy, you have pretty much hit the medical industry's rock bottom. This is, after all, medicine specifically designed to be toxic (to cancer cells). It is rough treatment. But there's a bright side: There is nowhere to go but up! The fundamentals of a plant-based diet, such as the one in Chapter 7, can be a big assist to your body's strength and resilience. (Supplements are disallowed during chemo.) When it is all over, you'll be free to regain your best health by eating the very best food and adapting the lifestyle choices that truly support your glowing wellness. The Detox Prescription can help you get there.

into proaction mode. We can work to cultivate a state of optimal health. Doing the Detox Prescription plan is a giant first step toward that goal.

As with the medical symptom questionnaire, this one is organized into particular areas of focus—do it, and you will quickly see where you might need to make lifestyle changes. Some will be simple swap-outs—for instance, if you're using a chemical-based air freshener, you can simply replace it with one that's based on natural essential oils. Others will require a sacrifice in service of the greater good—if you're using a lawn service that relies on chemical pesticides and fertilizers, for instance, you'll need to stop for your own health as well as that of those around you. In some cases, you may need professional help to make healthy changes—to stop smoking, if you've been at it for years, or to explore the possibility of reducing or eliminating a toxic medication.

You may have to do some investigation to answer these questions accurately. You may honestly not know whether the food you're buying contains herbicides or pesticides, or whether that furniture polish is made using harmful chemicals. In general, unless you've purchased a product that overtly states its wholesomeness and lack of toxicity right up front, it's pretty safe to assume the worst. This questionnaire refers to the standard-issue, conventional versions of consumer products—what you get if you don't specifically go looking for something safe and toxin free.

SELF-TEST #2: ENVIRONMENTAL FACTORS QUESTIONNAIRE

Scoring

0 = never (no)

1 = occasionally (yes)

2 = frequently

(Some exposures are so damaging, you'll need to add extra points where indicated.)

Cleaners

Do you use conventional chemical cleaners (furniture polish; disinfecting sprays; scrubs; or glass, surface, or metal cleaners) in any of these rooms?

• living room ___

• bedroom ___

• kitchen ___

• bathroom ___

Do you use conventional detergents, bleaches, or softeners for laundry? ___

Do you use conventional soap for dishwashing? ___

Do you use nonorganic room deodorizers like aerosols or plug-ins? ___

Is your shower curtain liner made of vinyl or plastic? ___

Do you use a conventional dry cleaner and remove the clothing from the plastic wrap less than 12 hours before wearing it? __

Ideal section score = < 2 __

Outdoors

Do you use chemical weed killers or herbicides on your lawn or landscape? __

Do you use chemical fertilizers? __

Have you treated your home or yard chemically for insect infestation? (ants, termites, etc.) __

Does your outdoor area feature older treated wood in decking, play structures, or landscaping materials? __

Ideal section score = < 2 __

Occupation

Does your work involve exposure to inhaled or skin-contact chemical agents (dentist, dry cleaner, shoe repairman, welder, industrial worker, etc.)? __

Ideal section score = < 2 __

Electromagnetic Fields (EMFs)

Do you use an electric blanket? __

Do you use a mobile phone next to your ear more than 15 minutes a day? __

Do you keep your mobile phone in a pocket or clipped to your body? __

Is there a powered electric device within 2 feet of your bed? __

Do you live within 50 feet of a mobile phone tower or high power line? __

Ideal section score = < 2 __

Air Quality

Have you renovated your home using any of the following?

• conventional paints __

• plasterboard __

• polyurethane (+1) __

• sanding __

• glues for carpet or flooring (+1) __

Are there outdoor-air-quality alerts where you live? __

Are you often exposed to automotive exhaust? __

Do you spend more than 2 hours a day in a car? __

Do you tend to travel by air? __

Do you own new furniture—purchased less than 2 years ago? __

Does your home contain cabinets made of pressed wood composites? __

Is there paint in your house that's cracking and more than 20 years old? __

Is there heavy accumulation of dust on furniture or drapes? __

Do you have wall-to-wall carpet? __

Do you have a damp or musty basement? __

Is there visible mold in your home? __

Does anyone in your household smoke? (+2) __

Ideal section score = < 8 __

(continued)

Water

Does your home have old pipes? __

Do you drink from untested
well water? __

Do you live in a building with a roof
tank? __

Do you have heavy water discoloration
in the morning? __

Ideal section score = < 1 __

Ingested Therapies and Over-the-Counter Medicines

Do you use antibiotics more
than twice a year? __

Do you use nicotine patches, gum, or
spray more than twice a week? __

Do you use acetaminophen (aka Tylenol)
more than 4 days a week? __

Do you use NSAIDs (such as aspirin or
ibuprofen) more than 4 days a week? __

Do you use antihistamines (like
diphenhydramine) daily? __

Do you use decongestants daily? __

Do you use stomach acid-suppressing
medications daily? (+1) __

Do you use nutritional or herbal
supplements that are produced with no
ostensible quality assurance? __

Do you drink grapefruit juice
(6 ounces) with your prescription
medication? __

Do you have silver mercury fillings in
your teeth? __

Ideal section score = < 4 __

Daily Prescription Medications

Do you use inhaled steroids? Or oral
steroids? (+1) __

Do you take anticonvulsing or
antipsychotic medication? __

Do you use tranquilizers, sleeping pills,
or antidepressants? __

Are you on hormone therapy? __

Are you undergoing
chemotherapy? (+1) __

Are you in radiation therapy? (+1) __

Are you on a biologic agent (e.g.,
TNF blocker)? __

Are you on other medications?
(+1 for each additional beyond 2) __

**Ideal section score = limit as much as
possible (see "The Medication
Equation," page 40)** __

Personal Care

How often do you use conventional (read:
not specifically organic nor free of
synthetic preservatives, fragrances, or
sudsing agents) versions of the following
beauty and personal care products?

• Soap (perfumed) __

• Antibacterial soap __

• Perfume __

• Moisturizers __

• Shampoo __

• Hair dye __

• Sunblock __

• Nail polish __

• Deodorant/antiperspirant __

- Conditioner —
- Hairspray —
- Foundation —
- Eye and cheek color —
- Lipstick —
Ideal section score = < 4 —

Food Quality and Quantity

Do you eat a lot (3 or 4 days a week)
of fried food? (+1) —

Do you eat a lot (3 or 4 days a week)
of red meat? —

Do you eat a lot (3 or 4 days a week)
of cheese or other full-fat dairy? —

Do you eat tuna, swordfish, or other
large predatory fish? —

Do you eat a lot of sugar or refined
carbohydrates? (+1) —

Do you charbroil your meat? (+1) —

Do you usually subject your
vegetables to long cooking times? —

Do you eat foods that contain
high-fructose corn syrup (such as
sodas or salad dressings)? (+1) —

Do you eat foods (such as drinks
or processed foods) that contain
preservatives or colorants? —

Do you eat less than 50 grams of
protein a day? —

Do you eat less than 25 grams
of fiber a day? —

Do you eat less than eight servings
of fruits and vegetables a day? (+1) —

Ideal section score = < 4 —

Drinking

Do you drink less than 8 cups
of water a day? —

Do you drink more than 4 cups
of coffee a day? —

Do you use artificial sweeteners such as
aspartame, saccharin, or sucralose? —

Do you drink sugary soda daily? (+2) —

Do you drink more than two alcoholic
drinks a day? —

Do you drink alcohol more than
5 days a week? —

Ideal section score = < 2 —

Grocery Shopping

Do you usually buy conventional rather
than organic produce? (+1) —

Do you buy meat, eggs, or milk that is not
labeled antibiotic or rBGH free? —

Do you buy fish that may contain
mercury/heavy metals? (+1) —

Do you accept and handle paper
shopping receipts? (+1) —

Ideal section score = < 3 —

Cooking

Do you use Teflon-coated nonstick pans? —

Do you store food in plastic containers? —

Do you reheat food in
plastic containers? (+1) —

Do you use plastic wrap? —

Do you use canned foods? —

Do you microwave popcorn in prepared
bags? (+1) —

Ideal section score = < 4 —

(continued)

Exercise and Rest

Do you sleep less than 7 hours a day? __

Do you wake more than twice
a night? __

Do you have a job that requires you to
sit more than 4 hours a day? __

Do you exercise less than 3 hours
a week? __

Do you exercise more than 2 hours
a day? __

Do you fail to take one rest day a week
away from exercise? __

Ideal section score = < 2 __

Stress

Do you experience continuous daily
stress? (+1) __

Do you have episodic, high-intensity
stress? (+1) __

Do you suffer from chronic anxiety? (+1) __

Are you depressed, or do you have a
feeling of hopelessness? (+1) __

Are you a caregiver for someone who is
chronically ill? (+1) __

Do you smoke? (+2) __

Ideal section score = < 4 __

GRAND TOTAL __

Scoring the Environmental Factors Questionnaire

0 to 50: Supportive Surroundings

If you totaled 50 points or less, you are living pretty clean. Don't rest on those laurels, though. Everything you do to nudge that number toward zero will benefit your health in the long term.

Also, look carefully at your results to see if the questionnaire has revealed one or more areas of your life that need your serious attention. I've indicated what I believe to be the healthiest range for each lifestyle area. If you scored very high in any one or two areas—say, your kitchen equipment needs updating or you haven't been buying organic personal care products—you should address it as soon as you can. If you can see that a little of this and a little of that environmental toxin is sneaking in, hopefully your awareness is raised enough to tighten up the ship. (Ever heard the expression "nibbled to death by ducks"? Don't let that be your fate.)

50+: Toxins All around You

If you scored over 50, consider this a wake-up call: You need to make changes to your lifestyle and your environment, because your lifestyle and/or your environment are putting your health at risk. If you haven't already, you may soon start to feel the onset of symptoms related to toxicity. Read this score in conjunction with the results of your medical symptoms questionnaire, and take the appropriate action.

The higher the score, of course, the higher the need to make changes. And you may require professional help. A qualified functional and/or integrative medical doctor can help you deal with problematic lifestyle behaviors like sleeplessness, smoking, or dependency on drugs (be they recreational or pharmaceutical). For guidance in making lifestyle changes, a practitioner of traditional Chinese medicine or naturopathic medicine can be just as, or sometimes more, helpful and hands-on in this area than a conventional MD. A nutritionist can educate you about how to read food labels, navigate the grocery store, and make your kitchen a healthier place. A sports trainer can help you adjust your level of exercise so that you're getting just enough, but not too much. A specialist in mind-body medicine techniques (such Transcendental Meditation, imagery, biofeedback, etc.) can give you tools to help you deal with stress significantly better. Also, don't overlook the possibility that a mental health professional could help—with behavioral issues (why do you need that third glass of wine?), dysfunctional attachments (does that green lawn really matter?), and stress (why keep a job when your boss is an explosive jerk?).

> Don't put your own best health off for even one more day: Get help now.

I recognize that even within the realm of toxic elements that can be controlled, you may not be able to change quickly, either for personal or monetary reasons. You may need to care for an ailing spouse or parent—that's just life. You may not be able to replace home furnishings or fittings right now. You might be stuck with those silver mercury fillings for a while.

What you *can* do is set an intention to steadily steer your life into clearer, less toxic territory—when you find yourself facing an opportunity to change, change for the better. You've already started the process; just reading this book, being willing to assess your life, is a huge step. Now keep going—you have the power to transform your symptoms and your lifestyle with the Detox Prescription.

the detox continuum

First of all: Don't panic. Chances are, having taken the quizzes in Chapter 2, your eyes have been opened to just how many risk factors you have to contend with—and maybe just how poor you're feeling as a result.

You are not alone—exposure to toxins isn't a matter of being a "good" person or leading a "healthy" life. The most conscientious among us carry on doing what we've always done to create good health—getting our exercise, enjoying time outdoors, keeping our houses clean, drinking lots of water, eating what we've been taught is a nutritious and balanced diet. Only the benefits we expect to reap are elusive. If we're doing everything right, why don't we feel good? Are we doing it wrong after all?

No. Those *are* the right things to do for health. Only the game has changed because the world around us has changed. Today that outdoor air we're breathing is likely to contain all sorts of unhelpful particles, from exhaust to pesticides to particulate matter from coal-burning power plants. The fresh produce and lean meat we buy have been raised in an industrial system that has left them tainted with herbicides, pesticides, and traces of growth hormones and antibiotics. Home cleaners have come a long way from the days of grandma's vinegar-water solutions. But today's highly effective multitaskers, cocktails of powerful chemicals, exact a steep bodily toll for getting the job done so effectively and efficiently. Even water is no longer a sure bet for good health: Numerous studies have found that the cleanest sources of tap water contain traces of perchlorates (rocket fuel), pesticides, arsenic, heavy metals, and a whole host of low-level pathogens. And bottled water is not always a safer bet—it can contain the same toxic brew, with the unwelcome bonus of BPA particles leached from the plastic bottle.

It's not you, in other words. It's *them*—the toxins that have slowly crept into every aspect of our modern lifestyle. It is not your fault.

It all seems like heavy, bad news—and in general, it is. But there is a bright side. With a little bit of education and willingness to make changes to your life and, especially, to your diet, you can detoxify effectively and quickly. You can restore your health in the midst of the toxic chaos around you. And you can feel not only well again, but better than ever.

The first thing you may want to do is clean up your home environment. Once you understand what those odor-eliminating, mildew-slaying, scrubless scrubbers are really made of, you'll want to replace them with products that use more natural ingredients. Beyond cleaning up your cleaners, you'll want to sort through your cabinets and look for other opportunities to make your home safer and less toxic. You don't have to do everything at once, but over time you may want to make positive changes. Install a water filter if you can afford one. Get rid of your kids' flame-resistant-coated pajamas (and flame-retardant anything). When it's time to replace your shower curtain liner, skip the PVC vinyl (which is softened with hormone-disrupting phthalates) and opt for eco-friendly PEVA. As you work in the kitchen, assess the state of your plastic containers and nonstick cookware, replacing what's questionable or worn with glass, ceramic, or stainless steel as you can.

If you can't afford to make big changes quickly, here's how to prioritize: If it is off-gassing wildly (that is to say, you can smell chemicals emanating from it), you're applying it to your body or spraying it into the air, or you heat your food in it, it bears immediate action. Assess, and eliminate if you think there's a toxic danger. Everything else is much less urgent. Just do what you can to upgrade to eco-friendly material when you can. The next chapter will help you take some sensible steps toward clearing out what's not needed or wanted in your new toxin-free life.

> Eating well and clean is the single most powerful step you can take to detox your body and restore it to wellness.

Once the coast is clear, you'll naturally turn your attention to your diet. Here is where you have a chance to not only make better choices for the future but to use food in such a way that it can undo years of unwitting exposure to environmental toxins, and even past deliberate mistakes (such as drinking too much, smoking, or doing recreational drugs).

The diet is an all-powerful detoxification tool, one that can do so much to nourish the body as it treats disease. It is just one part of a bigger picture of wellness (that includes exercise, sleep, connection, and stress relief), but it is a major part. Eating well and clean is the single most powerful step you can take to detox your body and restore it to wellness.

Three Steps to Feeling Great

How much you detox, and for how long, depends on you. How toxic *are* you? How bad are you feeling? Are you officially sick? How much time are you willing to commit? Are you motivated to change now? For the foreseeable future? Forever?

Looking at where we are and how we are living now in light of a future ideal can be discouraging if there seems to be too much ground to cover. We are mostly creatures of habit, and we know this about ourselves. Anytime we are faced with radical change, or feel we have to deny ourselves or "give up" something, we rebel—whether on a conscious level or not.

At the same time, we want results and we want them now! The human brain is hardwired to prefer swift reward to long-term benefit—it's part of our primitive survival instinct, a relic of our caveman days when a missed opportunity (*Look! A peach!*) was an opportunity lost forever.

On the face of it, it's a conundrum: How can you create the deep and lasting change your highest self desires while satisfying the innate drive for the pleasure of immediate results?

The answer, of course, is to take it one step at a time. If those steps feel (and taste) fantastic, so much the better!

The plan outlined in this book offers a cumulative approach that can bring phenomenal results in as little as 3 days and continue to achieve benefits over the course of 7 or 21 days. My promise is this: Each increment allows the body to rest, recharge, and rebuild. Move through all three phases and you will have mastered the fundamentals necessary to eat in a way that truly nourishes the body—not just for a limited "detox time-out," but for an entire lifetime of balance and wellness.

STEP ONE: **THE 3-DAY TURBO CLEANSE**
A Quick-Results Cleanse That Kick-Starts Your Energy

The liquids-only part of the cleanse works hard and fast. It's a time-out for bad habits and a chance for your body to detox and recoup, providing nourishment through fresh fruit and vegetable juices, smoothies, and homemade nut milks, which specifically include all the fiber of whole food. It is absolutely the best way I know to get real results quickly.

Multiple studies conducted in Scandinavia in the 1990s proved irrefutably that juice cleanses could powerfully reduce inflammation in the body and even heal tough conditions, including the notoriously debilitating rheumatoid arthritis. More recent studies conducted in the United States and published in *Nutrition Journal* have added to those results, showing that an all-liquid diet also lends cardioprotective benefits and improves weight loss. Both studies were based on longer-term plans, but I've found that 3 days is just right for most of my patients. This is short enough so that anyone can muster the willpower to do it, yet it is long enough to interrupt toxic inputs, infuse the body with nutrition, and call attention to cravings—a major side benefit. It's an effective detox that works on multiple levels.

During the 3 days, you'll be resting your digestive tract and easing its workload by reducing the amount of input. At the same time, you'll be spoon-feeding (rather, straw-sipping) every major phytonutrient your detox system needs to heal and recharge itself. Recalling how the detox process works (see page 4), you'll be ingesting far fewer toxins, reducing the number of toxic intermediaries created during phase I detoxification, and boosting the effect of each of the detoxification pathways used for phase II. You'll be giving your body time to play catch-up and nourishing it in a way that may even help it get ahead of the game.

Fewer toxins + more detoxifying nutrition = a net win for your health

Patients often ask me if this is a fast. No, it is *not*. You're not abstaining from anything your body truly needs, especially since we include two protein-rich and delicious nut milks as part of each day's menu. You are, in fact, bathing your system with the leanest, cleanest, and most powerful source of pure nutrition—you're mainlining health, in a sense.

What you lack in texture—and I know, it can be hard to go 3 days without really digging your teeth into something—you gain in flavor. In fact, I believe you'll be surprised at just how alive your taste buds begin to feel within the first 24 hours. Within 48 hours, you'll really start to feel as well as taste the difference—you'll discover a new inner buoyancy, perhaps a sense of freedom stemming from the ease with which your body is working now. And within 72 hours, you'll feel energized, enlivened, engaged—and completely enabled (in the best sense of that word).

> Fewer toxins + more detoxifying nutrition = a net win for your health

Beyond better energy and enhanced taste, my patients report an uplifted mood and sense of clarity—what psychologists call "subjective well-being." On a physical level, they notice decreased puffiness, especially in the face, but also in the hands (rings are less tight) and ankles. Dark circles fade. And bloating disappears—pants feel a little looser! (They love that.) Creaky joints are less stiff, skin is clearer, sinuses feel clearer . . . in fact, a lot of the little complaints you might have ticked off on the Medical Symptom Questionnaire from the last chapter may have gotten better already. Plus, it's easier to get up in the morning, no joke. Hopefully, you'll see all of the above with the 3-Day Turbo Cleanse and be motivated to keep on going . . . and reap even more benefits.

STEP TWO: **THE 7-DAY IN-DEPTH DETOX**

A weeklong juice-and-food plan that will deepen your detox results and reset your health

In the next step, you'll add 4 days of completely vegan eating for a 7-Day In-Depth Detox that supports the body as it continues to detoxify and rebuild. This idea, again, was inspired by the impressive Scandinavian studies that showed healing for rheumatoid arthritis patients. Those who followed their juice cleanses with 3 weeks of an all-vegan diet—meaning completely free from all animal products, including eggs and dairy—were able to stay symptom free and off medication not only during the course of the study, but for a full 2 years afterward, even after they returned to their old habits. Incredible.

For some, the "V-word" may be off-putting—especially to those who perceive it as a great letting go of their favorite foods. But it's worth doing this for 4 days, because the ongoing benefits it extends will allow your body to continue to deeply detox—especially if you choose all-organic fruits and vegetables. Believe me, this is not a hardship diet. Rather, the recipes we've developed for our program are designed for real food lovers—they are luscious, delicious, even a little indulgent.

Science is proving over and over again that a plant-based diet is the healthiest in the world. Thanks to the pioneering work of cardiologist Dean Ornish, MD (author of *Dr. Dean Ornish's Program for Reversing Heart Disease* and *The Spectrum*), who proved heart disease can be partly reversed by a healthy lifestyle, and Nobel-winning geneticist Elizabeth Blackburn, PhD, who showed how food choices can lengthen the telomeres in the DNA, we know that a vegan diet–based approach is able not only to prevent disease but stop it in its tracks and even, in some instances, reverse it. In fact, Dr. Ornish demonstrated in a study published in the *Journal of Urology* that a vegan-based diet can arrest the growth of prostate cancer cells—and his program actually "turned off" 500 cancer-causing genes through epigenetic changes. He is currently reviewing results of using his vegan diet-based program to significantly improve diabetes. (For more on epigenetics, see Chapter 9.)

Incontrovertibly, nutrition that comes from organic plant foods can have a direct positive effect on our very genetic code—turning on helpful genetic tendencies and turning off harmful (even cancerous) ones. Meanwhile, conventionally grown and processed foods that are high in pesticides, salt, sugar, preservatives, food dyes, trans fats, or saturated animal fat can have just the opposite effect—encouraging debility, discouraging resilience, and sabotaging our genetic destiny to tilt toward disease.

By choosing what you eat, you directly intervene in your own long-term health picture. When you make the best choices and focus on clean, plant-based foods that look and taste as nature intended them to, you take charge of your own health outcomes, influencing them in the very best way. Think of it like this: Every bite you eat will flip one of your genetic switches. What aspects of yourself would you like to turn on or off?

During the 7-day cleanse, you'll have an opportunity to become a kind of programmer, writing a new future software program for the hardware that is the human body. Plus, you'll expand your repertoire of fruits, vegetables, and grains. You'll learn to combine them in new ways that maximize nutrition, satiety, and flavor. And you'll be able to experience for yourself how energizing and completely satisfying a plants-only diet can be. Perhaps you'll love it so much you decide to stay vegan. Or perhaps you'll make vegan the core of your diet and begin to add some other healthful foods in a constructive way during the extended cleanse.

STEP THREE: **THE 21-DAY CLEAN AND LEAN DIET**

Three weeks to cleanse your mind and body, gain great new eating habits, and lose weight in a sustainable way

To me, the ideal detox plan isn't a 3-day affair, or a 7-day one, though both of those are incredibly effective and helpful. The ideal detox is a way of life. It is taking the time to adopt new habits that mean never getting toxic in the first place. And 21 days is the perfect amount of time to do that. Add just 2 more weeks of clean eating for a 21-day cleanse designed to not only detoxify and rebuild the body but also rewire the brain so that living clean can become your new normal (rather than an occasional pit stop on the road to health deterioration). In these 14 additional days, we add a few safer animal foods back to the diet in a controlled way, with emphasis on both quality and quantity.

I'll stick by what I said about a vegan diet being the healthiest; it really is. But I'm not "vegangelizing." I know that, in reality, some of my patients will struggle with veganism—either personally, because they continue to crave animal foods, or in the face of social pressure from carnivorous friends or family. Unless you are facing serious illness and desperately need the life-changing benefits of an all-vegan diet, it's okay to be a "flexitarian." (I am aware that many vegans would take issue with that statement, but I'm a pragmatist who has found that a gentle push toward plant-based foods yields better results than a good hard shove every time.)

You can eat "clean" and still enjoy occasional dairy, eggs, and fish. That would make you mainly an ovolactopescovegetarian (OLPV), if you want to attach a label to it. In fact, these OLPV (especially non-land-meat) foods can be beneficial for the body. But the challenge is making the best and healthiest choices you possibly can, and really making them count in terms of satisfaction and flavor. Such a diet—*especially* in service of optimal detoxification—requires self-education, planning, and enough willpower to resist what's most easily attained in our unhealthy food environment and to choose what's optimally healthy.

On days 8 through 14, we'll expand our scope, adding limited amounts of dairy, eggs, and fish. Though again, I stand by my conviction that a vegan diet is powerfully healthy for anyone who has already developed a disease process such as high blood pressure or diabetes. For the rest of us, lean yogurt (the healthiest and least irritating form of dairy), eggs, and fish can be healthy additions to the diet.

Overloading on dairy and cheese is common in our culture. The average American eats *33 pounds* of cheese a year (versus a mere 8.5 pounds of broccoli). This is problematic because studies show that many of us are actually mildly intolerant or allergic to components of dairy, either the lactose (dairy sugar) or casein (protein). There is much less of both of these in cheese than in other forms of dairy—but, of course, cheese is mainly saturated fat! The numbers of dairy-sensitive sufferers are thought to be high—as many as 90 percent among those of Asian descent, 75 percent among African Americans, 60 percent among Eastern Europeans, and even 40 percent of Northern Europeans. Even if you aren't sensitive to dairy in some way, studies published by the Physicians Committee for Responsible Medicine suggest that whole milk and cheese are of very limited usefulness as a vehicle for bone-building and heart-boosting calcium, in part because the saturated animal fat interferes with calcium absorption. Nonfat milk is an effective source of lean protein, but full-fat dairy and cheese provide way too much fat and calories. Neither can compete with a basket full of produce, in terms of nutrition.

Yogurt, however, offers something else: probiotics, which are beneficial to the gut. Bacteria are an integral part of our digestive system. I like to tell my patients this shocking truth: We are born 100 percent human, and we die 90 percent bacteria. That is a fact of life, part of the body's design. We think of bacteria as harmful, but truthfully they can also be beneficial—especially in our intestines, where the good stuff helps our bodies to break down and process food, strengthen our immune system, and even provide nutrients (such as vitamin B_{12}). We call the "good stuff" probiotics, or beneficial bacteria, because it helps to keep the digestive tract healthy and running well so that toxins are eliminated normally. There are bad bacteria, too, of course, which can work to undermine intestinal function and erode the lining of the gut—sometimes allowing toxins to leach back into the body rather than be eliminated. These "bad guys" are implicated in many systemic illnesses, including heart and autoimmune diseases and even obesity. You can influence this balance of good-and-bad bacteria (called the *microbiome* in science) by eating organic, low-fat yogurt a couple of times a week, and/or boost the benefit by taking a good probiotic supplement. (For recommendations on this, see "Pump Up the Probiotics" on page 301.)

Eggs have long been a dietary bogeyman of sorts, shunned first by dieters for their cholesterol and then for their potential to harbor salmonella. The bad, sad news is that salmonella is born into the eggs because of all the toxic substances the mother hens are exposed to in the farming process; when you buy conventionally raised eggs, you *do* run a risk of exposure (you can eat them, but you have to cook the heck out them to make sure you're safe). Fortunately, organic eggs are much safer. The latest meta-analysis, published in the *British Medical Journal*, found that there is absolutely no correlation—zero, zilch, nada—between eating eggs and elevated incidence of heart disease and stroke.

True, an egg and a half a day adds up to 1 day's worth of cholesterol, about 300 milligrams. But it also offers beneficial amounts of the carotenoids lutein and zeaxanthin, both needed for healthy eyesight, as well as choline, an essential nutrient that promotes cardiovascular and brain health. Eggs also contain an array of essential fatty acids, including the brain-boosting omega-3 DHA and arachidonic acid, which supports the skin and muscle tissues. I eat them occasionally and consider them a very good, complete food.

Finally, the 21-Day Clean and Lean Diet includes fish—and this is one animal protein I do recommend. We now know that because of the healthy omega-3 fatty acids it offers, fish—especially cold-water, fatty fish, like wild salmon and sardines—is a true health food and lives up to its moniker of *brain food*. The omega-3s protect not only brain function but also heart health, and quell inflammation throughout the body. Fish is commonly consumed throughout the "Blue Zones"—regions that boast the largest population of people who live to be 100 or more. It is arguably the healthiest of all animal-based foods

Unfortunately, due to environmental factors, it's not so simple to buy the best and safest fish. Because our water is polluted, so are the fish that swim in it. Farmed fish may be riddled with antibiotics and pesticides; large wild predator fish, like tuna and swordfish, may contain dangerous levels of mercury, arsenic, and PCBs. Eating fish requires a little research and a serious cost-benefit analysis. For pregnant women, I recommend avoiding fish altogether; I also steer everyone away from most freshwater fish, especially those caught in lakes or rivers near cities, which are likely to be polluted. But for everyone else, I recommend getting one or two servings a week of the cleanest fish you can find.

Wild salmon, herring, sardines, and mackerel are all great sources of omega-3s . . . but know what you're buying before you buy. Wild-caught Alaskan salmon is among the cleanest choices; farmed salmon, on the other hand, is likely to be contaminated with antibiotics, PCBs, and even artificial dyes to make their flesh pink! With trout, just the opposite is true—US farm–raised trout and shrimp are best. It can be confusing—and the advice is ever-changing. But I refer my patients who choose to eat fish to the best resource I know: the Environmental Defense Fund, which keeps an updated Seafood Selector that lets you check out your catch before you reel it in (metaphorically speaking). The site (and app) considers both environmental and health factors and presents the best and worst choices for every kind of seafood. Find them at edf.org.

I am okay with yogurt, eggs, and fish—if eaten in moderation. But don't mistake my message here: You don't *need* to eat these animal-based foods to enjoy good health; you can get everything you need from plant foods. Stick to a vegan diet if you prefer it. If you want to rotate in some of your more carnivorous urges, you can do it a couple of times a month if you must. Meat from hooved animals (cows, pigs, sheep) is hard on the body—its saturated fats are among the most difficult for the body to process and/or use efficiently and contain many substances that increase inflammation throughout the body. Coincidentally, these meats are the hardest on the planet, contributing up to 18 percent of our global warming emissions. (Beef production in particular requires a huge amount of energy—it takes 13 pounds of grain to produce 1 pound of beef.) Whatever you choose to eat, be sure to do it consciously—and in a way that will keep both your health and that of the planet in mind.

Conscious Carnivorism

If you must eat meat, some choices are better than others. Focus on free range and organic, always, and buy local when you can. Keep intake low, ideally no more than once or twice a month, until it becomes something your body and palate no longer crave. Until then, make the best choices you can afford.

Poultry: From a health standpoint, chicken and turkey are a relatively clean source of protein. Most of the fat is just under the skin, but there is still fat in the meat. Buy organic and cook poultry skinless to avoid most of the saturated animal fat. The bird with the lowest fat of all is the ostrich or emu. Fifteen years ago, ranchers starting raising these livestock, expecting they would take off. The meat is actually delicious (it's somewhere between chicken and veal, which should be off your menu forever), but the yuck factor in the public perception derailed all this. If you can find them, try them. You just might like them.

Bison: The true all-American meat, bison is very lean and clean—we don't factory farm the stuff, so it's nearly always free range and free of growth hormones and antibiotics. Because it is also grass fed, bison contains more omega-3s than beef because it lives off the land and eats a natural diet, which beef too often does not. If you must have a steak to feel satisfied, make it a bison steak. Also, you can substitute bison for hamburger in any dish. Still, it is not a "health food."

Game: Elk, quail, deer, pheasant, wild boar—if it lives in the wild the way nature intended it to, it's probably a relatively healthy meat choice. Game meats tend to be

Principles behind the Detox Prescription

As I've mentioned before, these three plans are the culmination of my life's work in nutritional approaches in integrative medicine. I believe that an informed person is more likely to be successful, so let me outline some of the fundamental tenets of this plan:

ORGANIC IS ALWAYS BEST

The nutrition community has long debated whether it's more important to go organic or to eat your fruits and veggies wherever and however you can

lean and often have a higher ratio of good fatty acid than animals raised in captivity (though some are farm raised now, which may result in the use of additives in their feed, a more sedentary existence, and higher saturated inflammatory fats). Use common sense, though—if the animal was snagged on a superfund site, you might want to pass; if you're just not sure where it came from, play it safe.

Pork: Don't go "whole hog"; pork can be very lean or ridiculously fatty. Certain preparations can be high in sodium and nitrates, too, which are a chemical preservative—sorry, bacon lovers. Skip the ham and sausage and choose lean pork loin for your occasional indulgence, if you absolutely must.

Beef: This is the worst choice from a personal health perspective, even if, for many, it's the most delicious one. If my patients can't live without it, I tell them to buy local, grass-fed beef—which will be easier on their bodies and on the environment—or at least bison, if they can. There's no defending factory-farmed beef—beef raised in close quarters, fed an unnatural diet (corn, in this case), and routinely treated with antibiotics to prevent the spread of disease in these horrible circumstances are toxic. Period. Veal? Even worse—take all of that and factor in confinement, forced feeding, and an early, horrible death for the animal. Don't eat veal, ever.

Lamb: Lamb is so marbled with fat that I recommend you skip it altogether or eat it very, very rarely.

most easily and conveniently get them. For the majority of Americans, the consensus has been the latter. Because we don't, as a group, eat enough plants, period, the thinking is that the benefits of the phytonutrients outweigh the risks associated with commercial produce, which include exposure to pesticides and herbicides as a matter of course.

For the purposes of detoxification, let me be clear. Always try to eat organic.

There is now no question that pesticides harm human health. They are known neurotoxins, associated with cognitive impairment, Parkinson's disease, and other neurodegenerative disorders. They have been found in study after study to interrupt the human endocrine system—interfering in particular with reproduction. The jury is still out on whether or not they are carcinogenic; even the Environmental Protection Agency has it down as an open question. But why take the risk?

Two seminal medical studies, both of school-age children, have clearly proven their value. The first showed that children who ate conventional produce had six times the level of pesticides in their urine when compared with those who were fed a wholly or mostly organic diet. The second study, supported by the EPA's Science to Achieve Results program, demonstrated two things. First, it established that food ingestion does, indeed, represent the primary source of exposure to pesticides among children. Second, more helpfully, it showed that replacing conventional with organic produce had what the study's authors called "a dramatic and immediate protective effect against exposures to . . . pesticides that are commonly used in agricultural production" after only 5 days. Although a much-talked-about 2012 study out of Stanford University claimed that organic produce was no more nutritious than conventional, researchers missed one crucial point of eating organic: It is drastically less toxic.

> For the purposes of detoxification, let me be clear. Always try to eat organic.

Food can be a poison or a cure. Why would you choose to ingest the toxins when you could be taking the world's best detox medicine? You wouldn't—and now that you understand what is at stake, you shouldn't.

That said, I do realize that organics can be expensive and, in some regions, difficult to find. For those with limited financial resources, I suggest spending the money it takes to get the produce that truly matters most. If you can't have it all, at least buy organic versions of the infamous "Dirty Dozen," the most pesticide-laden fruits and vegetables established by the Environmental Working Group (EWG), which usually includes apples, celery, bell peppers, peaches, strawberries, grapes, and other thin-skinned fruits (see the list on page 63).

The EWG's "Clean Fifteen"—the produce that tends to have the *lowest* amounts of pesticide, including onions, sweet corn, pineapples, and avocado—is also a helpful reference for making decisions when resources are limited. However, don't assume these crops are all truly clean. They are better only in the relative sense that most other conventionally grown crops are even worse. Avoid them if you can afford to—especially if you're detoxing!

If access is truly an issue, explore the freezer section—which can be a great source of organic produce. It is picked at the peak of ripeness and flash frozen foods—retaining virtually all of its nutritional value. (Even organic produce in your local grocery store is probably picked 7 to 10 days before you buy it—and often before it was fully ripened with its maximum nutrients.) Some canned organic produce can also work in a pinch, so long as you make sure the cans are not lined with BPA! (Eden Foods has removed BPA from their can linings; if a label doesn't specify otherwise, assume the worst.) These less-than-fresh fruits and vegetables can't be juiced, of course, but can easily be added to smoothies, compotes, or some cooked dishes. One caveat about frozen—you should wash these fruits and veggies, just as you would if they were fresh, as they may still contain microbes from the soil on their skins.

My bottom line is: Do the best you can to get fresh, organic fruits and vegetables. Think of them as a direct investment in your health.

DIETARY DIVERSITY IS AS IMPORTANT AS EATING WELL

Over the years I've noticed that in many of my patients who've unsuccessfully tried other detox or diet plans, their approach has been to choose one or two healthy foods and eat them to the exclusion of everything else. This keeps things simple, of course. But a menu limited to only a few items also robs the body of all the nutrients it needs to function at its best. For our health in general, as well as to keep the pathways of detoxification working optimally, we need to eat a rainbow of foods.

The current food fad is to put food under the microscope, to identify all the chemical constituents that make it "work." In a very real sense, what works is visible in living color. Broadly speaking, you can think of yellow and orange foods as the best source of carotenoids, which protect eyesight; they also offer large amounts of potassium and vitamin C. Red foods contain high amounts of lycopene, anthocyanins, and resveratrol—all powerful anticancer agents. Blue and purple foods are rife with antioxidants and phenolics, which protect against cancer. White, tan, and brown foods, such as garlic and onions, aren't the most colorful, but contain anti-inflammatory substances such as quercetin, along with powerful detoxifying sulfur compounds. And green foods are rich sources of chlorophyll, sulforaphane, and indoles and contain loads of B vitamins—needed to boost immunity and pump up the detox system. They all provide substrates (nutrient building blocks) needed to make our phase I and phase II detoxifying chemicals—and to help eliminate them once detoxified.

> Your goal: Try to eat at least one representative of each color group every day.

Nowadays, not just vitamins and minerals but many phytonutrient ingredients are available in supplement form, and many people take them religiously. But why the heck would you? Whole foods offer so much nutrition beyond what science has already revealed and whatever can be extracted and squirted into a capsule, which is why they are more potent than any supplements. When you eat an entire rainbow each day, you nourish your body with many more nutrients than we are even aware of. Science is just scratching the surface of what these nutrients are and what they can do. What we do know, thanks to incredible new studies, is that the dietary diversity of a rainbow plate protects the heart and prevents mutations within the human genome. Food is the best medicine, and you intervene in your health with every bite—for good or ill—from the time you are conceived (or maybe even before) until your ripe old age.

Your goal: Try to eat at least one representative of each color group every day. Once you're able to manage that, focus on eating broadly within each color spectrum. Not just kale, in other words, but kale and broccoli and chard and kiwifruit. Not just carrots, but pumpkin, tangerines, butternut squash, and organic bell peppers. There are three good reasons for this.

(continued on page 66)

The Dirty Dozen/Clean Fifteen

The Environmental Working Group, an ecological watchdog organization that puts human health at the top of its priority list, does a fantastic job of keeping us informed about levels of pesticides in produce. Their Dirty Dozen and Clean Fifteen Shoppers Guides to Produce are ones I endorse, use, and recommend to nearly everyone. (You can read more about them, and even download a related app, at ewg.org.) My only caveat is that the word *clean* here is relative; these are only the best of the worst. Go organic whenever you can—especially if you are making an effort to detoxify.

THE DIRTY DOZEN
(FROM MOST TO LEAST CONTAMINATED)

1. Apples
2. Strawberries
3. Grapes
4. Celery
5. Peaches
6. Spinach
7. Bell peppers
8. Nectarines (imported)
9. Cucumbers
10. Potatoes
11. Cherry tomatoes
12. Hot peppers

THE CLEAN FIFTEEN
(FROM LEAST TO MOST CONTAMINATED)

1. Pineapples
2. Papayas
3. Mangoes
4. Kiwifruit
5. Cantaloupes
6. Grapefruit
7. Sweet corn
8. Onions
9. Avocado
10. Sweet peas (frozen)
11. Cabbage
12. Asparagus
13. Eggplant
14. Sweet potatoes
15. Mushrooms

In general, the thicker the skin, the lower the pesticide levels that penetrate the produce from spraying. But studies show skin thickness isn't the only determining factor—some produce absorbs high levels of pesticide from the soil. And some seeds, such as corn, are coated with a pesticide before planting; once the plant starts to grow, it spreads throughout the plant.

Detox Spectrum and Powerhouses

Yellow-Orange	Red	Green	White-Tan-Brown
Apricots	Beets	Artichokes	Bananas
Butternut	Blood oranges	Arugula	Brown pears
squash	Cherries	Asparagus	Cauliflower
Canteloupe	Cranberries	Avocados	Dates
Carrots	Guava	Broccoli	Garlic
Corn	Pink grapefruit	Broccoli rabe	Ginger
Dandelion	Pomegranate	Brussels sprouts	Jerusalem
greens	Radicchio	Celery	artichokes
Golden	Radishes	Chayote squash	Jicama
kiwifruit	Raspberries	Cabbage	Kohlrabi
Grapefruit	Red apples	Cucumbers	Mushrooms
Lemon	Red chile	Endive	Onions
Mangoes	peppers	Escarole	Parsnips
Nectarines	Red grapes	Green apples	Potatoes
Oranges	Red onions	Green cabbage	Shallots
Papayas	Red pears	Green grapes	Turnips
Peaches	Red potatoes	Green onions	White corn
Persimmons	Rhubarb	Green pears	White
Pineapples	Strawberries	Honeydew	nectarines
Pumpkin	Tomatoes	Kiwifruit	White peaches
Rutabaga	Watermelon	Kale	
Sweet potatoes		Lettuces	
Tangerine		Limes	
Yams		Okra	
Yellow bell		Spinach	
peppers		Sugar snap	
Yellow squash		peas	
		Watercress	
		Zucchini	

Blue-Purple

Blackberries
Blueberries
Currants
Dried plums
Eggplant
Elderberries
Grapes
Pomegranates
Prunes
Purple
   cabbage
Purple carrots
Purple figs
Purple grapes
Purple peppers
Raisins

Detox Powerhouses: Cruciferous Vegetables

Arugula
Bok choy
Broccoflower
Broccoli
Broccoli rabe
Brussels
   sprouts
Cabbages (all)
Cauliflower
Collard greens
Daikon
Garden cress
Horseradish
Kale
Kohlrabi
Land cress
Maca
Mustard
   greens
Mustard seeds
Radishes
Rutabaga
Turnip root/
   greens
Wasabi
Watercress

Detox Powerhouses: Allium Vegetables

Chives
Garlic
Leeks
Onions
Scallions
Shallots

Detox Powerhouses: Citrus Fruits

Blood oranges
Clementines
Grapefruit
Lemons
Limes
Kumquats
Oranges
Tangerines
Ugli fruit

Reason One: Eating broadly maximizes your exposure to and consumption of beneficial phytonutrients, which naturally vary from one plant species to the next (you can flip forward and peruse the recipe notes in Chapters 5, 6, and 7 to get an idea of just how much variety there can be). *Reason Two:* Dietary diversity has been conclusively demonstrated to decrease the incidence of cardiovascular disease, cancer, obesity, and, in fact, all causes of mortality. *Reason Three:* Insomuch as some toxicity is likely to creep into some crops these days, even the organic ones, when you maximize your menu options, you minimize your risk. (Just FYI, foods have naturally occurring toxins, such as alkaloids in nightshade vegetables, lectins in legumes, and even goitrogens in broccoli. These are all healthy foods, and the benefits far outweigh the risks—unless you OD on them.) Eating around, in other words, plays the odds heavily in your favor.

Moreover, don't settle for the usual grocery store lot; seek out heirloom fruits and vegetables when you can get them. It's worth a little extra effort. When you find them, they're likely to be raised locally and organically (they're often hard to produce with industrial farming methods). They'll add even more diversity to your diet. And eating them will be a way to help preserve our agricultural heritage and keep these beautiful and healthy foods alive and available for future generations. Although there are estimated to be 20,000 edible plant species on Earth, right now only fewer than 20 comprise 90 percent of the American diet. And four—soy, corn, wheat, and rice—provide 50 percent of the human diet. Scarier, the FDA estimates that about three-quarters of the genetic diversity of agricultural crops have been lost over the last century. That's a pretty big hit. If we keep moving toward efficiency and away from diversity, we may face a future in which our options for healthful living are truly limited. Embrace beautiful, colorful, wild, and wonderful diversity with all your (disease-free) heart.

If you eat clean and colorfully, you're guaranteed to receive health-promoting benefits that up your odds of living a long, happy, and disease-free life. It's a beautiful system, and thinking in colors makes it easy to cover all your dietary bases. It's not rocket science to visualize a rainbow, though it does put a very beautiful, simple face on the complex artistry of nature. Truthfully, even our smartest rocket scientists couldn't do any better.

EATING CLEAN CAN [HELP] SAVE THE PLANET

In setting out to write this book, I intend to change the planet, one life at a time. It's a big job to get from where we are—a toxic, congested environment with rising global temperatures—to a life of planetary stability. We all yearn for a world in which Mother Nature can take care of us. But more and more, with our politics and our economic actions, we distance ourselves from that reality.

Business and industry are much to blame, as is our constant demand for energy. But underlying all of those is an agriculture system gone very, very wrong. We've increasingly moved away from nature and tried to outsmart her with synthetic pesticides, antibiotics, herbicides, growth factors, and energy-intensive farming and transportation equipment. Should we be surprised that she is fighting back in ever-more-creative and unpredictable ways? We now know that genetically modified foods developed to be more hardy are requiring ever-higher levels of pesticides, partly negating the advantage they were supposed to have in the first place. Nature adapts; what a surprise (think drug-resistant bacteria)!

As I mentioned above, Americans' appetite for meat—now being replicated around the globe—has created an untenable amount of greenhouse gas. The World Health Organization estimates that livestock alone accounts for 18 percent of all greenhouse gas emissions—more than the transportation sector.

But there are even more global consequences. Experts estimate that it takes 13 to 15 pounds of vegetables to create 1 pound of edible meat. Steak, it turns out, is one of the least-energy-efficient foods in the world! This is nothing new, of course. Pioneering researcher Frances Moore Lappé first reported on this phenomenon in her seminal 1971 book *Diet for a Small Planet*. In it, she tackled the issue of global hunger, concluding that there would essentially be no such thing if we distributed all the grain we are raising to humans rather than using it as livestock feed.

Even she couldn't imagine the crises we are seeing today. Though we all know better now, the situation is getting worse. People are hungry, and the environment is toxic. Anna Lappé has taken up the mantle of her mother's work, advocating a vegetarian diet as the cure for climate change in her book, *Diet for a Hot Planet*. The subtitle to this book says much about her hopes and dreams: *The Climate Crisis at the End of Your Fork and What You Can Do about It*.

She's pointing our attention back to the most powerful tool we have for our personal health and political action: the fork. (This is something that functional medicine expert Mark Hyman, MD, also does in his many excellent books.) When you use yours to eat plants, sustainably raised dairy and eggs and fish, you are voting, in a sense, for a healthier environment . . . one that will support you more. When you eat organic, you vote for more farmers practicing organic, sustainable farming. When you eat local, you vote for a thriving agriculture scene in your community. When you vote for free-range or organic dairy or eggs, you vote for kinder treatment to the animals who are providing for you. When you opt to skip factory-farmed meat, you are making a strong statement *against* the abuse and misuse of animals and the continued ill effects of industrial livestock production—whether you know it or not.

DOABLE DIETS HELP EVERYONE WIN

Have you tried umpteen diet plans meant to make you feel and look better, drop weight, and boost health? If so, you've probably failed umpteen times.

> Every time you yo-yo, a bigger percentage of you turns to fat. Literally.

The faster and harder you tried to make a change, chances are the faster and harder you failed (or succeeded and bounced back).

In my experience, extreme diets do more harm than good—whether they are aimed at weight loss or detox. If you are eating in a way that is not sustainable for a lifetime, you *will* regain what you've lost—and even if you bounce back to the same weight, you will regain most of those pounds in fat. That's because rapid weight loss comes off more evenly (fat and muscle). But then when you regain, especially quickly, you gain more fat than muscle.

This effect grows more pronounced as you age, and may be especially problematic for women. In a study of postmenopausal women at Wake Forest Baptist Medical Center sponsored by the National Institute on Aging, researchers found that when participants lost weight, they lost 67 percent fat and 33 percent muscle. When they regained, they regained 81 percent fat and only 19 percent muscle. What can we extrapolate from this one study? Every time you yo-yo, a bigger percentage of you turns to fat. Literally.

Also, any plan that causes your body to burn its fat reserves quickly will overload your system with toxins. Unprocessed toxins from food, air, water, etc., are stored in body fat by your overloaded system (and recent research has shown that in addition to their other unintended consequences, pesticides and many other toxins act as *obesogens*—they actually act to prevent weight loss). Later, when you're less overloaded, those toxins can be gradually released and processed. It's a natural solution. But when you force fat and all that is stored within it to be processed quickly through more drastic, restrictive eating patterns, your detoxification system will be forced back into overload. As a result, you will feel worse . . . and run a chance of causing yourself some unnecessary health problems, such as headaches, fatigue, joint pain, digestive complaints, and skin flare-ups.

Low and slow, sure and steady, nice and easy . . . these are my watchwords for diets. Yes, of course, especially if you are one of the more than 65 percent of Americans who are overweight or obese, the best thing you can do to help yourself is to lose weight. But why run the risks associated with doing it in a reckless, unsustainable manner? Take the time you need to add two extra elements to your plate: consciousness and nutritional abundance.

What Doesn't Work . . . and What Does

I grew up in Northern California in the 1960s and '70s, eating what today would be considered an unusually healthy diet—a milk truck, baker, fishmonger, and produce vendor used to stop by our house to offer the freshest and best foods. We ate from our small seasonal backyard garden or shopped for fresh produce at a nearby farmers' market. We ate in season and ate simply. We didn't rely on cans or freezer bags, or fast-food meals. Looking back, it was such an incredibly ideal diet, I can't believe it.

But every step I took away from that idyllic approach was a step in the wrong direction. In college, I tried macrobiotics, and invested in a small rice steamer I could use in my dorm room (brown rice was hardly a staple on college cafeteria lines then). I made my own and augmented the brown rice with the pans of steaming vegetables on offer from the college food service.

As the weeks wore by, I began to feel lousy and ended up in the college's infirmary with a wicked, bone-crunching, fatiguing virus. It became obvious that the fault for this unfortunate incident lay with the veggies on the college buffet, sourced from freezer bags or giant cans and prepared to feed the masses with a scant vestige of their original nutrition. Add to that a lack of sufficient protein (there was no tofu back then, and peanut butter was considered a child's food) and you have a recipe for imbalanced eating. I was literally sick from malnutrition.

I didn't quit experimenting, though. I have tried out many diets over the years, including the original Atkins Diet: all fat and protein, no grains or other carbohydrates. My body went into fat-burning ketosis the plan had prescribed, but I felt horrible. I had no energy; I couldn't think. Moreover, the idea of all the saturated fat coursing around my bloodstream worried me. The body needs carbohydrates to think, to act, and to perform all of its functions adequately— that doesn't mean refined carbs like doughnuts and candy, but it does require smart selection of whole foods, including adequate vegetables, fruits, beans and lentils, grains, nuts, and seeds.

Later, I tried the so-called Master Cleanse—a strict regimen of drinks consisting of water, maple syrup, lemon juice, and cayenne pepper—for a few days, just to see what my patients were doing. I could see no real scientific justification for it, but I was curious. Sure enough, I felt weak and spacey and horrible on it. I am always shocked when any of my patients say they have tried it for weeks—I cannot see how they don't land in the hospital as a result.

Ultimately, I've come to see that any "diet" that works cannot be a short-term plan—it has to be a way of life. I've done what I can here to create a lifetime plan for eating that includes a kick-starter at the beginning, and a few targeted upgrades throughout, but that is ultimately a way of living.

I've lived through a lot of trends, and personal and professional research has come full circle. Eat whole fresh food, in season. Buy organics when you can. Stick to fresh fruits, vegetables, and grains when you can. Limit poultry, wheat, dairy, and eggs, and try to stay away from meats, using fish instead. Use our guide to combine them in new ways to new effect, and you'll begin to see a diet you can not only live with for a long time, but absolutely learn to love.

This is just a snapshot of the food plan we've created. In the best-case scenario, you'll combine the diet with a few simple mind-body changes we'll suggest. When you get to day 1, don't worry—it will all be laid out for you; just follow the steps. Meanwhile, if you're ready, let's get started.

get ready, get set ... go!

N ow that you understand the basics, we're down to tactics. They're not supercomplicated. In fact, if you are feeling superconfident— and you already own a juicer and blender—you can skip directly to page 93, and the instructions for day 1, and jump right in. Because it's based on real food, everything you need you can get at a good market. Start tomorrow, if you like.

That said, I firmly believe that with a bit of planning and preparation you can set yourself up for longer-lasting success. You probably already know which plan you want to use—the 3-, 7-, or 21-day Detox Prescription. But I advise almost everyone who goes into day 1 to approach it with an open mind and in the best possible shape. That means not only being ready with all the right equipment and produce on hand, but mentally, emotionally, and physically prepared to make the most of their detox.

I've hinted at the fact that you'll experience some new energy and face some new feelings—I wasn't exaggerating. Some are exhilarating, some are challenging. All are just part of the process, which in the end will leave you slimmer, healthier, and recharged. If you can embrace this new, optimally healthy way of living, you'll also feel empowered, knowing you have made a truly positive change in your own life. That is my wish for every reader of this book. That's why this chapter is dedicated to helping you get ready not only physically but also mentally and emotionally.

Prepare Your Kitchen

There's plenty to shop for in the Detox Prescription, if that's your thing—most of it gloriously colorful, fresh produce. Once you begin to get a sense of how good great food can make you feel, the hunt for the best can be as satisfying—or more so—than any quest for the perfect shoe or power tool. Trust me, if you let yourself get into it, you'll begin to view artichokes, endive, and Lacinato kale with the eye of a true connoisseur.

Thanks to the popularity of juicing, it is pretty easy these days to minimize the work of days 1 through 3 of the plan. Many midsize to large cities have juice bars that can make everything you'll need; some even offer juice delivery services and will bring an entire day's menu right to your doorstep—Juice Press, Fresh Press, Organic Avenue, and Juice Generation are all reliable and organic. One national delivery service—Blueprint Cleanse—does an excellent job of providing everything you need for the full 3 days. Just pick your start date, place your order, and drink your way through the six daily juices.

However, it's fresher and less expensive if you can do it yourself. With the right equipment, juicing is fast and easy—and once you get the hang of it, you will have developed skills that will last a lifetime.

If you're going the DIY route, you may want to invest in a little hardware to underpin the plan: You absolutely need a juicer and a good whole-foods blender to get through days 1 through 3 of the plan and to support your detox efforts throughout the entire plan. Everything else you probably already have on hand, though I do suggest a few upgrades that can make it practically irresistible to stick to an optimally healthy plant-based diet.

As for what you spend, that's up to you—you can keep it cheap or spend like crazy. There are plenty of options at practically every price point. Here, Mary Beth Augustine, MS, RDN, and I offer our insights on a few favorites.

1. INVEST IN A WHOLE-FOODS BLENDER

Smoothies are among the healthiest options for providing the body with easy-to-digest nutrition. All you need to do is wash and roughly chop whole fruits and vegetables, drop them in a decent blender, and give them a whir. Then you get a healthy whole-foods drink that includes the whole package of nutrition—the way nature intended, with all its parts, including fiber and enzymes.

A standard-issue kitchen blender *can* do the trick . . . though you'll be happier if you get a heavy-duty model cut out to process whole foods (rather than simply whip up frozen drinks). These are characterized by their powerful motor and relatively wide blade. I have two personal favorites.

If you're on a budget, or cooking for one, consider the NutriBullet (about $100), which features a 600-watt motor. This compact blender comes with several cups that screw onto one of two blades—one intended for grinding nuts and seeds, the other for processing whole foods into smoothies. Throw the ingredients in, screw on the blades, invert onto the blender mechanism, and you can be drinking your smoothie out of the blender cup in a matter of seconds. It is low muss and low fuss, and pretty cool. There are also less expensive versions, for as little as $50 (see page 78).

If you have the money to spare and/or are cooking for a crowd, consider investing in a Vitamix. These are the blenders favored by professional chefs, for good reason: They can handle virtually anything. Whereas other blenders express their strength in watts, Vitamix works in horsepower—no joke. A Vitamix blender can liquefy virtually anything, creating some of the smoothest smoothies on the planet—to say nothing of soups, sauces, purees, pâtés, and spreads, and even frozen foods/drinks.

There are several models, and they are expensive—ranging from $375 to $500. But they are elegantly made, are built to last forever, and will indeed see you beyond the Detox Prescription and through the rest of your life.

2. GET A GOOD JUICER

In addition to a blender, you'll ideally want a juicer to create drinks in which the fiber is removed, creating a straight shot of detoxifying nutrition that can be absorbed by the body very quickly.

What makes a good juicer? That can be a loaded question. If you discuss it with a real juice nut, you can be at it for days, and everyone has an opinion. There are juicers that grind fruits and vegetables to remove the juice, that use centrifugal force, and that hydraulically press them; there are juicers that combine two or more of the above functions. Should you spend $2,500 to get the Norwalk 280—the very top of the line? Or should you cheap out and just drop $20 on the Black and Decker Hand Juicer at Walmart? No and no.

If you have a strong preference, by all means, follow it. But for the purposes of this plan, I recommend a simple and serviceable centrifugal machine along the lines of the Breville Compact Juice Fountain 700-Watt Juice Extractor or the Juiceman All-in-One Juicer. These have been favorites among my patients—they both work great, are easy to operate and to clean, and feature wide chutes, which means that you don't have to go crazy with chopping before you can use them. Best of all, you can easily buy either model online for around $100.

Fans of masticating (literally "chewing") juicers claim they do a better job of getting more juice from fruits and vegetables; certainly, they are more powerful machines. I have a Champion Juicer and can testify that the thing dims the lights in my house when I run it. Like the Vitamix, it will process nearly *anything*—the downside is that it takes up lots of space and can make a bit more of a mess, as the fiber may at times spew out of the machine and onto the countertop.

For the purposes of the Detox Prescription, it doesn't much matter which kind of juicer you choose, since there is no strong evidence to show that the method itself affects the quality of the nutrients from the food, as some self-educated juice nuts might claim. When we drink fresh juice, we deliver a powerful shot of concentrated nutrition to the body—one that it can absorb quickly and easily. Make the process of juicing as easy and pleasurable as you can for yourself by choosing a juicer that makes you happy.

3. DETOX YOUR CABINETS

Once you have your primary tools in place, turn your attention to everything else in your kitchen. You'll want to take some time to purge everything that might work against you—that is to say, all the toxins lurking in your cabinets.

Start with the hardware. Assess your cookware with a keen eye and toss anything that features a nonstick coating, which may contain perfluorooctanoic acid (PFOA). PFOA is a toxic chemical that has been linked to potential birth defects, heart disease, and kidney problems and has been declared by the Environmental Protection Agency "likely to be carcinogenic to humans." The evidence connecting PFOAs to human health concerns through the cooking process is not clear at this point—but exposing yourself to this chemical is not a risk worth taking—especially if the surface of your pans has already begun to break down. Replace nonstick pans with simple stainless steel or ceramic-coated pans.

Next, look at what you store your food in. All those plastic storage containers may be easy, sentimental favorites, but we know now that they may also contain bisphenol A (BPA), an endocrine disruptor that mimics the action of estrogen in the body. Check the bottoms of your containers for the recycling codes; if you see number 7, an indicator of the likely presence of BPA, recycle it immediately. For other codes, assess the condition—if the containers are old and worn, the plastics are more likely to be breaking down, releasing other chemicals into the food (even if BPA is not present). Trash those too. Replace them with new BPA-free plastic containers, or—better yet—glass ones, which are safe for reheating. (Never, ever heat food in plastic, no matter how safe and green you think that plastic might be.)

Finally, turn an eye to the area around your sink. Here, you may have to grapple with some chemicals. For the duration of the Detox Prescription, please put away chemical-laden scrubs, soaps, and cleaners—why expose yourself to toxins, especially around your food-preparation area, while you're working so hard to eliminate them and recover from their effects? Read labels and reject any product that contains the carcinogens diethanolamine (DEA), triethanolamine (TEA), or ethoxylated alcohols; the neurotoxin ethylene glycol monobutyl ether; the respiratory antagonists ammonia or chlorine; or the hormone disruptor alkylphenol ethoxylates (APEs). Ditto triclosan, the agent found in many antibacterial soaps, which is found to have deleterious effects on the immune and endocrine systems of both humans and animals in the environment after it has passed through waste-treatment plants. That is the very short list of problematic chemicals—there are many others, which may be hidden behind the catch-all term "fragrance."

As a rule of thumb, you should be able to read the label and have a pretty good idea of what every ingredient is. If it sounds toxic, it probably is. If it's not found in nature or you can't pronounce it, ditch it. It's just not worth it.

Instead, invest in ecofriendly kitchen soaps (for hands, dishes, and dishwasher) and cleaners (for sink, floor, and surfaces) that rely on glycerin or another natural soap for their power (and essential oils for their scent and antibacterial properties). Good brands include Seventh Generation, Eco Nuts, GreenShield, Greenology, Earthsavers, Ecover, and Biokleen. These can be just as effective as anything cooked up in a laboratory, with no net-negative health effects. That's a big positive.

4. CONSIDER GREAT GADGETRY

Beyond a blender and juicer, a knife and a cutting board, clean storage containers, and a couple of pots and pans, you don't really *need* anything else to succeed on the Detox Prescription. But you may want a few things to make your new way of eating easy and appealing. Kitchen gadgets can be a revelation, taking the work out of onerous tasks and making them outright fun. Here are a few tools that may come in handy, if you have them:

• **FOOD PROCESSOR:** Not necessary by any means (especially if you have a Vitamix), a food processor can nonetheless take over a lot of kitchen tasks: chopping, mincing, slicing, shredding, kneading, and whipping. Most come with multiple blades and attachments for different chores and can be operated at different speeds, allowing for more nuanced preparation. Full-size models can handle anything and everything, but miniature versions are also available and are a good choice if your main tasks are mincing garlic and chopping onions, or if you're cooking for just one or two.

• **IMMERSION BLENDER:** Essentially a blender on a stick, an immersion blender can work a very special kind of magic: It can be inserted into a boiling-hot pot of soup or stew and used to blend it until smooth without splattering. If you have ever tried to transfer a Dutch oven's worth of potato soup to a blender or food processor (and back again), you'll appreciate this nifty trick. New moms will love it—it works its magic on baby food, too.

• **MEZZALUNA:** This is one of the most satisfying kitchen tools to use; I defy you to use it and not have fun. The double-handled blade lets you make short work of chopping or mincing greens, garlic, ginger, and other aromatic herbs and spices—some of the most powerful weapons in the detox arsenal.

• **SALAD CHOPPER:** Anything you can do to make salads easier and more appealing . . . you should do. Salad choppers allow you to cut and toss fresh greens right in the salad bowl. After day 3 of the Detox Prescription, you can have a salad every day, if you like. Make it irresistible and easy.

• **CITRUS SQUEEZER AND ZESTER:** Research continues to mount supporting the detoxification power and health-promoting benefits of bioflavonoids and citrus pectin. That's why so many of the recipes in the Detox Prescription call for a squeeze of lemon juice. You can DIY manually, of course, but specially designed tools save you the strain and let you get the most juice from your fruit. Likewise, a zester lets you scrape off just the most aromatic portion of the peel to add the powerful flavors and colors to your food.

• **MUDDLER:** Muddlers have achieved fame in recent cocktail culture as the force behind the mojito, the caipirinha, and the newly fashionable old-fashioned. Of course, we're not indulging in mixed drinks during the Detox Prescription, but we are indulging in flavor—something the muddler delivers in spades to all drinks, with or without the kicker. (Think "like a virgin.") Muddle a little mint and add it to the Green Goodness Smoothie (page 111) to keep your inner lounge lizard happy.

• **PIZZA CUTTER:** No, we're not having hot, cheesy Italian pies during the Detox Prescription. But pizza cutters come in handy for all kinds of jobs. They are the best tool for cutting up messy, open-faced sandwiches, quesadillas, breakfast tortillas, and one of my favorite brunch dishes, the Zucchini and Sweet Potato Frittata that appears on page 211.

• **SHAKER BOTTLE:** Thanks to weight lifters and their obsession with protein powders, shaker bottles are easy to get nearly anywhere. With a screw-on lid, pop top, and nifty little whisk ball, they make mixing liquids incredibly easy. They work great to reblend made-ahead juices. But they also work well on any kind of cold sauce or salad dressing. A little citrus juice, olive oil, sea salt, and ground black pepper . . . shake, shake, shake . . . genius. Put it to use with recipes like our Kale, Pecan, and Dried Cherry Salad with Rosemary Quinoa (page 251). Just be sure to get a BPA-free model, such as Blender-Bottle (blenderbottle.com).

• **CHEESECLOTH:** Okay, this isn't really a gadget, but it is a handy thing to have on hand if you like your nut milks smooth and creamy. Cheesecloth lets you strain out lumps and bumps, and in the case of Raw Almond Milk (page 112), skins. If you like your nut milk chunky, you can keep the texture—it won't hurt anything. But cheesecloth affords a more refined experience.

Shopping for Kitchen Equipment

Shopping for good kitchen equipment can be exhausting—or elating, if you think of it as an investment in your good health. The right tools can make cooking and eating healthy a simple pleasure. There are no right or wrong purchases—whatever works for you is just fine. That said, you'll have the best success if you make a moderate investment in quality equipment that is sturdy and effective. This list of options was compiled by Mary Beth Augustine, MS, RDN. Prices are approximate. All equipment can be ordered online.

Equipment	Brands
Blender, full size	Vitamix Blenders ~$375–$500
	Blendtec Blenders ~$375–$500
	DeLonghi Food Processor/Blender ~$150
	KitchenAid Blenders ~$100–$150
	Cuisinart Blenders ~$75–$150
Blender, compact/bullet size	NutriBullet ~$100
	Cuisinart Compact Blender/Chopper ~$75
	Original Magic Bullet Express ~$50
Blender, immersion	KitchenAid 5-Speed Hand Blender ~$100
	KitchenAid 3-Speed Hand Blender ~$60
	KitchenAid 2-Speed Hand Blender ~$40
	Cuisinart Smart Stick ~$35

Get Your Body Ready

Once you have everything you need on hand, you can improve your chances of success by getting yourself ready, too. You can take five key steps to improve your chances of making it through the entire 21 days successfully

Juicer	Champion Juicer Household Models ~$250
	Breville Juicers ~$100–$300
	Jack LaLanne Power Juicer Pro ~$150
	Juiceman Juice Extractor ~$100
	Waring Pro Juice Extractor ~$60
Food processor, full size	DeLonghi Food Processor/Blender ~$150
	KitchenAid Food Processors ~$100–$150
	Cuisinart Food Processors ~$100–$300
Food processor, mini-chopper	Cuisinart Mini-Prep Processors ~$40
	KitchenAid 3.5-Cup Food Chopper ~$40
Salad chopper/mezzaluna	Guy Fieri Double Blade ~$20
	Silvermark Toss and Chop ~$20
	Fox Run Stainless Steel Mezzaluna ~$15
	Chef'n SaladShears Lettuce Chopper ~$10
	Mezzaluna Chopper ~$10
Mortar and pestle	CHEFS Natural Granite Mortar and Pestle set ~$40
Citrus squeezer	Oxo Good Grips ~$15
Citrus zester	Oxo Good Grips ~$10
Muddler	Oxo Good Grips ~$10
Pizza cutter	Oxo Good Grips ~$10
Cheesecloth	Any ~$5
Shaker bottle	Any ~$5

(or 3, or 7, if you're doing a shorter cleanse). I offer this advice up front simply to help end-run the rebound effect that sometimes occurs if you go from one extreme (a very toxic lifestyle with poor food choices paired with lots of other unhealthy habits such as high stress, lack of sleep, and alcohol or drug use) to the other (a superclean diet and healthy new habits).

I call this "retox" and caution my patients that this yo-yoing between detox and retox doesn't help in the long term. What *does* help is taking it one step at a time, setting and reinforcing doable health habits, and committing to a less toxic way of living and being in the world. And that means thinking a little bit beyond *what* you eat and looking at the circumstances in which you eat . . . how you eat, where you eat, with whom you eat. Just the process of editing out a few key foods will introduce you to some of your most ingrained habits—and triggers. Pay close attention now, and you will be ready to make better decisions in the future.

To set yourself up for success in the Detox Prescription and beyond it, take a few days—perhaps a week—before you begin the program to do the following—some steps are easy, some are a little more challenging. All will help you increase your chances for success, optimize your experience, and maybe even break the vicious detox-retox cycle once and for all. They are:

1. STOP SMOKING

This is highly charged emotional territory, so I'll just stick to the facts: We know that cigarette smoke contains more than 4,000 different chemicals. We know for sure that 43 of them are carcinogens and that 400 others are toxins. The list includes nicotine, tar, carbon monoxide, formaldehyde, ammonia, hydrogen cyanide, arsenic, lead, styrene, benzene, phenol, and DDT.

I put this item first on the detox to-do list because it is of utmost importance. If you are smoking, you are subjecting your body to incredible toxic stress, and the number-one thing you can do to promote your own health—and protect the health of everyone around you—is to quit. Smoking doesn't make you a bad person; I'm not judging character. It does make you a toxic one. That's just a fact. It makes you toxic to everyone around you, too—many, many studies have now proven the deleterious health effects of secondhand smoke.

I know it's not easy to quit. Very few people can successfully quit cold turkey. Nicotine patches can be helpful (only as a transitional agent to help prevent nicotine withdrawal while eliminating most other toxic chemicals found mainly in the smoke) but work best in conjunction with strong social support and/or cognitive therapy. Most of all, you have to want to quit—that is, you have to want what you get as a nonsmoker (energy, healthfulness, acceptance) more than what you get as a smoker (immediate gratification, a quick buzz, or—worse—relief from withdrawal symptoms). You might need to do a little inner exploration to find out exactly what it is you do get from a cigarette—try to be honest with yourself. Make a list of all the benefits and positive associations you have in connection with smoking. Then, only then, will you be able to weigh whether it is worth the cost. If you find—and I think you will, if not now then later—that it is not, you will finally be properly motivated to quit for good.

When you know what cigarettes represent for you, you'll know how to support yourself—if they were your nerve soother, you can try yoga or meditation. If smoke breaks with friends were your social connection, you can join a reading group or explore a new coffee hangout. Whatever the case, please know that you can get what you need in a way that does not bombard your body with toxins—and that does leave you free to embrace vitality.

Don't go it alone. Enlist the help of friends and family—you may be surprised by how many of them are eager to help you (if they haven't already been nagging you for years). If you need to reach out and don't feel comfortable with your close friends and acquaintances, I wholeheartedly recommend checking out Smokefree.gov, a stop-smoking Web portal established by the National Cancer Institute. It offers a wealth of resources—including the most precious one of all, live human connection via phone or Web chat.

I also recommend ear acupuncture for many of my patients, who report that it significantly eases the symptoms of physical withdrawal. To find a qualified acupuncturist in your area, check out the Web site for the National Certification Commission for Acupuncture and Oriental Medicine at nccaom.org. Hypnosis has also proven helpful for those who report that aberrant thought processes lead them to irresistible cravings. For a qualified practitioner, try the American Society of Clinical Hypnosis (asch.net).

Get at least a smoke-free day or two under your belt before you start the plan, but then go ahead. It will support your newfound energy, unlock a new lease on your sense of smell and taste, and—I hope very much—help you really feel in your bones the benefits of a healthy, smoke-free life.

2. ELIMINATE SUGARY AND PROCESSED FOODS

In case you haven't gotten the picture yet, foods are best enjoyed as close as possible to the way nature designed them. The Detox Prescription relies solely on whole foods with minimal added sweeteners. That is the healthiest diet on the planet. But it can be a shock to the system for anyone who is used to eating highly processed, highly refined food out of boxes, bags, and cans. If you are used to eating a high-sugar diet especially, it can be a thorny transition.

Here's what you need to know, though, if you're absolutely addicted: It's all in your head. Functional studies show that sugar does light up the dopamine-fueled reward centers in the human brain, setting up a cycle of craving—we eat sugar, the brain registers a reward, then blood sugar levels soar, then we crash, then we want more sugar, so we eat more . . . *ding, ding, ding, ding!* You can easily see how the cycle of craving and reward gets out of hand, as the more we get the more we want.

Plus, if you overindulge, you become inured to sugar's effects over time. The more you eat, especially if you are overweight, the more resistant you become to its impact (this is quite literally the insulin resistance that underpins diabetes), and the more sugar it takes to set off the reward bells in your head. Because we weren't designed to encounter a sugar motherlode like a frosted doughnut or an Oreo, the body has a hard time processing them.

The good news is that every day you get a do-over. That is to say, you wake up in the morning with a clean physiological slate, free from the reward-craving cycle. And if you make good food choices, you'll never have to go down that rabbit hole.

On the other hand, if you start the day with a cup of coffee and a pastry, you'll send your blood sugar levels soaring and nervous system jangling—only to crash again a couple of hours later. At this time you'll be running solely on fumes (you've had no real nutrition), your energy will flag, and you will crave more sugar. If you cave to that craving, you'll send your levels soaring again, only to crash again an hour or two later . . . then more craving, crashing, craving, crashing, craving, crashing. You get the picture.

Tomorrow get up and have a healthy whole-foods breakfast combining a healthier, low-sugar mix of carbs, fat, and protein—perhaps a banana and some nut butter mixed into a bowl of steel-cut oats. You'll be giving your body some real fuel to run on and minimizing your chances of getting caught up in the sugar cycle.

If you find yourself fantasizing about chocolate or cookies or cake, eat a piece of whole fruit instead. You'll get some natural sugar (and a nice fiber boost), plus an array of phytonutrients and antioxidants.

3. DELETE THE WHEAT

Who can argue with a hot, crusty loaf of sourdough bread? Or fresh, hand-made pasta? Or a chewy pizza crust? I can, that's who.

In my practice I clearly see that about 50 percent of my patients over the age of 40 have developed some kind of problematic sensitivity to wheat. They aren't allergic to it, per se, and so aren't manifesting hives, wheezing, fainting, swelling up, or vomiting. Neither are they suffering from the hellish celiac disease, an immune disorder in which the body reacts to the wheat protein molecule gluten by attacking the lining of the small intestine.

Nonetheless, for this unfortunate 50 percent, wheat has become poison, no different in its effects than any other toxic substance, undermining the body's proper functioning. Their symptoms are all over the map: They might suffer from headaches or joint pain; they might have something like chronic fatigue or fibromyalgia. They may have gained (or more rarely lost) weight, and not know why. Or they might have a digestive-system condition, like irritable bowel or gastroesophogeal reflux disorder (GERD). Nothing life-threatening, mind you, but enough to undermine quality of life.

So what's the problem? Often part, or even all of it, is simply the nature of the new American wheat, a highly homogenized, hybridized, and genetically modified strain that includes molecules that have never been found in wheat before. To this add the factor of processing, which removes the natural fiber from the grain and transforms it into something that functions very much like a simple sugar and sets the body up for the cycle of craving and crashing described above.

This new wheat may be good business for makers of processed foods, but from the look of my patient pool it is hard on the human body. And yet we eat it all the time—for many of us, all day, every day.

There is no way to know whether wheat is toxic for you, personally, except to go off the stuff altogether and see how you feel. That's exactly what we'll do during the Detox Prescription—*the entire 21 days are wheat free*. Getting a jump-start on eliminating wheat will let you notice where and what it is, so that if you choose to add wheat back to your diet after the cleanse, you can do so slowly and consciously. Make the best choices you can make—opt for whole wheat so that you get the entire grain, including fiber.

If you later do choose to eat wheat, watch carefully during the first 4 or 5 days after you add it back to your diet. How is your digestion? How are your joints? Are you having any unusual headaches? Are you feeling run down? If you experience a recurrence of some symptoms that had waned during the cleanse, wheat may well be the culprit. Take it back out of your diet and add back your energy and good health.

4. WEAN YOURSELF FROM COFFEE AND ALCOHOL

Americans lean on coffee and alcohol to keep the old lifestyle going. We use coffee to wake up in the morning and alcohol to wind down at night. Both drinks have an upside and a downside. Let's start with coffee. The bitter brew is the leading source of antioxidants in the American diet—a benefit that is negated by the heart-racing effects of caffeine, often associated with frazzled nervous systems and afternoon crashes. More recent science, however, suggests that caffeine actually does boost brain function (the reason we drink the stuff in the first place) and may in fact prevent depression and protect against Alzheimer's disease. That's all good news.

But for the purposes of detox, there's some bad news. For all its beneficial properties, caffeine still needs to be processed by the liver, and it uses the same detox pathway as some of the toxins we are working to get out of our system, including mercury and PCBs. Also, caffeine blocks the brain's receptors for the sleep-inducing chemical adenosine. And good sleep is essential for proper detoxification. Some of us are simply slow detoxifiers, which means that the caffeine we drank in the morning might still be hanging around in the evening. There's no way to know for sure, but why take a chance? Sleep is the time for the body to rest and recover, and it's the only time your liver gets to do its job unharassed. It needs its beauty rest—don't mess with it.

You'll need to come off coffee—slowly, if you've been using it for a long time, or drinking more than two cups a day, so that you do not trigger caffeine headaches. (Cut back by a cup a day until you're able to quit.) If you must have a little caffeine, try a half-caff blend, then move to a quarter-caff blend. Or for an even better "fix," try getting your lift from green tea. You'll be swallowing a much milder dose (about 10 to 30 milligrams, as opposed to 100 to 150 milligrams); you'll also receive the benefits of catechins, some of nature's most potent antioxidants and essential to the process of detoxification, as well as the calming amino acid L-theanine, which naturally counteracts caffeine's stimulating effects by producing calming neurotransmitters in the brain.

That's a win-win . . . and when the detox starts, you'll be ready to have your morning cuppa green supplanted by an even-more-healthy juice or smoothie packed with spinach and kale. That may be hard to imagine right now, but trust me—you'll be hooked within the space of a week.

As for alcohol, well . . . the dose makes it medicine or poison. When consumed in small quantities, alcohol—even the hard stuff—offers anti-oxidant protection. Red wine is especially healthful, and much has been written about the health-boosting benefits of resveratrol, which may protect the brain, improve insulin resistance, and fight both heart disease and cancer. However, when alcohol is tossed back in large doses, it is poison to the body—impairing the nervous system (that's what we call "drunk"), undermining sleep, slowing respiration and cardiovascular response, and overloading the organs of elimination and detoxification. It is especially harmful to the liver and is, in fact, considered to be a liver toxin—leading to cirrhosis and even to death in the case of hard-core alcoholics.

How much alcohol is too much? The Centers for Disease Control and Prevention recommends no more than two drinks (12 ounces beer; 5 ounces wine; 1.5 ounces distilled spirits or liquor) per day for men, and no more than one for women. (I also encourage everyone to take 1 or 2 alcohol-free days each week to rest the liver completely.) This seems sensible to me. I am not a teetotaler, and I counsel my patients that an occasional glass of wine with dinner is fine. But during the Detox Prescription, our express purpose is to rest and recharge the liver. No alcohol allowed. Drown your sorrows (or your stress) in a tall glass of water instead. (See "Why You Need More Water," page 90.) If you are tempted, whip up one of the delicious juices from days 1 to 3 and serve it in a highball glass. I like the Hot Tomato! Juice (page 129) with a dash of hot sauce and a celery stick. You'll never miss the vodka.

5. DIAL BACK DAIRY, EGGS, AND MEAT

You'll be off these entirely for the first week of the plan, but it can be a little shocking to give them up all at once. Instead, I suggest going at it step-by-step—which can be a learning process if you do it with real attention.

Often my clients tell me, "Oh, I really don't even eat that much meat." But when they set out to scale back or eliminate everything that includes the flesh of any animal—not just the hooved ones—they realize that they actually do. They have a little bacon at breakfast, a turkey sandwich at lunch, a steak for dinner once or twice a week, and chicken in their soup. It doesn't seem like much—but it adds up.

Try first just going vegetarian—cutting out animal flesh. Notice when you're tempted to order meat, and *what* you're tempted to order. Moreover, where are you tempted to order it? Do you know much about the quality of the meat? Where it came from? How it's been treated? This will be useful information later, should you decide to rotate animal products back into your diet. For now, just make vegetarian substitutions where you can. When you get ready to add back meat, you can be a lot more conscientious about what it is and where you get it.

Next, tackle eggs. This should be a little easier, unless you are hooked on omelets. It may, however, require you to look carefully at the baked and processed foods you are eating. Do they contain eggs? If so, edit them out for now. Again, when you put them back, do it with awareness. Eggs can be a healthy part of a diet provided they are organic and you eat them in balance.

Finally, bring your focus to dairy. Swapping cow's milk for a nut- or plant-based alternative is pretty easy to do, as soy, almond, coconut, and even hemp milks have gotten so good that most people can find a product they like as much, if not better, than regular milk for most purposes, including cooking. The same is true with butter—and if you don't believe me, I suggest you get down to the organic foods section of your nearest grocery store and try a product called Earth Balance. It is that good.

More difficult to replace is cheese. What comfort food isn't slathered or covered with cheese? It also happens to be ubiquitous in our diet and culture. It's hard to resist it, I understand. I used to like the stuff, too. To do it myself, I have to appeal to my own higher mind: Though it is delicious in taste and texture, cheese takes a heavy toll on health and offers almost nothing in the way of nutritional benefit. It's high in calories and saturated fat—a cup of Cheddar has 532 calories and 44 grams of fat, 28 of them saturated (that's 139 percent of your recommended Daily Value). It's also pretty inflammatory.

And though cheese does offer some vitamin D and calcium, it's not offering it in a way that makes it easy for your body to use those nutrients—in fact, studies conducted by the Physicians Committee for Responsible Medicine have found that the animal fats in dairy products may actually cause calcium to leach from bones. The jury's still out, in my opinion, but there's simply no justification for including full-fat dairy in the diet. When you are ready to reintroduce dairy to your diet, it will be far easier to decide in favor of better stuff—high quality, hormone free, and cultured.

Get Your Mind Ready

No detox plan can be successful if it moves your body forward and leaves your mind behind. Yes, you might flush out a few toxins. Yes, you might feel better for a little while. But if you don't reset your head and put your healthy new dietary habits in the context of a wellness-oriented lifestyle, they won't be sustainable over the long haul.

Plus, as we've already demonstrated, unbearable stress and negative emotional states can be as toxic as any of the worst man-made chemicals, wreaking absolute havoc in the body. How you respond to your environment and care for yourself within it—even amidst the burden of chemical, dietary, and emotional toxic exposure—can often make the difference between health and disease.

If you are living, as many of us are, in a highly reactive state, just getting by as best you can from day to day, it may seem like a stretch to think that within the course of the 21-day Detox Prescription you will become calm, collected, and in control of your responses to your world. *But you will.*

The distance between where you are and that place of greater wellness is not so vast, even if it does feel that way. Throughout the plan, I offer lifestyle tips designed to help ease stress, promote connection, facilitate rest, and help you discover for yourself what is most meaningful to you in the hope that you might pursue more of it.

These are not cumulative; there will not be 21 more things on your to-do list at the end of the plan. Rather, they are invitational—play with each idea on the day that it is offered and see what you think. I'll bet that by the end of the plan you will have encountered five or six ideas that really work for you and that are keepers. This is a tremendous success. Keep those things, and keep doing them for life.

Meanwhile, to get ready for the Detox Prescription, you can do a little planning ahead—get a jump-start on the lifestyle of wellness. All the dietary changes you'll be making are beneficial and designed to help you feel and actually *be* better. But they are still changes, and therefore somewhat stressful. Taking these four preparatory steps will help you be ready.

1. PRACTICE ADEQUATE REST

There is no doubt about it. We are a society that values doing—we like to achieve things, explore things, know things, research things, experience things, watch things, taste things, go out and get things. And we are willing to give up our rest—which we don't value nearly so much—in service of that.

Sleep is critical to good health. Without it, we don't have energy, as we well know. We can't think straight. Memory and problem-solving skills start to lag, the efficiency of the immune system starts to decline, and it becomes harder and harder for us to lose weight. We go down in flames, in other words, and still so many of us are up Googling and e-mailing into the wee hours. We're still trying to "do," dragging our poor bodies down in the effort—getting less and less done effectively.

To detoxify and heal the body, it is *absolutely essential* that you set aside the doing in favor of a solid 7 or 8 hours of sleep. Sleep provides the body a needed metabolic slowdown, allowing it time to clear out the cell-damaging free radicals produced by a day's worth of activity, as well as any additional toxins it has encountered during the day, such as heavy metals. This is also the time when the subconscious mind works through our mental and emotional problems and stressors, which can also have toxic effects on the body. Moreover, during sleep, the body produces thyroid and growth hormones and cortisol. Without sleep, you cannot rejuvenate or recharge.

> To detoxify and heal the body, it is *absolutely essential* that you set aside the "doing" in favor of a solid 7 or 8 hours of sleep.

To get a jump on good sleep, start by simply penciling it in. Figure out when you need to get up, count back by 8 hours, and allow yourself to be in bed by then. Let other priorities fall away—nothing is more important to your health and well-being, and nothing can be accomplished without it.

When it's time for bed, observe good sleep hygiene. Turn off all your screens an hour before bedtime—that means TV, iPad, computer, *and* mobile phone. Make sure your room is cool and dark (get rid of any night-lights, digital clocks, or other devices that might be emitting light pollution) and that your bed is used only for sleeping (no eating, planning, or problem solving in there, no matter how tempting). If you're still awake after 20 minutes, get up and move to another room to do a quiet activity, such as reading or stretching, until you're ready to try again. If the mind yearns to return to the day's problems, try focusing it on a peaceful thought or mantra, such as "Everything is taken care of." Don't turn on any screens. Don't panic about not sleeping, either. And when it's time to get up, get up. Even if you had a bad night's sleep last night, waking on time is the best chance you have for a better night today. When bedtime comes, try again. Practice makes perfect—after a few days, you will get the hang of it.

2. LEARN A SIMPLE DE-STRESSING TECHNIQUE

Stress creates endogenous toxins in the body—the natural by-product of spending too much time in fight-or-flight mode—generating hormones like cortisol and adrenaline. We were designed to cope with these—when we meet a saber-toothed tiger in the wild, say. We were not meant to be flooded with stress hormones around the clock.

It is essential to the process of detoxification that you embrace a stress-reduction technique. Without de-stressing, detox doesn't stand a chance. There are many viable options: meditation, dance, yoga, massage, exercise, psychotherapy, tai chi, art, music, knitting, cooking, sports, hiking, nature time, journaling, talking with friends, or spending time with a child. If you love to do it, it fully absorbs your attention, and it comes with little pressure to perform, it can work to relieve stress.

But the most simple and immediate tool I know of to calm down quickly is the breath. I teach nearly everyone who comes to me a simple breathing technique designed to create instant focus, calm the mind, and shift the emphasis from the sympathetic nervous system (that's the adrenaline-driven fight-or-flight mode) to the parasympathetic nervous system, which helps you calm down, reduces heart rate, and promotes digestion.

Here's how it works: Inhale to a count of four. Pause for a count of one, retaining the breath. Exhale for a count of five. Pause for a count of one, suspending the breath. (That's a 4:1:5:1 pattern.) Do it again, and again, and again . . . for 5 or 10 minutes, if you can. If you can only get through three or four cycles, that's fine. Every little bit will help.

Anyone can do this breathing technique—it gives the mind just enough to focus on, without overwhelming it or introducing it to anything abstract or esoteric. The slight emphasis on the exhalation—what yogis call *lang-hana* breathing—quiets the body quickly and effectively, displacing the kind of panting or shallow breathing we all do when we are stressed out.

Why You Need More Water

Dehydration is the enemy of detox. When the body is dehydrated, it compensates by pulling water away especially from the organs of elimination—namely the kidneys, bowels, and skin—so as to keep a ready supply available to the cells. The liver will continue its work apace, but you won't be able to efficiently excrete the toxins it is processing for disposal through urine, feces, and/or sweat. As a matter of fact, the toxins may have a hard time getting from the cell to the veins and lymphatics that need to drain them off. The fluid outside cells acts as a reservoir for nutrients (coming in) and waste products (going out) becomes more like a sludge, impeding movement through it. And that's not good.

Food is 70 percent water. But you need more. If you're comatose in a hospital bed, your body needs at least a liter of water just to stay alive. For good basic health, you need to get about a liter and a half every day—about six glasses. That's not much, but you'd be surprised how many people are walking around without this most fundamental nourishment.

Since you wake up dehydrated after a night's worth of detoxifying sleep, drink at least two glasses of fluid in the morning. Have another two glasses around lunchtime and another two in the afternoon—before 3 p.m., especially if night waking is a problem (if you drink them later, you might need to get up in the night to use the bathroom).

Filtered water is a great choice, but any decaffeinated beverage counts toward your overall goal—including decaf coffee, herbal and decaf teas, smoothies and juices, and sparkling water. (Decaffeinated sodas also provide fluids but aren't worth the body burden of the chemicals they contain. If you are hooked on the bubbly stuff, transition to flavored club soda or seltzer.) To minimize your toxin load *and* your carbon footprint, carry your own beverages in a stainless steel bottle rather than buying them in plastic—as a bonus, you'll save money, too.

Of course, you can always drink more than 1.5 liters—and definitely should if you are exercising vigorously or spending time outdoors in high heat. But it is also possible to drink too much water, which can dilute the sodium in the cells of body and result in a condition known as hyponatremia, or water intoxication. This mostly happens if you are drinking too much, too fast—generally more than 4 cups in an hour. For safety's sake, keep your fluid intake slow and steady.

Anytime you start to feel uncomfortable during the Detox Prescription—especially during the early days, when you might be feeling like you don't know what to expect or you're unsure whether you can stick with it, or you're just feeling an overwhelming craving for a burger and fries—you will be able to come to your breath immediately. Even three or four cycles will help—often you won't remember what you were thinking about by the fourth breath. It will literally be your lifesaver.

3. START MOVING

If you are already exercising, good for you; stick with it. If you are sedentary, you'll need to start moving to make the most of the Detox Prescription.

You don't have to join a gym, or train for a 5-K, or go out for a yoga class—all you need to do is take a brisk walk, three times a week, for 30 minutes. This is what has been shown in recent studies to be effective for protecting health and reducing the risk of heart disease and increasing longevity. If you like, you can break that up into two 15-minute segments.

I'm not talking about putting on a special outfit or hitting the track or doing some crazy power walk; indeed, we're not aiming for the aerobic zone here. You should be able to carry on a conversation as you exercise.

If you can possibly manage it, get your exercise out in nature—a healing force indeed. I like to tell the story of one of my personal heroes, former justice William O. Douglas, who served on the Supreme Court for 45 years. Douglas took an hourlong walk in the woods every day at lunchtime and credited that time in nature—during which he allowed his mind to float—for many of his clear-thinking decisions.

If you just can't find the time to get out, then get up and get moving, stretching if only just a little (see "Stand Up for Yourself," page 92). Something is always better than nothing—and more is even better—but every little bit helps.

4. JOURNAL YOUR TOXINS AND ANTIDOTES

About a week before you start the plan, begin a journal. Take 5 minutes each evening to write down everything you encountered that day that was toxic and everything that day you felt was a life-enriching antidote.

Start by writing down all the bad stuff. Toxins can be quite literal—yes, you can include bad air, bad food, and random encounters with chemicals, such as walking into a cloud of hairspray at a salon or a blast of exhaust from a tailpipe. But also consider the broader sense of the term. Are there people, places, and things that feel toxic to you? Are there situations that drive you nuts? Are there relationships that are sapping the life out of you? Do you have daily to-dos that are literally making you ill? Write them all down—everything that happened or that you encountered that made you feel stressed or sad or sick. Write down exactly what happened, and—more important!—exactly how you felt about it. Getting it all down on paper means getting it out of your head.

Next write down everything good that happened to you—that gave you

Stand Up for Yourself

Sitting around is a toxic habit with real health consequences. Studies show that sitting more than 4 hours a day—and face it, lots of us do that, just moving our hands and eyeballs—can significantly increase your risk of developing heart disease and diabetes and shave years off your life—regardless of whether you exercise at other times! Think about it—add up your computer time, TV time, drive time. Are you at risk?

If so, take action! Try the following:

Fidget: Forget what your mom told you, go ahead and fidget—fidgeting is good! Bounce your foot, cross and uncross your leg, squirm in your seat . . . it's all movement.

Take a break: At least once an hour, get up and leave the scene. Get a cup of tea or a glass of water, use the restroom. Walk around a little. Get outside if you can.

Stretch: Sitting for long periods takes a toll on the muscles of the body, too. Stretching can offset some of the damage. Reach the arms wide to the sides to open the chest, twist to the right and the left using your chair for light leverage, then stand and take the left foot in the left hand to stretch out the quadriceps and hip flexors. Repeat the last action with the right hand and the right foot. Stretch out in any other way that feels good.

Sit on a ball: Sitting on an exercise ball rather than a chair is better, as it requires you to use your core muscles to maintain balance. This is active sitting.

Stand at work: Consider converting your workspace to standing. At the Continuum Center, we have equipped our offices with Humanscale wall-mounted monitors and keyboards so that we can stand during patient consultations. If you can't swing such an investment, maybe you can put your monitor on a kitchen bar instead of a desk—or on top of a box, even. Just standing, rather than sitting, will encourage you to move much more.

pleasure. What made you smile? What made your heart sing? Who lit you up? Where were you happiest? Were there things you did or said that felt joyful or somehow really right? Were there moments that felt spiritual to you—when you felt connected to something greater than yourself? Put your thoughts, feelings, and insights in your journal. This is the good stuff. These are your antidotes.

When you are done with your two lists, review what you have written. Then take a few moments to set an intention for tomorrow. What will you do more of? What will you do less of? Don't just think about it . . . say it. Then write it. Writing is a powerful way to intention, making it palpable, in a sense, to the mind. It is also an incredible tool for shoring up will-power—a key ingredient in any plan for self-improvement, which the health-promoting Detox Prescription most certainly, unapologetically, is. (It belongs, in fact, on your antidote list.)

Get Ready for Day 1!

Once your kitchen, body, and soul are prepared and in alignment, you only have to handle some simple practicalities before you get started. That means shopping for the produce you'll need to make your nut milks, juices, and smoothies and doing some simple prep work so you can just jump in on day 1.

Certainly, you can shop your list one day at a time—and you may well want to do that for certain fresh fruits and veggies to get them at their peak of ripeness, especially if you're able to source them from a local farmer.

However, for most of us, it's more practical to shop for a few days at a time—in this case, you can get everything you need for the 3-day cleanse in one shopping trip. You'll still be getting all the benefits of fresh produce—the vitamins, minerals, and phytonutrients, as well as naturally occurring plant enzymes—even if you have to keep it on hand for a few days.

Although I'm no fan of plastics in general, it's okay to store produce in the refrigerator in plastic bags if you need to—the cool temperatures will minimize the chances that chemicals will leach into your food. (Never heat your food in the plastic bags, of course.) Store sturdier, thicker-skinned fruits and veggies in glass containers if you can; for leafy greens and delicate produce, keep air circulating by leaving bags open. But best, consider using cloth bags, or one of the new reusable vegetable storage bags, such as

Debbie Meyer GreenBags (debbiemeyer.com), Evert-Fresh (evertfresh.com), or Natural Home Produce Bags (naturalhomemerchandise.com). These keep greens together, minimize the risk of developing microbes, and feature small holes that allow air to flow freely so that rot is less likely. Some refrigerator crisper drawers may also offer the additional advantage of minimizing humidity, which can cause fermentation (think moldy berries).

Buy everything organic if you can, or refer to the Dirty Dozen list on

Buddy Up

Often we see detox as a solitary pursuit, something we have to muscle up for and go it alone. But the truth is that it will be easier and healthier if you find a way to integrate your friends and family into the experience.

Social isolation is toxic in the extreme; science is now producing study after study showing that the loneliness, depression, and anxiety that disconnection breeds contribute to heart disease and dementia and shave years off what would otherwise be healthy and fruitful lives. Indeed, in a definitive study published in the *Proceedings of the National Academy of Sciences of the United States* in 2013, isolation was linked to all causes of mortality among both men and women. You can do everything else right—you can eat right, sleep right, exercise right, and be incredibly pure—but if you are not connected to something or somebody outside yourself, you can easily still suffer the consequences of ill health. That's just a fact.

If you can persuade a friend or family member to do the Detox Prescription with you, that's fantastic—you'll enjoy sharing the food and good health and having someone to compare notes with along the way. But if you don't have that—and you may well not, as the Detox Prescription does require a willingness to not only follow the plan but to do a little self-education—you can find other ways to incorporate connection.

• **Cook for others.** Even if your loved ones are still going about their business 90 percent of the time, you can offer them a healthy vegan meal once or twice a day. Everyone loves a Bravocado! Smoothie for breakfast (page 123); even the most skeptical co-workers have been won over by the delicious Curry Butternut Squash Soup with Cayenne-Roasted Butternut Squash Seeds (page 151); and our Kale,

page 63 to help you make some key decisions if you can't. It is essential that the apples be organic, as these are one of the most highly toxic conventional crops (they can easily contain up to five pesticides/herbicides per fruit)—no exceptions to this rule. The same is true for other thin-skinned fruits, and for celery. If you are juicing, and including the skins in the juice, make organic mandatory. Always wash produce to remove dirt and microbes. Everything else is negotiable.

Pecan, and Dried Cherry Salad with Rosemary Quinoa never fails to stop the show at casual dinner parties (see page 251).

• **Find a walking buddy.** Walk at a pace where you can maintain the ability to carry on a conversation—then chat it up. Taking a friend with you on a short walk reinforces your commitment to exercise and adds the bonus of connection. If you walk out in nature, you'll hit the trifecta of stress relief.

• **Join a support group.** If you've had to give up some bad habits—say smoking, drinking, or overeating—chances are there's a support group around to encourage you—at a local community center, church, or even online. If you connect with other people who are committed to the same goal, you'll feel empowered to succeed.

• **Ask lots of questions.** For many people, the Detox Prescription will be an opportunity to learn about a world of new fruits, vegetables, and spices. When you go out to shop for them, get curious. The stores that stock the best often have employees who really care and who are happy (or even thrilled) to connect with you to answer your questions. So ask them! Where did the food come from? How do you pick the best? What seasonal tips can they offer?

• **Tell a friend.** Even if you can't persuade anyone to join you on your detox journey, find a friend or two to talk to about what you are doing. In particular, see if you can find someone to talk with about your daily journaling exercise. When you are able to not only formulate a positive intention to limit your toxins and introduce more antidotes into your life, but then actually express that intention to another human being who can support you, then you have taken a giant step toward success.

Proceed with Caution

Days 4 through 21 of the Detox Prescription, which emphasize maximizing nutrition, are safe and effective for almost everyone. However, some patient populations should approach the 3-day juice cleanse with caution. Talk to your doctor before you undertake this plan if you:

Are pregnant: There's nothing harmful here for mother or baby, but gestating mothers need more protein and calories than the plan provides, especially in the first weeks.

Are undergoing chemotherapy: Because this plan is ultrarich in antioxidants, it may work directly against chemotherapy drugs, which pointedly use the process of oxidation to kill cancer cells. Eat as your oncologist advises (though some of them may not have a full nutritional understanding); you can do the Detox Prescription when you are done with your treatment to help fully return your body to good health. Also, some people who lose an enormous amount of weight during chemotherapy may need more calories than the Detox Prescription provides.

Suffer from inflammatory bowel disease (Crohn's disease or ulcerative colitis): Any inflammatory bowel disease creates unique nutritional needs and deficits, as the body's ability to absorb nutrients is compromised. During a flare-up you may need to use a specific medical food or observe specific dietary restrictions not

If you do end up using some conventional produce, scrub the produce with diluted soap and water and rinse well before using. Then I recommend using one of the citrus-based sprays—such as Swanson's Citrus Magic Veggie Wash—which may mitigate any remaining pesticide residue. These contain essential oils, are safe to eat, and are a good idea even if you are eating organic, as they kill naturally occurring microbes, too.

Most large grocery stores, health food stores, and food cooperatives now carry a good selection of organic produce, so it shouldn't be hard to find everything on this list. Some large cities also offer fresh produce delivery services, such as FreshDirect in New York (freshdirect.com). However, if you simply can't turn something up, don't stress too much, or go crazy driving all over town. Instead make a smart swap in the same color family. For instance, if you can't find a papaya, swap for mangoes or peaches, which

accounted for here. If you are in remission and doing well, this plan should be okay—especially the first 7 days. However, the soluble fiber content during days 8 through 21 can be problematic for some patients. Talk to your primary care provider before you start this plan.

Have unstable or low blood pressure: A selling point of this plan is that it can reduce hypertension. However, it's also possible that blood pressure can drop precipitously. If you take blood pressure medication, you might want to monitor your blood pressure regularly. There is a chance you may be able to—or need to—reduce your medication.

Have unstable blood sugar: The Detox Prescription is low in carbohydrates and may cause blood sugar levels to drop. If you are prone to spells of hypoglycemia or are diabetic and taking insulin or medications designed to lower blood glucose levels, you will need to use caution. There is a chance you may be able to—or need to—reduce your medication.

Are significantly underweight: Though the Detox Prescription isn't foremost a weight loss plan, most people who do the plan will lose pounds. This can be dangerous if you are extremely underweight when you begin. If this is the case, any kind of weight loss can be dangerous; do the plan working in conjunction with your doctor or nutritionist.

are still in the orange family. If you can't find cranberries, use strawberries or raspberries, both in the red family. If you can't find good spinach, opt for another leafy green, such as romaine lettuce or arugula.

Fresh ingredients are absolutely essential for the juice recipes. However, frozen organic fruits and veggies can work just as well as fresh in the smoothies and are nearly as nutritious, so use your judgment. Such brands as Cascadian Farms, 365, and Wild Harvest are widely available; many supermarket chains also offer an organic house brand, so it may pay to investigate the freezer section with some interest. FYI: Frozen fruits and veggies can be used in cooking, too.

The bottom line is, you don't have to be absolutely perfect in order to get the most from the Detox Prescription; you simply have to be willing to commit to the plan and do the best you can. No stressing.

the 3-day turbo cleanse

A re you ready to feel better than you have in a very long time? Fire up the juicer, because it's time to do the all-liquid 3-Day Turbo Cleanse. There is no doubt that this will be an intense 3 days—though most of the challenge you will face will be psychological. You may think you feel hungry on the first day, but part of that may be psychological, too. In truth, you're getting plenty of calories and taking in nourishment frequently enough to get you through the day just fine. What you are really facing is an interruption of your habits and the rearing up of your personal cravings. Simply observe your reactions when you find yourself automatically reaching for a bag of chips or a cup of coffee, recommit yourself to the Detox Prescription, and refuse to cave in to the craving. To overcome a sneaky and persuasive cycle of self-talk ("You *need* that coffee," perhaps, or "You deserve a cookie!"), craft yourself a supportive phrase you can repeat to affirm your purpose and help yourself stick to the plan. (See "Make Yourself a Mantra" on page 162 for suggestions on how to do this.)

Everything you put in your body for these 3 days will be in liquid form, so you may be tempted to just chug it. But slow down—take your time. Savor. I am even going to go so far as to say: Chew your juices! Yes, that's right: Chew your juices and smoothies and nut milks. Bite down on them, roll them around in your mouth. This will let you really taste these incredible drinks, but even more important, it will jump-start the digestive process. Digestion begins in the mouth—a fact we too often overlook. Your saliva contains valuable enzymes that help break down food. When you take a few moments on the front end to activate these enzymes, not only will you enjoy your taste experience more, you'll *literally* get more out of it. A few extra moments in the mouth help optimize digestion, nutrient absorption, and even detoxification. It might sound silly, but do it anyway: Chew, chew, chew.

Each day of the 3-Day Turbo Cleanse starts with a green drink—a great replacement for the bitter flavor we usually get in a morning cup of coffee. Rather than getting revved up from a jolt of caffeine—which stimulates the nervous system to start firing but doesn't really add energy to the body and therefore just depletes our reserves—we get a boost of *real* nutrition, including the detoxifying power of cruciferous vegetables like kale, spinach, and broccoli (yes, broccoli for breakfast!). There's not much added sugar here, by design—these smoothies and juices are meant to get your day started well without kicking off the dysfunctional cycle of sugar craving. Drink this first thing in the morning—perhaps after a cup of fresh, filtered water. By day 3, you'll be craving your daily cuppa green.

You'll follow that with a midmorning snack. Have this whenever you want; I time mine for about 10 a.m. Here, we recommend a delicious and satisfying nut milk, whose heavy texture satisfies the mouth, and a bit of protein to boost stamina. The raw nuts and seeds used in the recipes offer beneficial essential fatty acids, which support heart and brain health.

Our two phytonutrient powerhouse juices—the red and the yellow-orange—are scheduled for midday and provide the fuel you need to keep going as well as an incredible dose of antioxidants to nourish your body as it begins to work through some of the old toxins it is releasing. The ingredient list reads like a who's who of power foods: sweet potatoes, tomatoes, cranberries, beets, and pineapples all play starring roles and are rounded out by an interesting array of anti-inflammatory herbs and spices.

Make these in the a.m. if you like, carry them in shaker jars, store them on ice, and mix them just before drinking. You can also order a fresh juice or smoothie with the same ingredients at a local juice bar or grab one of the premixed juices that are increasingly available in health food stores, Whole Foods, and even local supermarkets (they aren't all organic—so look carefully—most of these should be, with no sugar added). Have one drink right around lunchtime (noon or 1 p.m.), then another whenever you feel your afternoon slump beginning to come on—for most of my patients this happens around 3 p.m.

For a late-afternoon snack—we're talking 4 or 5 p.m.—you'll have another green smoothie, to provide even more phytonutrient vegetable power. This late-day dose will fuel the liver for its important overnight work.

Finally, you'll have another rich nut milk in place of your evening meal. I suggest having this around 7 p.m.—a late dinner. This will soothe both nerves and body, especially if you have it at room temperature or even slightly warmed. (Remember that warm milk mom used to soothe you with when you were a child?) The protein will stabilize blood sugar and the texture will satisfy you as you settle in for a good night's sleep—an important factor in any detox plan.

These 3 days are designed to deliver phytonutrients straight to the gut as efficiently as possible—in liquid form, they can be absorbed nearly instantaneously. There is relatively little fat, fiber, or protein here—by design. The nutrition information might look a little high in carbs (and in sugars) as a result. Juices contain sugar; that's just a fact. Nature has packaged some of its most powerful healing phytonutrients—the very substances your body needs to fuel phase I and phase II detoxification—along with naturally occurring sugars. Note, however, that fruit accounts for only 2.3 percent of total caloric intake for the typical American adult (and 4.8 percent of total carbohydrate intake), so clearly it's not the sugar in fruit that's responsible for obesity, diabetes, heart disease, or other diet-related chronic diseases.

And as we introduce solids in day 4 and add more complex carbohydrates, these naturally occurring sugars will be reduced.

It's optimal for the 3-Day Turbo Cleanse to try a little bit of everything (you never know what you might love, and each fruit, vegetable, or nut offers its own panoply of nutritional benefits). But you can make substitutions among these recipes based on your personal taste preference or on what's most readily available or convenient for you. All of the nut milks are interchangeable—drink what you want, when you want. Just know that different nuts offer different nutrients, and when you vary the recipes you get broader nutrition. With the juices and smoothies, you can swap within the same color family, though we also recommend you stick with the type of drink recommended. Drink yellow juice when it's time to drink yellow juice—but choose whichever yellow juice works best for you. When it's time for a green smoothie, you have several good options.

The basic plan starts on page 109. In the pages between, we offer some of our best advice for tailoring the nutrition to your needs. There's even a shopping list ready for you on page 107. The basic idea? Maximum results, minimum fuss.

Take It to Go

Making and taking has never been easier, thanks to the ready availability of shaker bottles, cooler bags, and mini blenders. If you want to juice in the morning and carry your midday juices and smoothies, just keep them on ice to preserve nutrients and blend them in a shaker bottle (or with a whisk or immersion blender) just before drinking. Better yet, load everything you need into your NutriBullet (or other portable juicer), screw on the carry lid, and mix up your smoothie right at work.

If neither of those options works for you, take your juice recipe with you to the nearest juice bar and see how close you can get. You don't have to have an exact match, but aim for the same mix of colors—stay green or red or yellow, swapping celery for spinach, say—or mango for peach.

Boost Your Juice!

The recipes in this chapter are designed to give you everything you need for 3 days of optimal detoxifying nutrition. However, you can add some smart, food-based "boosters" to any of our juice, smoothie, or nut milk recipes to bump up the flavor, protein, fiber, essential fatty acids, or even detoxifying power. In some cases, you can add them to a glass of water or herbal tea to include a beverage with your daily menu. These are purely optional—though I do recommend that you get a high-quality protein powder if you are very active, as having one on hand makes it easy to meet your protein needs. We've offered some rough guidelines for how much of each powder to use, though you should also rely on package information—and your own taste buds.

Protein Powders

Protein powders aren't meal replacements—but they are a good way to bump up the protein content of any juice, smoothie, or nut milk. They come in whey, soy, rice, and hemp formulas, as well as in vegan blends. You might have to try a few to find one you like. Add 10 to 20 grams of protein (generally a half or full scoop) per serving.

ORGANIC WHEY PROTEIN

Jarrow Formulas
Designs for Health
Xymogen

ORGANIC NON-GMO SOY PROTEIN

Now Foods
Wegmans

RICE PROTEIN POWDER

Sun Warrior
Nutribiotic

HEMP PROTEIN SEEDS AND POWDER

Manitoba Harvest
Nutiva

VEGAN PROTEIN BLEND

Essential Living Foods
Life Time Life's Basics Plant
   Protein
Garden of Life Raw Protein
Vega

Energy Boosters

If you're coming off of coffee and find you need a little something extra to help you get going in the morning, consider adding one of these natural energy boosters to an a.m. juice or smoothie. Use 1 to 3 teaspoons per serving (see note under matcha), adjusting for flavor and effect.

Cacao powder and unsweetened nibs: The seed of the tropical cacao fruit, cacao is the primary ingredient in all chocolate and is high in antioxidants, magnesium, theobromine, and phenethylamine. The taste is bitter and chocolaty.

Maca powder: Maca root is a Peruvian superfruit in the cruciferous mustard family traditionally used by indigenous cultures for energy, endurance, and libido. The powder has a sweet, nutty taste with hints of butterscotch.

Matcha green tea: Matcha green tea is a finely ground, powdered, high-quality green tea from Japan known for its anticancer properties and typically used to boost metabolism and relieve stress. It is high in catechins, chlorophyll, antioxidants, and L-theanine. Matcha green tea has an intense sweetness and deeper flavor than standard grades of green tea due to its high amino acid profile. *Note:* Matcha is relatively high in caffeine (about 70 milligrams per teaspoon), though it does deliver L-theanine, which helps eliminate the jagged buzz. If you know you are sensitive, stick with only about a quarter or a third of a teaspoon with this one. That will give you about the amount of caffeine of a cup of green tea. (Going caffeine free for at least the first week is optimal.)

Rainbow Superfood Boosters

Want to add even more color and botanical diversity to your diet? You can play around with these exotic superfood powders, many of which are among the most antioxidant-rich plants found on the planet. They are purely optional—but do add vibrant colors and interesting new flavors to both juices and smoothies. Add 1 to 3 teaspoons per serving.

Acai pulp or powder (red): Pronounced *ah-sigh-ee*, acai is an Amazon forest superfruit that is superhigh in antioxidants, polyphenols, and flavonoids, which have been studied for their anticancer, anti-inflammatory, and antiaging activity. Acai has a dark, chocolate-like berry taste.

Alfalfa juice powder (green): Alfalfa powder, cultivated from a plant in the pea family, is used to aid digestion and detoxification and is high in phytoestrogens. Alfalfa powder has an earthy aroma and is slightly bitter, with a subtle, grassy flavor.

Camu powder (red/yellow-orange): Camu is an Amazon forest superfruit that's high in antioxidants and carotenoids, with a tart berry taste.

Goji berries and powder (red): Also known as wolfberries, goji berries are Asian superfruits that have been studied for their immune-enhancing effects. They

(continued)

Boost Your Juice!—*Continued*

are high in antioxidant carotenoids, vitamin A, vitamin C, and iron. Gojis have a tart berry flavor.

Goldenberries and goldenberry powder (yellow): Goldenberries are a Colombian superfruit, high in antioxidants, carotenoids, bioflavonoids, and vitamin A, with a tart berry taste.

Lucuma powder (yellow): Lucuma is a Peruvian superfruit high in antioxidants and carotenoids, with a sweet, aromatic, almost maple-like taste.

Mangosteen powder (yellow-orange/red): Mangosteen is a tropical superfruit high in antioxidant xanthones, The rind is a deep purple and the flesh is white. The powder is typically made up of both ground rind and flesh and contains antioxidant catechins, anthocyanins, tannins, and polyphenols. Mangosteen has been studied for its anti-inflammatory and antimicrobial activity.

Maqui powder (purple-blue): Maqui berries are a tart Chilean superfruit that's rich in antioxidants, flavonoid anthocyanins, and polyphenols.

Mulberry powder (purple-blue): A superfruit berry native to Turkey, mulberries contain iron, vitamin C, fiber, and resveratrol and offer a rich, fig-like taste.

Pomegranate powder (red): Tart pomegranate is high in vitamin C, vitamin K, folate, antioxidant polyphenols, and phytoestrogens. Pomegranate has been studied for its anti-inflammatory and anticancer activity.

Spirulina powder (green): Spirulina is a marine algae superfood. It contains proteins, essential fatty acids, amino acids, and B vitamins. It is used for immunity, digestion, and energy. Spirulina has a slightly bitter and strong mossy flavor.

Fiber Boosters

Fiber is critical to the detoxification process—helping to bind toxins coming into the intestines in food and then absorbing detoxified substances that come out of the gall bladder and liver. Generally 25 grams of daily fiber (or 14 grams per every 1,000 calories of food) is sufficient—through a mix of soluble fiber (e.g., oat bran, beans, psyllium) and insoluble fibers (e.g., wheat bran, flax, and legumes). While the Detox Prescription includes plenty of fiber each day—including the juices, which contain all the fiber of whole food (juicing typically minimizes fiber)—you may need to supplement. If constipation sets in, there is a greater chance that some of the detoxified substances will be reabsorbed into the body before they are eliminated, allowing a longer time for harmful substances to be in contact with the bowel wall. This can result in some pretty unpleasant bloating, cramping, and gas. Fiber also helps to maintain proper pH in the intestines and delays sugar absorption. If you know you have been exposed to heavy metals, scored high on the toxicity questionnaires in Chapter 2, and/or are prone to constipation, aim to add approximately 5 grams of one of the following supplements per juice serving, adjusting up or down for taste and tolerance.

Brown rice bran: Brown rice bran is the brown part of the brown rice kernel that is removed from the germ. It is high in antioxidants, vitamins, minerals, fiber, and essential fatty acids and has a mild, nutty flavor.

Chia seeds: Chia seeds have anti-inflammatory and antioxidant properties, and both slow and lower the blood sugar rise. Chia seeds form a gel when added to water and have a mild, poppy-seed taste.

Psyllium husks: Psyllium husks are portions of the seeds of an Indian plant called *Plantago ovata*. Psyllium is used for cholesterol lowering and bowel regularity. Psyllium husks have a bland taste and expand in water. They are known as a mucilaginous fiber because of the mucus-like consistency; this helps stool softening and bulking.

Essential Fatty Acid Boosters

Most Americans are deficient in essential fatty acids—especially heart- and brain-boosting and anti-inflammatory omega-3 fatty acids—so adding more to the diet is always a good thing. Most people think of omega-3s as coming from fish—and they do—but there are some excellent vegan sources as well. Another essential fatty acid, gamma-linolenic acid (GLA: an omega-6), also has anti-inflammatory properties and has been studied for its usefulness in treating skin conditions (such as eczema) and for its anticancer potential. Do consider using one of these vegan, nonfish sources of beneficial essential fatty acids if you had been eating a meat-heavy diet prior to starting the Detox Prescription, or if you suffer from an inflammatory condition, such as arthritis, atherosclerosis, or colitis. Use approximately 1 to 2 tablespoons for the seeds and meals and 1 to 2 teaspoons for the oils per serving. Adjust as needed.

Almond meal (omega-3): Almond meal and almond flour add both protein and magnesium. They are high in antioxidants and nutrients that contain omega-3 fatty acids for inflammation. Almond meal has a strong, nutty flavor.

Chia seeds (omega-3): Chia seeds were cultivated from the Aztecs for their many health benefits. A top plant source of omega-3 fatty acids, chia seeds are very anti-inflammatory and have a mild, poppy-seed flavor.

Flax seed, flax meal, golden flax seed (omega-3): Flax seed is from a fibrous plant that is native to Ethiopia and Egypt. Flaxseed is high in omega-3 fatty acids and lignans that have been studied for their anti-inflammatory and anticancer activity. Flax meal is ground fine and has a nutty taste.

Flax oil (omega-3): Flax oil is cold pressed from flaxseed. It is also high in omega-3 fatty acids and lignans and has a mild, sweet, and nutty taste.

(continued)

Boost Your Juice!—*Continued*

Evening primrose oil (GLA: omega-6): Evening primrose oil is cold pressed from a plant native to North America and has a slightly nutty taste.

Borage oil (GLA: omega-6): Borage oil is cultivated from the starflower plant native to the Mediterranean region; it is one of the highest forms of GLA and has a slightly nutty taste.

Hemp oil (GLA: omega-6): Hemp oil is obtained by pressing hemp seeds from North America. High in GLA, it has a pleasant and very mild, nutty flavor.

Detox Boosters

These special-circumstances boosters chelate heavy metals in the gut. Use them if you know (or highly suspect) you have been exposed to mercury, lead, arsenic, cadmium, hexavalent chromium, or beryllium. (To learn this definitively, have your doctor do a panel of heavy metal tests—see page 35.)

Modified citrus pectin (5 grams; Pectasol-C, Econugenics.com): Citrus pectin, a fiber compound found in the skins and peels of citrus fruits, is used commercially to thicken food. *Modified* citrus pectin has been reduced in size (a smaller polysaccharide) so instead of remaining within the intestine, it can be absorbed. Its actions within the body have been shown to have anti-cancer, heavy-metal binding, and detoxification properties. It has a mild bitter and citrus flavor.

Apple pectin (5 grams; Solgar Apple Pectin Powder, solgar.com): Apple pectin is a fiber compound found in the skins and flesh of apple. Apple pectin has heavy metal–binding chelation abilities and detoxification activity. Its flavor is slightly sweet and fruity.

Chlorella (2,500 milligrams; Vega, myvega.com): There are studies of chlorella that find mixed effectiveness in enhancing immunity and binding with heavy metals in the gut. Additionally, it is a nutritionally dense green food with a slightly bitter taste.

Thickeners

If you like a little more body to your drink, you can add one of these to thicken things up. Use 1 or 2 tablespoons per serving and adjust as needed until you achieve the desired texture.

Lecithin granules: Lecithin is a fatty acid found in egg yolks and soy. Lecithin has the ability to break up cholesterol and prevent it from building up in artery walls. Lecithin granules have a slightly natural and nutty flavor.

Flaxseed: Flaxseed is from a fibrous plant that is native to Ethiopia and Egypt. Flax seeds are high in omega-3 fatty acids and lignans, which have been studied for their anti-inflammatory and anticancer activity. Ground flaxseed thickens and emulsifies, and when used soaked in water, it can replace egg whites in vegan recipes.

Shopping Lists

EVERYTHING YOU NEED FOR DAY 1

3 cups spinach

3 large cucumbers (or 2 large English cucumbers)

1 avocado

2 limes

1 lemon

3 Granny Smith apples

1 red apple (such as Gala, McIntosh, Red Delicious . . . your choice)

¾ cup cranberries (or substitute ¾ cup raspberries)

½ cup mint leaves

4 or 5 carrots

½ papaya (freeze ½ for later use or substitute equal parts peach or mango)

Honey

EVERYTHING YOU NEED FOR DAY 2

1 cucumber

4 or 5 stalks celery

1 Granny Smith apple

5 or 6 carrots

1 small beet

1 lemon

1 small sweet potato

1 McIntosh apple

½ cup So Delicious or Trader Joe's coconut milk beverage

½ avocado (freeze ½ for later use)

1 pear

Fresh ginger (2 inches)

Coconut oil

Pumpkin pie spice

EVERYTHING YOU NEED FOR DAY 3

2 cups kale

2 green figs

1 banana

3 large tomatoes

2 cucumbers

3 or 4 celery stalks

¼ cup basil leaves

1 fresh pineapple

1 carrot

1 cup baby spinach

½ cup broccoli florets and stalks

1 Granny Smith apple

1 garlic clove

Fresh ginger (2 inches)

Cinnamon

Cayenne pepper

(continued)

Shopping Lists—*Continued*

EVERYTHING YOU NEED FOR NUT/SEED MILKS FOR ALL 3 DAYS

2 cups raw almonds

2 cups raw cashews

1 cup raw walnuts

1 cup shelled hemp seeds (aka hemp hearts)

3 whole vanilla beans, or small bottle vanilla extract*

*Vanilla extract: substitute 2 teaspoons extract for 1 vanilla bean, 1 teaspoon vanilla extract for ½ vanilla bean, ½ teaspoon extract for ¼ vanilla bean

OPTIONAL INGREDIENTS FOR NUT/SEED MILKS

Cinnamon

Lecithin granules, 1–6 tablespoons

Medjool dates, to sweeten and thicken

Optional boosters (see list on page 102)

About the Recipe Notes

All the recipes in the Detox Prescriptions were created by integrative nutritionist Mary Beth Augustine, MS, RDN, to provide the optimal mix of nutrient-dense as well as detoxifying foods for every part of the plan. You can trust that each day includes a balanced mix of nutrients that will meet your body's basic needs and tilt all mechanisms—digestion, assimilation, elimination—toward better detoxification. The recipe notes and tips she's written reflect her deep understanding of nutritional science—as well as her enthusiasm for the power of particular ingredients. Enjoy.

3-DAY TURBO CLEANSE MENU

	Day 1	Day 2	Day 3
Breakfast	Green **Green Goodness Smoothie**	Green **Get-Up-and-Go Juice**	Green **Kale-icious! Smoothie**
Mid-morning Snack	Nut Milk **Raw Almond Milk**	Nut Milk **Raw Cashew Milk**	Nut Milk **Hemp Milk**
Lunch	Red **Cranberry Supreme Juice**	Red **Just Beet It Juice**	Red **Hot Tomato! Juice**
Afternoon Snack 1	Yellow-Orange **Sunburst Juice**	Yellow-Orange **Carotenoid Smoothie**	Yellow-Orange **Pineapple Sizzle Juice**
Afternoon Snack 2	Green **Limetastic! Juice**	Green **Bravocado! Smoothie**	Green **Crucifer Crusader Smoothie**
Dinner	Nut Milk **Raw Walnut Milk**	Nut Milk **Raw Almond Milk**	Nut Milk **Raw Cashew Milk**

Day 1 Menu

BREAKFAST: Green Goodness Smoothie

MIDMORNING SNACK: Raw Almond Milk

LUNCH: Cranberry Supreme Juice

AFTERNOON SNACK 1: Sunburst Juice

AFTERNOON SNACK 2: Limetastic! Juice

DINNER: Raw Walnut Milk

BREAKFAST

Green Goodness Smoothie

Avocado has gotten an undeserved bad rap for its fat, but it's all good—literally. In fact, avocados lower cholesterol and lipids and have been studied for their anti-cancer potency. The D-glucaric acid, beta-carotene, and sulfur in the spinach and the toxin-binding citrus pectin contribute to the detoxifying activity of this recipe. Interestingly, one study found that spinach-supplemented diets reversed age-related declines in brain cells, cognition, motor skills, and behavior in rats. Like Popeye, you'll be saying, "I'm strong to the finish, 'cause I eats my spinach!"

MAKES 1 SERVING

3 cups loosely packed baby spinach leaves
1 large cucumber, peeled and seeds removed
1 avocado
½ lime, peel and white pith removed
12–16 ounces cold water

Combine the spinach, cucumber, avocado, lime, and water in a blender.

Blend on high speed for 1 to 2 minutes, or until smooth. Turn off the blender and check consistency. Add water as needed.

Pour into a chilled glass, stir, and serve.

Can be refrigerated in a blender jar, shaker cup, or Mason jar for up to 12 hours. Blend briefly or shake well before serving.

Per serving: 51 calories, 0 g total fat, 0 mg cholesterol, 53 mg sodium, 422 mg potassium, 12 g total carbohydrates (8 g sugar), 2 g fiber, 2 g protein

TIP: Buy avocados in three stages of ripeness: ripe, almost ripe, and unripe, and you'll have avocados all week. If the lime's too strong for you in this recipe, next time blend all ingredients and just finish off with ½ lime squeezed with a citrus squeezer (no pulp or pith gets in this way). Also, if you're feeling adventurous, try a variation with a little muddled mint for the mojito lover in you!

MIDMORNING SNACK

Raw Almond Milk

Almonds are chock-full of omega-3s, fiber, zinc, magnesium, antioxidants, chlorogenic acid, terpenoids, resveratrol, ellagic acid, and quercetin and have been studied for their anti-inflammatory, cholesterol-lowering, cancer-fighting, and weight loss properties. These nuts also provide steadying protein, so blend up and power up!

MAKES 4 SERVINGS (12 OUNCES EACH)

1 cup raw almonds
Water for soaking nuts
3–4 cups water
½ vanilla bean, split, and seeds scraped and reserved, or 1 teaspoon vanilla extract
3 Medjool dates, pits removed, optional
1 tablespoon lecithin granules, optional (to act as an emulsifier)

Combine the almonds with just enough water to cover. Soak overnight in the refrigerator (or 10 to 12 hours during the day).

Drain the soaking water and discard (to remove phytic acid).

Combine the almonds, water, vanilla bean seeds, dates (if using), and lecithin (if using) in a blender. Using 3 cups of water makes a creamy milk (whole or 2% milk consistency) and using 4 cups of water makes a thin milk (1% or fat-free milk consistency). Blend on high speed until smooth.

Strain the almond milk through cheesecloth to remove any lumps or almond skins. Serve immediately or refrigerate in an airtight jar for up to 3 days. Tastes best after chilled for several hours. If separated, it may require shaking, a quick pulse in a blender, or a quick spin with a handheld immersion blender.

Per serving: 180 calories, 13 g total fat (1 g saturated), 0 mg cholesterol, 2 mg sodium, 0 mg potassium, 8 g total carbohydrates (0 g sugar), 0 g fiber, 8 g protein

TIP: You'll be surprised by the tender, plush texture of Medjools—order organic American dates online at medjooldates.com.

LUNCH

Cranberry Supreme Juice

Although it's better known for its effectiveness in fighting bladder infections, cranberry also has demonstrated anticancer and anti-inflammatory power, and glucuronidation detoxification activity, too. (For more on this critically important detoxification pathway, see Chapter 9.) It might be a bit of an acquired taste, but cranberry is a berry that deserves a more prominent place in the diet … and not just on Thanksgiving Day.

MAKES 1 SERVING

2 Granny Smith apples
1 red apple
¼ cup mint leaves
¾ cup cranberries
1 teaspoon honey, optional

Cut the apples to a size that will fit in the juicer chute.

Add the mint to the juicer first, followed by the cranberries and apples.

Pour into a chilled glass, stir, and serve. If it is too tart, dilute with water or stir in honey. Tastes best iced or chilled.

Can be refrigerated in a shaker cup or Mason jar for up to 12 hours. Shake well or use a handheld immersion blender before serving.

Per serving: 195 calories, 0 g total fat, 0 mg cholesterol, 28 mg sodium, 120 mg potassium, 48 g total carbohydrates (32 g sugar), 3 g fiber, 0 g protein

TIP: You can dilute this juice with water and/or sweeten it a bit more with honey. Over time, as you grow to love the bittersweet flavor of the natural fruit, decrease the water and sweetener.

AFTERNOON SNACK 1

Sunburst Juice

This carrot-based juice is exploding with carotenoids and more: According to the American Cancer Society, carrots have more than 100 beneficial phytochemicals. The anti-inflammatory papain in the papaya and the toxin-binding citrus pectin in the lemon amp up the power and electricity in this yellow-orange juice.

MAKES 1 SERVING

4–5 carrots
½ ripe papaya, peeled and seeded
½ lemon, peel and pith removed

Cut the carrots and papaya to a size that will fit in the juicer chute.

Add the lemon to the juicer first, followed by the carrots and papaya.

Pour into a chilled glass, stir, and serve.

Can be refrigerated in a shaker cup or Mason jar for up to 12 hours. Shake well or use a handheld immersion blender before serving.

Per serving: 180 calories, 0 g total fat, 0 mg cholesterol, 23 mg sodium, 330 mg potassium, 46 g total carbohydrates (28 g sugar), 3 g fiber, 0 g protein

TIP: If the lemon's too strong for you in this recipe, next time blend the carrots and papaya alone and just finish off with ½ lemon squeezed with a citrus squeezer (no pulp or pith gets in this way). For a delicious flavor variation, add ¼ cup of mint to this recipe.

AFTERNOON SNACK 2

Limetastic! Juice

Citrus pectin and apple pectin chelate heavy metals, while the cucumber acts as a diuretic. The mint is a carminative, which means it works as a general digestive tonic, increasing intestinal movement and decreasing bloating and gas. This juice just happens to taste great, too.

MAKES 1 SERVING

2 large cucumbers (or 1 large English cucumber)
1 lime, zest and pith included
1 Granny Smith apple
$\frac{1}{4}$ cup packed mint leaves

Cut the cucumbers, lime, and apple to a size that will fit in the juicer chute.

Add the mint to the juicer first, followed by the cucumbers, lime, and apple.

Pour into a chilled glass, stir, and serve.

Can be refrigerated in a shaker cup or Mason jar for up to 12 hours. Shake well or use a handheld immersion blender before serving.

Per serving: 152 calories, 1 g total fat (0 g saturated), 0 mg cholesterol, 11 mg sodium, 652 mg potassium, 34 g total carbohydrates (24 g sugar), 2 g fiber, 1 g protein

TIP: If the lime's too strong for you in this recipe, next time repeat the recipe with most of the bitter zest removed or juice all ingredients and just finish off with $\frac{1}{2}$ lime squeezed with a citrus squeezer (no pulp or pith gets in this way). Refrigerate the zest for future use.

DINNER

Raw Walnut Milk

Walnut's ellagic acid, melatonin, arginine, glutamic and aspartic acids, vitamin E, and alpha-linolenic acid put the "fight" in phytochemical. Walnuts lower cholesterol, improve the blood-pumping action of the heart, reduce inflammation, and improve blood clotting. They even boost levels of the sleepytime hormone melatonin—so try warm walnut milk sprinkled with cinnamon before bedtime.

MAKES 2 SERVINGS (12 OUNCES EACH)

1 cup raw walnut halves
Water for soaking nuts
3–4 cups water
½ vanilla bean, split, and seeds scraped and reserved, or 1 teaspoon vanilla extract
3 Medjool dates, pitted, optional
1 tablespoon lecithin granules, optional (to act as an emulsifier)

Combine the walnuts with just enough water to cover. Soak overnight in the refrigerator (or 6 to 8 hours during the day).

Drain the soaking water and discard (to remove tannins).

Combine the walnuts, water, vanilla bean seeds, dates (if using), and lecithin (if using) in a blender. Using 3 cups of water makes a creamy milk (whole or 2% milk consistency) and using 4 cups of water makes a thin milk (1% or fat-free milk consistency). Blend on high speed until smooth.

Strain the walnut milk through cheesecloth to remove any lumps. Serve immediately or refrigerate in an airtight jar for up to 3 days. Tastes best after chilled for several hours. If separated, it may require shaking, a quick pulse in a blender, or a quick spin with a handheld immersion blender.

Per serving: 273 calories, 23 g total fat (2 g saturated), 0 mg cholesterol, 0 mg sodium, 0 mg potassium, 10 g total carbohydrates (0 g sugar), 3 g fiber, 6 g protein

TIP: Inspect your walnuts closely to make sure none are rancid or molding (with a white coating). You know what they say: One bad walnut spoils the milk.

Day 1 Mind-Body Detox

ENERGIZE WITH THE BREATH

There's no sugar-coating it: Day 1 can be a challenge. About halfway through the day, you'll stop feeling hungry and start feeling great. That doesn't help much, though, during the first few hours. If your energy or commitment feels like it's flagging, take a few minutes to practice an energizing breathing technique. Here's how to do it:

Find a comfortable sitting position, either cross-legged on the floor with the hips supported on a cushion or on the edge of a chair with your feet planted firmly on the floor. The important thing is that you feel at ease in your body and able to keep the spine relatively erect—slouching collapses the lungs and diaphragm and defeats the purpose of breathwork, which is to funnel lots of oxygen into the body. Place your hands palms down on your knees and pull your chin in slightly toward the back of your head. Next place your tongue lightly on the ridge behind your front teeth.

Take a deep inhalation through your nose and exhale forcefully through your mouth, making a loud "SHHHHHH!" sound. Pull the abdominals in strongly on the exhalation, as though working a pump. Make absolutely no effort whatsoever to inhale, but allow the abdominal muscles to totally relax, naturally drawing air into the lungs. The inhalation happens reflexively, almost like a rebound. Then contract the abs again forcefully and exhale, repeating the cycle. Do this 10 to 20 times, working at a pace that feels comfortable to you. Then just rest and allow your breathing to return to normal.

If you'd like, you can also contract your lower abdominal muscles and pull up on the pelvic floor as you exhale. If you add these factors, you are doing the yoga technique known as *Kapalabhati*, or Skull-Shining Breath. This is believed by yogis to be a powerfully cleansing breath. Certainly—as the name implies—it clears the head! Once you've learned to do this, you can do it anytime and practically anywhere. In fact, I recommend taking frequent "breath breaks" throughout the day to unplug from stress and recharge your energy.

Day 2 Menu

BREAKFAST: Get-Up-and-Go Juice

MIDMORNING SNACK: Raw Cashew Milk

LUNCH: Just Beet It Juice

AFTERNOON SNACK 1: Carotenoid Smoothie

AFTERNOON SNACK 2: Bravocado! Smoothie

DINNER: Raw Almond Milk

BREAKFAST

Get-Up-and-Go Juice

Celery is more than just a garnish for cocktails or chicken wings—it's a cancer-fighting powerhouse due to the activity of its isoflavones and the flavones apigenin and luteolin. Because of the electrolyte-replenishing power of the cucumber and celery and the detox-promoting activity of the apple pectin, this juice could also be a great revivifier when taken the morning after imbibing too much. Ginger is an all-purpose anti-inflammatory that enhances your intestinal motility. Altogether, this is a perfect morning get-up-and-go juice.

MAKES 1 SERVING

1 cucumber
1 slice (1") fresh ginger, peeled
1 medium Granny Smith apple
4–5 celery stalks

Roughly chop the cucumber, ginger, apple, and celery to a size that will fit in the juicer chute.

Add the cucumber to the juicer first, followed by the ginger, apple, and celery.

Pour into a chilled glass, stir, and serve.

Can be refrigerated in a shaker cup or Mason jar for up to 12 hours. Shake well or use a handheld immersion blender before serving.

Per serving: 149 calories, 1 g total fat (0 g saturated), 0 mg cholesterol, 161 mg sodium, 958 mg potassium, 32 g total carbohydrates (16 g sugar), 2 g fiber, 3 g protein

MIDMORNING SNACK

Raw Cashew Milk

Almonds and walnuts may hog the superfood spotlight, but don't think of the cashew as the underdog—it's super, too. Proanthocyanidins, phytosterols, quercetin, oleic acid, and copper are just a few of the nutrients responsible for the cholesterol-lowering, cancer-fighting, and blood-sugar-lowering benefits of cashews. And as with all nut milks, this one is a good source of protein.

MAKES 3 SERVINGS (8 OUNCES EACH)

1 cup raw cashews
Water for soaking nuts
3–4 cups cold water
½ vanilla bean, split, and seeds scraped and reserved, or 1 teaspoon vanilla extract
3 Medjool dates, pitted, optional
1 tablespoon lecithin granules, optional (to act as an emulsifier)

Combine the cashews with just enough water to cover. Soak overnight in the refrigerator (or 6–8 hours during the day).

Drain the soaking water and discard.

Combine the cashews, water, vanilla bean seeds, dates (if using), and lecithin (if using) in a blender. Using 3 cups of water makes a creamy milk (whole or 2% milk consistency) and using 4 cups of water makes a thin milk (1% or fat-free milk consistency). Blend on high speed until smooth.

If necessary (it's usually not), strain the cashew milk through cheesecloth to remove any lumps. Serve immediately or refrigerate in an airtight jar for up to 3 days. Tastes best after chilled for several hours. If separated, it may require shaking, a quick pulse in a blender, or a quick spin with a handheld immersion blender.

Per serving: 262 calories, 21 g total fat (4 g saturated), 0 mg cholesterol, 7 mg sodium, 259 mg potassium, 15 g total carbohydrates (2 g sugar), 2 g fiber, 7 g protein

TIP: For a great-tasting smoothie, blend 1 cup raw cashew milk with a banana, 5 or 6 ice cubes, and an optional pinch of cinnamon and serve immediately.

LUNCH

Just Beet It Juice

This recipe should be called phase I and phase II Beet Juice. It's that powerful. The lowly underground beetroot is a powerful detoxifier and cancer fighter. One study of rats given a cancer-causing compound (NDEA) found that beetroot juice enhanced liver detoxification and reduced liver injury and oxidative damage. PS: The zesty citrus pectin chelates metals and toxins, and the zingy ginger gives an anti-inflammatory boost.

MAKES 1 SERVING

5–6 carrots
½ lemon, zest removed and reserved, pith left on
1 slice (1") fresh ginger, peeled
1 small beet

Roughly chop the carrots to a size that will fit in the juicer chute.

Add the carrots to the juicer first, followed with the lemon, ginger, and beet.

Pour into a chilled glass, stir, and serve.

Can be refrigerated in a shaker cup or Mason jar for up to 12 hours. Shake well or use a handheld immersion blender before serving.

Per serving: 75 calories, 0 g total fat, 0 mg cholesterol, 0 mg sodium, 705 mg potassium, 15 g total carbohydrates (12 g sugar), 3 g fiber, 3 g protein

TIP: Wear an apron, your grubbiest clothes, or make this juice naked! Or be prepared for a little beet tie-dye, because the superpowered red pigment also stains.

Get a Jump on Day 3

Soak the cashews for Raw Cashew Milk and the hemp hearts for the Raw Hemp Milk (page 128). If you like, you can even make the milks ahead of time and refrigerate them overnight.

AFTERNOON SNACK 1

Carotenoid Smoothie

From a nutritional standpoint, this recipe gets an A+ for sweet potato's vitamin A, carotenoids, fiber, vitamin B$_6$, and manganese content. And if you're lucky enough to find a purple one, you can add anthocyanin to the phytonutrient cocktail. As always, apples add toxin-binding pectin and cholesterol-lowering soluble fiber to the mix. The spice makes this one taste like a decadent dessert. Drink it warm or cold—your choice.

MAKES 1 OR 2 SERVINGS

1 small sweet potato (about 6 ounces), peeled and quartered

1 small McIntosh apple, peeled, cored, and quartered

2 teaspoons coconut oil

$\frac{1}{4}$ teaspoon pumpkin pie spice

12–16 ounces cold water

In a 1-quart saucepan, boil the sweet potato until fork-tender, about 15 minutes.

With a slotted spoon, remove the sweet potato from the heat and add it to the blender.

Blanch the apple in simmering water for 1 to 2 minutes. With a slotted spoon, remove it from the heat and add it to the blender.

Add the coconut oil and pumpkin pie spice and blend on high speed for 1 minute.

Add 12 ounces of cold water and blend on high speed for 2 to 3 minutes, or until smooth.

Turn off the blender and check consistency. Add water as needed. This recipe may need as much as 16 ounces of water and may make 1 or 2 hearty servings, depending upon sweet potato and apple size. Serve warm or chilled.

Per serving: 219 calories, 10 g total fat (8 g saturated), 0 mg cholesterol, 23 mg sodium, 455 mg potassium, 35 g total carbohydrates (19 g sugar), 6 g fiber, 2 g protein

TIP: If you're getting tired of drinking juice after juice, try this one warm. Make it thick, serve it in a bowl, and eat it with a spoon. It's decadent with a little coconut yogurt either blended in or dolloped on top.

AFTERNOON SNACK 2

Bravocado! Smoothie

This avocado-pear smoothie is a crowd pleaser—adults and kids adore it. And what's not to love? Avocado is a rich source of heart-healthy, cholesterol-lowering good fats (move over, oats!) and cancer-fighting beta-sitosterol. But that's not all— carotenoids, vitamin E, glutathione (the body's master antioxidant), and oleic acid make avocado a super-duper superfruit. Add the toxin-binding power of the soluble fiber in the pear, and you've got a glass of detox delight.

MAKES 1 SERVING

8–12 ounces cold water
½ cup unsweetened coconut milk beverage (such as So Delicious)
½ avocado, pit removed, flesh scooped
1 pear, peeled and cored

Add 8 ounces of water, the milk, avocado, and pear to the blender.

Blend on high for 1 to 2 minutes, or until smooth. Turn off the blender and check consistency. Add water as needed.

Serve immediately, in a chilled glass if possible. This smoothie does not refrigerate well (avocado oxidizes).

Per serving: 288 calories, 18 g total fat (6 g saturated), 0 mg cholesterol, 11 mg sodium, 741 mg potassium, 34 g total carbohydrates (17 g sugar), 13 g fiber, 4 g protein

TIP: When buying avocados, use your sense of touch to establish the degree of ripeness. Buy avocados in three stages of ripeness—ripe, almost ripe, and unripe—and you'll have avocados all week. Freeze the remaining avocado half for future use in smoothies. Before freezing, remove the avocado from the peel and cut in chunks.

DINNER

Raw Almond Milk

See recipe, page 112.

Day 2 Mind-Body Detox

SALUTE THE SUN

You'll be feeling energetic today, so take the opportunity to get moving. In addition to your daily walk, try a little yoga. The classic Sun Salutation (aka *Surya Namaskar*) is a 12-pose series that is a great warmup for an extended yoga practice—or a complete practice in and of itself. It is energizing, so I recommend doing it in the morning (hey, that's where the name came from) or afternoon so you'll have plenty of time to wind down before bed. Doing the series all the way through, leading first with the right foot and then again leading with the left, constitutes one complete salutation. Do three to six salutations in total. You don't need a mat to do this (though if you have one, you can certainly use it); in fact, I often do this sequence of poses in my tennis shoes! Here's how to do it:

1. Standing at the top of your mat with your feet hip-distance apart, bring your hands together at your heart and take a second to balance your body weight evenly over your feet. Your shoulders should be relaxed, crown of the head lifting gently toward the ceiling, chin even with the floor. This is *Tadasana*, Mountain Pose.

2. On an inhalation, sweep your arms out to the sides and overhead, looking gently up. Allow your spine to arc gently backward, but don't strain; rather, focus on moving your breastbone up toward the ceiling. This is *Urdhva Hastasana* (Upward Salute).

3. On an exhalation, sweep your arms to the sides and down toward the floor, hinging at the waist and bending into a forward fold. You can rest your hands on the floor or on the ankles, or on the shins or knees. Allow the head to hang and the neck to be soft. Inhale and exhale again here. This is *Uttanasana* (Standing Forward Fold).

4. On another inhalation, step your right leg straight back into a lunge. Keeping your chest lifted, the right leg straight, and both hands on the ground on either side of the left foot, look slightly forward. This is High Lunge.

5. On the next exhalation, step the left foot back to meet the right foot, balancing your weight on the hands and toes. Keep the buttocks down, the head reaching toward the top of the mat, and the spine straight and in alignment. This is Plank Pose. Inhale here.

6. On an exhalation, lower to the floor. You can do this pushup style in the pose yogis call *Chaturanga Dandasana* (Four-Limbed Staff Pose), keeping the legs straight and bending at the elbows, drawing the arms back and close to the sides of the body. Or you can drop the knees, chest, and chin to the floor, channeling an inchworm in the pose called, appropriately, Knees-Chest-Chin.

7. As you inhale again, straighten your spine, drop your hips to the floor, push lightly through the hands, and roll the upper body very gently into the backbend known as Cobra Pose (or *Bhujangasana*). Don't strain in this pose. Keep your neck relaxed, arms slightly bent, and shoulders rolled down and away from the ears. Let your back do the work and use your hands for support.

8. As you exhale, pull your hips back, roll over the tops of the feet, and push through the hands to come into an inverted V. This is *Adho Mukha Svanasana*, or Downward Facing Dog, the most delicious yoga posture of them all. Distribute your weight evenly between your hands and feet, dropping your heels to the floor. Let your head hang like a ripe fruit from the vine, completely supported by your spine. Your weight should be spread across the palms, elbows lifted, shoulders drawing onto the back. Extend fully through the back—don't slouch or hunch your shoulders. Work toward straightening the legs, but don't lock the knees. As you relax into the pose, lift your hips more. You can stay here for several breaths if you like.

9. On an inhalation, step the right foot forward into High Lunge, keeping the left foot back.

10. On an exhalation, step the left foot to meet the right in Standing Forward Fold.

11. On an inhalation, sweep the arms to the sides and overhead, looking up and slightly back in Upward Salute.

12. On an exhalation, return to Mountain Pose with your hands in prayer position at the center of your chest. Take a few breaths to get centered. Then repeat the series again, this time stepping into High Lunge with the left foot first.

Day 3 Menu

BREAKFAST: Kale-icious! Smoothie

MIDMORNING SNACK: Raw Hemp Milk

LUNCH: Hot Tomato! Juice

AFTERNOON SNACK 1: Pineapple Sizzle Juice

AFTERNOON SNACK 2: Crucifer Crusader

DINNER: Raw Cashew Milk

BREAKFAST

Kale-icious! Smoothie

Kale is the Queen of Greens, and it is truly a power detoxifier. This recipe packs a whopping 10 grams of fiber, 24 percent of your daily calcium (move over milk!), 40 percent of B_6 (hello, brain power!), 712 percent of vitamin A, and 190 percent of vitamin C. Carotenoids, flavonoids, and glucosinolate phytonutrients make kale one of the super-est of the superfoods.

MAKES 1 SERVING

½ large banana (or 1 small banana)

2 fresh green figs

2 cups loosely packed curly kale leaves, stems removed

16–20 ounces cold water

¼ teaspoon ground cinnamon

Add the banana, figs, and kale to the bottom of a blender. Add 16 ounces of water and the cinnamon and blend on high speed for about 1 minute, or until smooth.

Turn off the blender and check consistency. Add water as needed. Pour into a chilled glass, stir, and serve.

Can be refrigerated in a blender jar, shaker cup, or Mason jar for up to 12 hours. Blend briefly or shake well before serving.

Per serving: 203 calories, 2 g total fat (0 g saturated), 0 mg cholesterol, 71 mg sodium, 1,061 mg potassium, 48 g total carbohydrates (27 g sugar), 10 g fiber, 6 g protein

TIP: Kale is available in curly, ornamental, and dinosaur (also known as Tuscan or Lacinato) varieties. Dinosaur kale is much more fibrous (woody) and much stronger flavored. If you're a kale novice, start with the mild curly variety to acquire a taste for it. Still too strong? You can substitute romaine lettuce or baby spinach for a milder taste. Freeze fresh figs to avoid spoilage and reserve for future use. You can also use dried figs; just soak them first for a couple of hours to soften them up. (If you like, you can use the soaking water in the recipe for natural sweetness.) Peel and freeze bananas in quarters (which will blend more easily and help smoothies stay cold) for future use.

MIDMORNING SNACK

Raw Hemp Milk

Though hemp is a member of the marijuana plant family, it is virtually free of THC (the psychoactive compound in marijuana). The only way it will get you high is through its nutrients! Hemp is a top source of the anti-inflammatory fatty acid GLA and a great source of the toxin-binding fiber inulin. Hemp can be an acquired taste but it's well worth learning to love this drink—with 13 grams per serving, it's got the highest protein of all the nut milks.

MAKES 4 SERVINGS (8 OUNCES EACH)

1 cup shelled hemp seeds

1 cup water for soaking seeds

3–4 cups cold water

½ vanilla bean, split, and seeds scraped and reserved, or 1 teaspoon vanilla extract

3 Medjool dates, pitted, optional

1 tablespoon lecithin granules, optional (to act as an emulsifier)

Combine the hemp seeds and 1 cup of water in a blender. Allow the seeds to soak for 10 minutes. Blend for 20 seconds.

Add the remaining 3 to 4 cups water, vanilla bean seeds, dates (if using), and lecithin (if using). Using 3 cups of water makes a creamy milk (whole or 2% milk consistency) and using 4 cups of water makes a thin milk (1% or fat-free milk consistency). Blend on high speed until smooth.

Strain the hemp milk through cheesecloth to remove any lumps or unblended seeds. Serve immediately or refrigerate in an airtight jar for up to 3 days. Tastes best after chilled for several hours. If separated, it may require shaking, a quick pulse in a blender, or a quick spin with a handheld immersion blender.

Per serving: 246 calories, 17 g total fat (2 g saturated), 0 mg cholesterol, 4 mg sodium, 4 mg potassium, 9 g total carbohydrates (6 g sugar), 4 g fiber, 13 g protein

TIP: Manitoba Harvest sells organic shelled hemp seeds (aka hemp "hearts")—along with a full line of other hemp-related products, including protein powder and oil—at manitobaharvest.com.

LUNCH

Hot Tomato! Juice

Tomato is best known for its prostate-protective lycopene but is also high in anti-inflammatory, detoxifying, and disease-fighting antioxidants, catechins, and carotenoids. The cucumber tones down the tomato and lends its cleansing, diuretic, and detoxifying support. Add the antimicrobial activity of basil and this drink is just rawsome.

MAKES 1 SERVING

3 large ripe tomatoes (or 4–5 small/medium tomatoes)
1 cucumber
3–4 celery stalks
¼ cup basil leaves
1 garlic clove
Pinch of cayenne pepper, optional

Roughly chop the tomatoes, cucumber, and celery to a size that will fit in the juicer chute.

Add the basil and garlic to the juicer first, followed by the cucumber, tomatoes, and celery.

Pour into a chilled glass, add the cayenne (if using), stir, and serve.

Can be refrigerated in a shaker cup or Mason jar for up to 12 hours. Shake well or use a handheld immersion blender before serving.

Per serving: 87 calories, 1 g total fat (0 g saturated), 0 mg cholesterol, 32 mg sodium, 1,190 mg potassium, 17 g total carbohydrates (10 g sugar), 4 g fiber, 4 g protein

TIP: For a raw Bloody Mary mocktail, stir in the juice of ½ lemon, ½ teaspoon of tamari or Bragg Liquid Aminos (bragg.com), and a pinch of horseradish to the finished juice.

AFTERNOON SNACK 1

Pineapple Sizzle Juice

The antiaging, antiwrinkle, and anti-inflammatory bromelain in pineapples will give you plenty of reason to want to commit to this sweet-tart tropical fruit. Say good-bye to water retention and puffiness with the diuretic action of cucumber and the added anti-inflammatory boost of the ginger. As for the carrots, well, they're a sweet carotenoid boost. You'll look better with every glass!

MAKES 1 SERVING

3 cups fresh pineapple chunks
1 cucumber
1 carrot
1 piece (1") fresh ginger, peeled

Roughly chop the pineapple, cucumber, and carrot to a size that will fit in the juicer chute.

Add the pineapple to the juicer first, followed with the ginger, cucumber, and carrot.

Pour into a chilled glass, stir, and serve.

Can be refrigerated in a shaker cup or Mason jar for up to 12 hours. Shake well or use a handheld immersion blender before serving.

Per serving: 166 calories, 0 g total fat, 0 mg cholesterol, 26 mg sodium, 578 mg potassium, 40 g total carbohydrates (37 g sugar), 3 g fiber, 2 g protein

TIP: Cut a whole fresh pineapple into 2" cubes, use what's needed, and freeze the rest in ½-cup servings for quick and easy future smoothies. If you want to add sparkle, mix ½ cup of juice with ½ cup of seltzer for a yummy, nutrient-packed fruit spritzer. This juice also works great when you add the texture and color of the seeds of ½ pomegranate.

AFTERNOON SNACK 2

Crucifer Crusader

How good is broccoli? The American Cancer Society printed diet and cancer prevention brochures with a head of broccoli on the cover. The cruciferous veggie is also a super detoxifier—as is the toxin-binding apple pectin.

MAKES 1 SERVING

1 cup loosely packed baby spinach leaves
½ cup broccoli florets and stalks
1 Granny Smith apple, peeled
1 piece (1") fresh ginger, peeled
16–20 ounces cold water

Combine the spinach, broccoli, apple, ginger, and 16 ounces of the water in a blender.

Blend on high speed for 2 to 3 minutes, or until smooth. Turn off the blender and check consistency. Add water as needed.

Pour into a chilled glass, stir, and serve.

Can be refrigerated in a blender jar, shaker cup, or Mason jar for up to 12 hours. Blend briefly or shake well before serving.

Per serving: 122 calories, 1 g total fat (0 g saturated), 0 mg cholesterol, 53 mg sodium, 802 mg potassium, 30 g total carbohydrates (15 g sugar), 4 g fiber, 3 g protein

TIP: Double the broccoli, leave out the apple, and squeeze in half a lemon at the finish for a hard-core green, alkalizing detox juice. You'll need all 20 ounces of water for this green giant.

DINNER

Raw Cashew Milk

See recipe on page 120.

Day 3 Mind-Body Detox

CLEAR YOUR HEAD IN THE MORNING

Did you know that Americans are likelier to have heart attacks in the morning than at any other time of day? (And that Monday mornings are twice as risky?!?) That's in part because we often wake with a sense of dread, allowing yesterday's stresses to rush back in and today's to-do list to overwhelm us. Rather than easing into the day, we sit bolt upright, grab a cup of coffee, and sprint out the door. You can interrupt this process, however, by creating for yourself an intentional morning ritual of clearing your thoughts.

Habitual thoughts may arise—that's just human nature—but rather than let them run the show, use them as a reminder to slow down and take a few moments to nurture yourself. As soon as you are awake and realize that you are thinking, remind yourself that it's time to do your morning ritual. Here's how:

Before you even set foot on the floor, call your attention to your breath. You don't have to change it—just notice how it flows freely in and out in the morning. You can also notice that when anxious thoughts come creeping in, the breath gets shallower or speeds up. Inhale deeply, and on an exhalation, release the thoughts—you might imagine them blowing away as a cloud might move through the sky.

When you're ready to rise, sit on the edge of your bed for a few minutes and clear your mind of all thoughts. Breathe deeply into your belly, keeping your attention on the breath. Again, if your mind starts to wander, simply return to the breath—over and over and over. This is like strength training for the brain. If you start the day in this way, it becomes easier and easier over time for you to wake up well—and to return to a peaceful place throughout the day. Once you've rested in stillness for 5 or 10 minutes, stand up, stretch, and move into your day from a calm, centered place. FYI: This is a basic practice of no-frills, ecumenical meditation. If you can do this regularly, you can do anything!

Check In with Yourself

Congratulations—you've finished the 3-Day Turbo Cleanse. Now it's time to check in with yourself and see how you're feeling.

First, do it in a very practical, tangible way by flipping back to Chapter 2 and retaking both the Medical Symptom Questionnaire (page 35) and the Environmental Factors Questionnaire (page 42). You should see marked improvement on both scales, as you have taken a big step toward a less-toxic lifestyle.

Second, get out that journal you started before the Detox Prescription (see page 91). Flip through to review what was making you feel bad then . . . and what was making you feel good. Then make a new inventory. How are you feeling now? What's your energy level? Do you see subjective changes in mood? In the way you look or feel or think? Do you feel that doing the 3-Day Turbo Cleanse has changed your perspective in any way? Will it change the way you eat from here on out?

Also write down any mental or emotional challenges or frustrations you encountered during the 3 days. The good, the bad, the ugly . . . put it all down.

When you're done, you can take a moment to sit quietly and reflect on what you've written. Add your own thoughts to the results of the Medical Symptom Questionnaire and the Environmental Factors Questionnaire. Do you need and want to go deeper?

If so, turn the page and get ready to start the 7-Day In-Depth Detox.

Get a Jump on Day 4

Tomorrow, you'll be transitioning to solid food. There's really nothing you *have* to do ahead of time, but because soup always tastes better the day after you make it and the flavors marry overnight, you can go ahead and make the Curry Butternut Squash Soup with Cayenne-Roasted Butternut Squash Seeds (page 151). It will certainly save you time during the day! Store the soup in the refrigerator overnight in a glass bowl or stainless steel pot and simply reheat before serving.

the
7-day
in-depth detox

Days 4 to 7–Continuing a weeklong juice-and-food plan that will deepen your detox results and reset your health

With the 3-Day Turbo Cleanse now under your belt, you're probably feeling great. Your head is clear, your energy is good—and your digestion is likely functioning better than it has for a long, long while. Take the opportunity to build on your good health by going with 4 more days of an all-plant-foods diet—that is to say, focusing solely on plant foods, such as fruits, vegetables, grains, beans, nuts, and seeds. Add 4 days of vegan meals to your 3 days of juices and smoothies, and you have a 7-Day In-Depth Detox that will truly deep-cleanse your system and give you additional time for long-needed repair and replenishment. Believe it or not, by the end of day 7, you'll feel even better than you do right now! You may also have lost a little weight.

You may be surprised when you look at the menu that it's not limited to a spartan assortment of raw salads and crunchy crudités. Rather, Mary Beth has created a luscious array of soups, stews, purees, and other soft, cooked foods to help the body continue to heal and perfect its digestive processes.

Digestion starts at the mouth—though we don't always acknowledge that. In Chapter 9 I'll explain the process in detail, but here's what you need to know for now: Saliva plays a critical role, as does chewing. For optimal digestion, food should be chewed well enough to allow the salivary enzymes to do their work helping to break down the food into a soft mush. (Bonus: Chewing boosts satiety, too.) But too many of us do an inadequate job of chewing our food, impatiently gulping it down in large chunks.

The body has mechanisms to deal with this, of course—it is incredibly intelligent and ever hard at work creating homeostasis. It begins to produce a whole range of secretions—called the "digestive cascade"—to compensate. To deal with these larger food molecules, the stomach cranks out more hydrochloric acid. The liver and gallbladder take note and begin to produce more bile to help you digest fat in the gut. The small intestine signals the pancreas to produce buffering salts (called bicarb) to help neutralize the excess acid from the stomach and keep the intestinal environment more alkaline. The pancreas also introduces a much wider range of enzymes than are in the mouth to continue chewing apart every possible kind of food group. If, despite all this, the food continues through the intestines in large chunks, intestinal bacteria will have to take over the job of breaking it down—which can lead to gas, cramping, bloating, and a whole host of other unpleasant symptoms, especially if the balance of your intestinal flora isn't optimal and there are more "bad" bacteria than "good" guys.

Your body will get the job done, but at a higher cost—when you swallow unchewed food, every organ must compensate for something that should have happened way upstream. You quite simply work the system harder.

During days 4 through 7, we've taken some of the chew factor out of the equation, creating small meals with a modified consistency. These are satisfying soups, stews, sautés, spreads, and compotes, featuring soft grains and nut butters. There are some crunchies here, don't worry—but the bulk of this menu is easy on the digestion so that the nutrients it contains can be

Why Not Raw All the Time?

The 3-Day Turbo Cleanse was a real fatigue buster, in part because it is so incredibly dense in phytonutrients. It certainly didn't hurt anything that those 3 days were also 100 percent raw. Raw foods deliver lots of live enzymes (see page 307) and ATP (adenosine triphosphate, see page 321)—the molecules used by every cell to produce energy in the mitochondrial energy factories. By day 2 you felt energized because you *were* energized—literally.

There are plenty of raw foods advocates out there, and they're fired up about the all-raw diet—because they feel great. Not only do raw foods deliver energy, but they also offer a very complete array of vitamins and minerals. (Heat can destroy enzymes and other nutrients beginning at about 140°F.) When you apply the three Cs of raw cookery—chop, crush, and chew—you release nutrients, break down hard-to-digest fiber, and in some cases even get a jump on the digestive process. Juicing, obviously, takes the three Cs to the max.

So why not all raw all the time?

The truth is that cooking offers big benefits, too. For one thing, it puts some incredibly nutritious foods that would be otherwise inedible—like beans and grains—on the menu. It kills molds and microbes, as well as naturally occurring toxins within the plant foods themselves (such as goitrogens, protease inhibitors, and saponins designed to act as built-in pesticides). Cooking transforms some of the insoluble fiber into detoxifying soluble fiber. And heat renders some nutrients—especially members of the carotenoid family, such as lycopene—more bioavailable.

The healthiest diet includes both the raw and the cooked, and that's what we offer in the 7-Day In-Depth Detox. Keep on having your daily juices and nut milks; dig in to fresh fruit and veggie snacks; enjoy the energizing, detoxifying benefits of a daily salad. But also enjoy the warm and satisfying pleasures of soups, sautés, and casseroles. Keep your diet balanced, and have the best of both worlds.

absorbed with minimum strain on the system. That doesn't mean you shouldn't chew well—you should. In fact, I recommend that you take some time to "chew" even your juices and smoothies, as allowing time for your saliva to interact with food leads to more efficient digestion, nutrient absorption, and detoxification. It's just that with this particular menu, you've got a little jump-start on the process.

7-DAY IN-DEPTH DETOX MENU, DAYS 4 THROUGH 7

	Day 4	Day 5	Day 6	Day 7
Beverage	Detox Tea (Dandelion, Chicory, or Burdock Root)	Detox Tea (Dandelion, Chicory, or Burdock Root)	Detox Tea (Dandelion, Chicory, or Burdock Root)	Detox Tea (Dandelion, Chicory, or Burdock Root)
Breakfast	Almond Butter Banana-Raspberry Tortilla	Coconut Yogurt, Berry, and Hemp Heart Parfait	Polenta with Granny Smith Apple Compote	Savory Green Tea–Buckwheat Cereal
Midmorning Snack	Any Nut Milk from 3-Day Turbo Cleanse	Any Nut Milk from 3-Day Turbo Cleanse	Any Nut Milk from 3-Day Turbo Cleanse	Any Nut Milk from 3-Day Turbo Cleanse
Lunch	Curry Butternut Squash Soup with Cayenne-Roasted Butternut Squash Seeds	Lentil-Cashew–Stuffed Peppers	Savory Mushroom Soup	Carrot-Rhubarb Soup
Midafternoon Snack	Snack from "Grab and Go Snacks" (page 139)	Snack from "Grab and Go Snacks" (page 139)	Snack from "Grab and Go Snacks" (page 139)	Snack from "Grab and Go Snacks" (page 139)
Dinner	Tahini-Buckwheat Tabbouleh with Middle Eastern White Beans and Salad	Roasted Lemon-Garlic Artichokes with Mediterranean Kidney Beans and Salad	Rosemary Celeriac and Root Vegetables with Southwestern Black-Bean Mash and Salad	Three-Bean Kale Sauté with Brown Rice and Salad

As with the 3-day cleanse, the focus is on fresh and (ideally) organic produce for the absolutely best nutrition. Each day includes the entire rainbow—red, blue, yellow, green, as well as some whites and tans. You'll also be at liberty now to choose a favorite nut milk as a midmorning snack and a health-boosting midafternoon snack. For this one, we offer a list of 12 choices—choose 2 each day. You can eat them separately—say, have a coconut or soy yogurt at 2 p.m. and a piece of fruit at 4. Or you can pair them up to create a more filling mini-meal—combine your crackers with hummus or avocado, have veggie slices with salad dressing, or enjoy veggie slices with salsa.

You'll come back to this list if you opt to continue through the entire 21-day Detox Prescription plan. After day 7 is done, you'll be able to add a little dairy, eggs, and even some fish back onto the menu. However, during the 7-Day In-Depth Detox, I recommend that you stick to the vegan plan—hold off on cheese and dairy yogurt for now and explore the vegan alternatives that Mary Beth has recommended (you'll be surprised how good they are—especially a few palate-cleansing days on an all-vegan diet).

Please note that days 4 through 7 are by design an intensive cleansing period—high in the phytonutrients that support both phase I and phase II of the detox process but also slightly low in protein in the basic menu plan. It's hard to say how much protein intake is adequate for you, as needs vary so much based on size and physical activity level: The RDA baseline level in adults of moderate weight is 46 grams for women and 56 grams daily for men. Most Americans on the typical meat-sweet diet may actually be getting too much protein. But if you're exercising vigorously during these 4 days, weigh close to 200 pounds and up, or feel the need to boost your stamina, you can choose additional protein-rich snacks (such as nuts or hummus), add an extra nut milk to the menu, or have a late-afternoon protein shake (see our recommendations for good protein powders on page 102).

To help keep both protein and nutrition steady—without introducing fat and calories—you'll be eating a lot of beans during the 7-Day In-Depth Detox (see "All about Beans," page 146). There's really no getting around the fact that in a vegan diet, beans take the center of the plate. That's a good thing—you simply can't get a healthier protein option. It's a shame that most Americans undervalue beans, consuming on average just 6½ pounds per person annually, less than 2 percent of their total protein intake and far less than the recommended 3 cups per week.

Sometimes my patients tell me, "I hate beans." I ask them what they are thinking about, and it's some kind of childhood memory they're replaying—overcooked lima beans, maybe, or baked beans covered in sickly sweet tomato sauce. They haven't had the good stuff you can get today—adzukis, edamame, chickpeas, cannellinis, favas, borlottis . . . the

Grab-and-Go Snacks

Eat any one of these snacks alone or pair two together. For the 7-Day In-Depth Detox, skip the Greek yogurt and keep to vegan cheese. When you move into the 21-Day Clean and Lean Diet, it's okay—if it agrees with you—to choose high-quality, low-fat dairy.

• Unlimited nonstarchy vegetables (25 calories, 0 g protein per serving). Serving size, nonstarchy veggies: 1 cup leafy greens, $\frac{1}{2}$ cup cooked or raw veggies

• 1 serving fruit (60 calories, 0 g protein). Serving size, fruit: 1 small fruit, $\frac{3}{4}$ cup berries or melon, 2 tablespoons dried fruit

• 1 serving nuts or seeds (170 calories, 6 g protein). Serving size, nuts or seeds: 1 ounce nuts or seeds or 2 tablespoons nut or seed butter

• $\frac{1}{4}$ cup bean spread (50 to 100 calories, 2 to 4 g protein). Try Trader Joe's black bean dip, Desert Pepper's white bean or pinto bean spreads

• 4 ounces plain coconut yogurt (110 calories, 0 g protein)

• 6 ounces plain almond yogurt (140 calories, 7 g protein)

• 6 ounces fat-free plain Greek yogurt (100 calories, 18 g protein) {after Day 7}

• $\frac{1}{2}$ cup shelled edamame beans (100 calories, 8 g protein)

• $\frac{1}{2}$ cup firm or extra-firm cubed tofu (90 calories, 10 g protein)

• $\frac{1}{3}$ cup unsweetened natural salsa (25 calories, 0 g protein)

• $\frac{1}{2}$ avocado (170 calories, 1 g protein)

• 6 high-fiber, gluten-free crackers (varies; read label). Try Mary's Gone Crackers flax quinoa crackers (6 crackers = 65 calories, 1 g protein)

• 2 tablespoons natural unsweetened salad dressing (varies; read label)

• 1 ounce vegan cheese (90 calories, 1 g protein). Try Daiya brand vegan "cheese" wedges

variety of colors, flavors, and textures available to us now is absolutely incredible. And so are the dishes you can create with them: Beans are great pureed and mashed and in chilis, soups, stews, salads, and spreads. The beans featured here are pretty simple, though they're used with some complex flavors, which illustrate a point—with beans you can create anything. All you need is a handful of spices and a little imagination.

More to the point of this book, beans are high in beneficial fiber, which is a big boon to detox. Not only are we helping the body do its job of releasing and processing toxins in the liver, we are ushering those bound-up bad

Morning Detox Teas

Most of us are used to starting the day with something hot—often coffee. For the rest of the Detox Prescription, try something new: These three herbal teas rehydrate the body, contribute phytonutrients and enzymes beneficial to both phase I and phase II detoxification, and are choleretics—which is to say that they stimulate the secretion of bile for better digestion. Dandelion, burdock root, and chicory are bitter in flavor, but don't give in to the temptation to add sugar—experiencing the bitterness may dampen cravings for sweets. Bitter is one of the essential flavors—along with salty, sweet, sour, and umami—and it should be experienced and savored as part of the spectrum of human sensory experience. The bitter taste is highly prized in other parts of the world, where it is incorporated with meals as a digestive tonic, but it's too often overlooked in America.

If the flavor truly puts you off, brew the tea for only a few moments at first and build up to a "deep steep" over time. By the end of the 7-Day In-Depth Detox, you may be surprised to find yourself craving these herbal teas the moment you wake up. Buy these teas loose or in bags at any health food store or order online from Tea Haven (teahaven.com) or Frontier Natural Products Co-op (frontiercoop.com).

DANDELION ROOT TEA

Dandelion contains a wide array of phytonutrients with biological activities. These have liver-protective, diuretic, antioxidant, antidiabetes, anticlotting, anti-inflammatory,

boys out of the body through elimination. I don't want to go too far on that topic now and get off the subject of all the yummy healing food on this well-crafted menu (you can read more about it in Chapter 8), but suffice it to say that fiber is a big asset to elimination. And if despite doing all the preparation of beans that we recommend, you still find them challenging to digest, you can take an enzyme (such as Beano) to help break down some of their harder-to-digest starches. Embrace beans for the next 4 days, and you just might find that you want to hold on to them for life.

During the 7-Day In-Depth Detox, you'll also be able to add a salad to your

and anticancer activity. The main active compounds in dandelion root are glycosides, carotenoids, and terpenoids. Dandelion leaves are used in salads or as a cooked green, and the flowers are used to make wine. The flavor is bitter, green, and earthy.

BURDOCK ROOT TEA

Burdock root is used in folk medicine and as a vegetable in Asian countries, especially Japan, Korea, and Thailand. Burdock roots have detoxifying, liver-protective, antioxidant, anti-inflammatory, antidiabetes, and anticancer properties. The main active compounds in burdock root are lignans, flavonoids, phenolic acids, luteolin, and quercetin. The flavor is earthy and woody, though somewhat cleaner than dandelion.

CHICORY ROOT TEA

Chicory root has been studied for its detoxifying, liver-protective, anti-inflammatory, anticlotting, and anticancer activity. The main active compounds in chicory root are phenolics, including caffeic acid (not caffeine), but chicory root is best known for its inulin content and prebiotic activity that helps balance intestinal bacteria. The flavor is so similar to that of coffee that chicory is often used as a replacement—or an adjunct, as it is in New Orleans, most notably at the famous Café du Monde.

dinner. This is something that's not so prescriptive—choose whatever greens you like. However, I do recommend that you think beyond iceberg lettuce, and even beyond romaine and spinach. A nightly salad is a great opportunity to practice botanical diversity, which yields nutrient diversity. So explore mesclun, arugula, watercress, dandelion, Bibb, radicchio, frisée, chard, tango, mâche, endive, escarole, and oak leaf lettuce. Explore at the farmers' market and be open to whatever is fresh and local. Add a few chopped onions or sunflower seeds or carrot shreds or mushrooms—whatever sounds good to you and is on hand (however, don't add croutons or cheese, please).

Dressing can be as simple as a squeeze of lemon or a dash of good vinegar blended with a small amount of a healthy oil (olive or sesame, etc.). Invest in an aged balsamic, and you'll enjoy rich, complex flavors that won't even necessitate the use of oil (find good ones online at avantisavoia.com or oliviersandco.

All About Lentils

Lentils are legumes that have a milder flavor than beans. Lentils are more easily digested than dried beans because they contain lower indigestible-sugar (oligosaccharide) levels. They also cook faster than dried beans and do not require soaking. Green, brown, and black lentils hold their shape best after cooking and are a good choice for additions to soups, stews, and salads. Orange and red lentils don't hold their shape as well and are a better choice for mashed and pureed lentils, spreads, and pâtés.

Nutrition

A half-cup serving of lentils contains 115 calories, 7 to 9 grams of protein, and 7 grams of fiber. Lentils are low in total fat and saturated fat and contain B vitamins, zinc, iron, magnesium, and antioxidants and phytonutrients such as isoflavones, phytosterols, saponins, and phenolic compounds.

Buying Lentils

Lentils are sold prepackaged in boxes or bags, or in bulk form. Shop for them much as you would for beans: Lentils should be uniform in size and color and free of insect

com). Try one of our four special dressings, which are specifically designed to amp up the flavor *and* the detox power (see Detox Dressings, page 144).

We're not promoting dessert . . . yet. If you feel that you need something sweet at the end of a meal, have a piece of fresh fruit. You might also unwind after dinner with a warm cup of chamomile tea and just a drop of honey, or better yet with a cup of naturally sweet licorice tea (though if you have uncontrolled hypertension, don't do this one, as it can raise blood pressure). Finally, although I want to go on record as discouraging you from indulging your sweet tooth, which can set you up for future cravings, go ahead and reward yourself on day 7 for a week of work well done. I can think of little better than one of nature's most enjoyable health foods: a small piece of dark chocolate. (See "Walk on the Dark Side," page 175, for more on the subject.)

damage pinholes. If they look particularly "dusty" in the package, they may be old or damaged by insects.

Cleaning and Cooking Lentils

1. Spread the lentils out in a single layer on a counter or tabletop. Check for and discard dirt, stones, or damaged lentils.

2. Place the lentils in a strainer and rinse under cold water.

3. Add 2 cups of water or broth for every 1 cup of lentils you're cooking to a saucepan and add desired spices, herbs, or oils. Do not add salt until the lentils are cooked, because salt will toughen the lentils if added at the beginning of the cooking time.

4. Bring the water or broth to a boil and add the lentils. Boil for 2 or 3 minutes and then reduce the heat to a simmer. Cook until tender. Cook green, brown, and black lentils for 25 to 35 minutes and red and orange lentils for 15 to 25 minutes. Test lentils for desired tenderness for use in soups, stews, salad, pâtés, and spreads.

Note: The soups and nut milks are perfect for "making and taking"—both store well in the refrigerator and are easy to carry to work (or play, for that matter). Carry nut milks in a shaker bottle so you can blend before drinking; carry soups in a Thermos bottle warm or cold. Accessorize the soup with gluten-free crackers, veggies, and nuts (one of your snacks) to make a bigger meal, if you like. You'll be so satisfied with the complex flavors and velvety textures of these soups, you'll never miss your usual sandwich.

Detox Dressings

Your nightly salad isn't just a side-dish afterthought—for your liver, it's a main event! Greens are arguably nature's most potent nutrient-containing foods and even have a positive impact on the way your immune system works in your intestine. They also provide plenty of antioxidants to quench the free radicals produced by phase I detoxification, as well as the phytonutrient inducers of the phase II enzyme reactions. Win-win.

You can make your salad an even more powerful detoxifying ally by dressing it well.

Here, Mary Beth offers four powerhouse options. Each one packs a unique flavor and nutrition punch. The zesty Citrus Zinger Detox Dressing offers bonus bioflavonoids and citrus pectin, which can bind with heavy metals in the body. The rich Lemon-Tahini Dressing introduces the antioxidant sesamin—as well as a luscious texture that works well as a sauce or dip, too. The sweet and pungent Honey-Mustard Detox Dressing contains thiols from the mustard seeds and linalool from the coriander, which have antioxidant and diuretic properties. And the spicy Sesame-Ginger Detox Dressing combines the anti-inflammatory power of ginger with garlic's sulfur compounds and lemon's quercetin to deliver a detox trifecta.

Each dressing makes eight to ten 2-tablespoon servings. Simply combine all ingredients in a Mason or shaker jar and shake well or whisk together thoroughly in a small bowl. Use an immersion blender, if need be, to achieve a smooth consistency. You can store these in the refrigerator for up to a week, but shake or whisk just before serving.

Citrus Zinger Detox Dressing

MAKES 10 SERVINGS (2 TABLESPOONS EACH)

½ cup extra-virgin olive oil

½ cup freshly squeezed lemon juice

¼ cup freshly squeezed orange juice

1 teaspoon freshly grated ginger

¼ teaspoon finely grated lemon zest

¼ teaspoon finely grated orange zest

½ teaspoon freshly ground black pepper

½ teaspoon sea salt

Per serving: 102 calories, 11 g total fat (2 g saturated), 0 mg cholesterol, 117 mg sodium, 29 mg potassium, 2 g carbohydrates (1 g sugar), 0 g fiber, 0 g protein

Lemon-Tahini Dressing

MAKES 8 SERVINGS (2 TABLESPOONS EACH)

4 tablespoons tahini

4 tablespoons extra-virgin olive oil

2 tablespoons apple cider vinegar

2 tablespoons freshly squeezed lemon juice

½ teaspoon wheat-free tamari

1 teaspoon lemon zest

2 teaspoons minced fresh ginger

2 garlic cloves, minced

1 tablespoon minced green chives

½ teaspoon sea salt

2–4 tablespoons water, as needed to adjust consistency

Per serving: 120 calories, 12 g total fat (2 g saturated), 0 mg cholesterol, 175 mg sodium, 77 mg potassium, 3 g carbohydrates (0 g sugar), 1 g fiber, 1 g protein

Honey-Mustard Detox Dressing

MAKES 8 SERVINGS (2 TABLESPOONS EACH)

½ cup extra-virgin olive oil

¼ cup apple cider vinegar

1 tablespoon organic mustard with
seeds (try Eden Organics Brown
Mustard)

2 tablespoons honey

½ teaspoon coriander

½ teaspoon orange zest

½ teaspoon sea salt

Per serving: 116 calories, 11 g total fat (2 g saturated), 0 mg cholesterol, 117 mg sodium, 25 mg potassium, 5 g carbohydrates (4 g sugar), 0 g fiber, 0 g protein

All About Beans

Throughout the Detox Prescription, you'll be eating lots of beans in the incredible recipes Mary Beth Augustine has customized for you, and also as a simple side dish. Beans are the best way I know to boost protein power without also boosting fat and calories, as nuts, seeds (due to their caloric healthy fats), and animal foods (due to their caloric *unhealthy* fats) do in a more pronounced way. During the 7-Day In-Depth Detox, days 4 through 7 in particular, you'll be eating them straight up—their protein and fiber content will nourish the body and help it in its cleansing and detoxifying tasks. This is a very good thing.

Nutrition

For each ½ cup serving of beans you eat, you get approximately 90 to 115 calories, 6 to 8 grams of protein, and 6 to 7 grams of fiber (it varies a bit from bean to bean). Beans are low in total fat and saturated fat and high in the methylation-supporting B vitamins thiamin, folic acid, riboflavin, and B_6. Beans are high in the minerals iron, zinc, and magnesium, and antioxidants and phytonutrients such as isoflavones, lignans, flavonoids, phytosterols, saponins, and phenolic compounds. Higher dietary bean intake is linked to lower rates of cancer, heart disease, diabetes, and obesity, and greater longevity. Good stuff!

Sesame-Ginger Detox Dressing

MAKES 10 SERVINGS (2 TABLESPOONS EACH)

½ cup sesame oil

⅓ cup rice wine vinegar

4 tablespoons minced fresh ginger

2 tablespoons minced celery

1 tablespoon freshly squeezed lemon juice

1 tablespoon honey

1 teaspoon minced garlic

½ teaspoon sea salt

Per serving: 107 calories, 11 g total fat (2 g saturated), 0 mg cholesterol, 118 mg sodium, 26 mg potassium, 3 g carbohydrates (2 g sugar), 0 g fiber, 0 g protein

Buying Beans

Beans are sold prepackaged in boxes or bags or in bulk form. When you are buying them, look for beans that are uniform in size and color and free of insect damage pinholes. One cup of dried beans produces about 3 cups cooked, so plan accordingly.

Why Soak Dried Beans or Rinse Canned Beans?

Beans are high in indigestible sugars, called oligosaccharides. These indigestible sugars are just that—indigestible—which is the reason beans are known as a "gassy" food. Adding a bay leaf (and discarding after cooking), the spices cumin or epazote, or a few strips of kombu when cooking beans may also help reduce their gassiness. Taking Beano when eating beans may help reduce gassiness, as it contains the enzyme oligosaccharidase, which is necessary to digest the indigestible sugars. Beano really works. If you are working with canned beans, rinsing them and draining them will also help to remove some of the starch content and reduce calories.

Cleaning, Soaking, and Cooking Dried Beans

1. Spread the beans out in a single layer on a counter or tabletop. Check for dirt, stones, or damaged beans and discard them if you find them.

2. Place the beans in a strainer and rinse under cold water.

(continued)

Cleaning, Soaking, and Cooking Dried Beans—*Continued*

3. Place the beans in a saucepan and cover with water. Remove any beans that float to the top. Soak for 8 hours or overnight in the refrigerator.

4. Drain the beans, discard the soaking water, and rinse with cold water.

5. Put the beans into a large pot and fill with water or broth to about 2 inches above the beans. Add desired spices, herbs, and/or oils. Do not add salt until the beans are cooked, otherwise salt will toughen the beans.

6. Bring the beans to a boil, skimming off any foam on the surface. Reduce the heat, cover, and simmer, stirring occasionally and adding more liquid if necessary, until the beans are at desired tenderness when fork tested. Cooking times vary with variety, age, and size of beans, but generally range from 1 to 2 hours.

Dealing with Setbacks

What should you do if you fall off the wagon? First thing: Don't freak out. It happens. We're all human. Forgive yourself and prepare to move on. Here's what to do:

• **If your slip-up happens during any day of the 3-Day Turbo Cleanse:** If you are slipping up on day 1, you need to stop, recommit, and restart the plan. If there is a one-meal slip, add an extra day to the end. If you completely go off for a day, you need to reboot and start over to get the best results.

• **If your slip-up happens during the 7-Day In-Depth Detox:** That's not a huge deal, especially if it was just a one-time lapse. I'd recommend adding another day of all-vegan eating to the plan to compensate. If you slipped up big-time—say, bacon and eggs for breakfast, a three-martini lunch, and steak for dinner—you should probably start over and recommit yourself to the process.

• **If your slip-up happens during the 21-Day Clean and Lean Diet:** In this case, the best thing you can do is simply move on and pick up where you left off. Nobody is perfect all the time. That's not a license to go crazy, but it is a license for you to acknowledge what happened with minimal muss and fuss and continue with your good habits. Everyone who succeeds at making positive change also succeeds at moving through setbacks. Don't let them derail you.

Day 4 Menu

BEVERAGE: Detox Tea (Dandelion, Chicory, or Burdock Root)

BREAKFAST: Almond Butter Banana-Raspberry Tortilla

MIDMORNING SNACK: Nut Milk from 3-Day Turbo Cleanse, Your Choice

LUNCH: Curry Butternut Squash Soup with Cayenne-Roasted Butternut Squash Seeds

MIDAFTERNOON SNACK: Your Choice (see page 139)

DINNER: Tahini-Buckwheat Tabbouleh with Middle Eastern White Beans and Salad

BREAKFAST

Almond Butter Banana-Raspberry Tortilla

Balanced in good carbs and good fats, this morning tortilla lowers levels of the appetite-stimulating hormone ghrelin and raises levels of the appetite-suppressing hormone leptin so you feel satisfied with plenty of energy to get through the morning slump with no coffee! This recipe is also an excellent source of vitamins B_6, C, and E; magnesium; riboflavin; and phosphorus.

MAKES 1 SERVING

½ teaspoon ground cinnamon

1 teaspoon coconut oil or extra-virgin olive oil

1 corn tortilla

2 tablespoons almond butter

½ large banana (or 1 small banana), sliced

¼ cup raspberries

¼ teaspoon cacao powder, optional

Mix the cinnamon into the coconut or olive oil. In a small skillet, heat the oil on medium-high heat.

Sauté each side of the tortilla for 2 to 3 minutes, or until golden.

Before removing the tortilla from the skillet, reduce the heat to medium-low, spread the almond butter on the tortilla, and allow to warm for 1 to 2 minutes, or until the almond butter is creamy.

Remove from the heat, top with the banana and raspberries, and sprinkle on the cacao powder (if using).

Per serving: 345 calories, 23 g total fat (6 g saturated), 0 mg cholesterol, 5 mg sodium, 695 mg potassium, 35 g carbohydrates (14 g sugar), 8 g fiber, 6 g protein

TIP: Don't confuse cacao powder with cocoa powder—they're made from the same plant, but cocoa powder is highly processed, often sweetened, and generally less flavorful. Navitas Naturals offers cacao powder, along with a range of other cacao products; navitasnaturals.com. You can substitute blueberries for the raspberries or any nut butter for the almond butter.

LUNCH

Curry Butternut Squash Soup with Cayenne-Roasted Butternut Squash Seeds

This recipe is an excellent source of vitamins A and C and a good source of zinc, magnesium, manganese, vitamin B_6, and copper. Butternut squash is chock-full of carotenoids, and the apple and pepper pack a flavonoid and antioxidant punch. Pectin in the apple, allyl sulfides in the onion, curcumin in the curry, and capsaicin in the cayenne boost the detoxifying and anti-inflammatory power of this recipe. They'll rock your taste buds, too! Say good-bye to day-old croutons and toss on the protein-packed, sizzling seeds for a spicy, crunchy energy boost and a little extra protein-packed nutrition.

MAKES 6 SERVINGS

SOUP

¼ cup extra-virgin olive oil

1 medium onion, chopped

1 Granny Smith apple, peeled, cored, and chopped

1 large red bell pepper, seeded and chopped

1 medium butternut squash (about 2 pounds), peeled, seeded, and cut in 1" squares, seeds reserved

6 cups low-sodium vegetable broth

2 sprigs fresh thyme

1 bay leaf

1 teaspoon curry powder

CAYENNE-ROASTED BUTTERNUT SQUASH SEEDS

Reserved butternut squash seeds, rinsed and patted dry

Extra-virgin olive oil

½ teaspoon cayenne pepper, or to taste

(continued)

To make the soup: In a 4-quart stockpot, heat the olive oil on medium-high heat. Add the onion and cook for 5 to 7 minutes, or until translucent.

Add the apple and red bell pepper and cook for an additional 2 to 3 minutes.

Add the squash, vegetable broth, thyme, and bay leaf. Bring to a simmer and cook for 15 to 20 minutes, or until the squash is fork-tender.

Remove the bay leaf and thyme sprigs and add the curry powder.

Transfer the soup to a blender or food processor. Blend until smooth (or until the desired consistency is attained).

Pour the soup into bowls and top with 2 tablespoons Cayenne-Roasted Butternut Squash Seeds.

To make the seeds: While the soup is simmering, preheat the oven to 275°F.

In a bowl, toss the butternut squash seeds with the olive oil to coat and sprinkle with the cayenne.

Spread the seeds in a thin, even layer on a baking sheet lined with parchment paper.

Bake for 15 minutes. Remove from the oven and allow to cool.

Per soup serving: 171 calories, 9 g total fat (1 g saturated), 0 mg cholesterol, 146 mg sodium, 409 mg potassium, 23 g carbohydrates (3 g sugar), 1 g fiber, 6 g protein

Per squash seed serving: 125 calories, 5 g total fat (1 g saturated), 0 mg cholesterol, 5 mg sodium, 257 mg potassium, 15 g carbohydrates (0 g sugar), 5 g fiber, 6 g protein

TIP: You can make your own veggie broth, or buy a good one: Imagine Natural Creations, Pacific Natural Foods, Whole Foods 365, and Trader Joe's all make excellent organic broths using just filtered water, organic veggies, organic spices, and a lot of good taste. Get your spices from Frontier Natural Products, whose organic herbs and spices are processed without radiation or ethylene oxide sterilization (frontiercoop.com).

DINNER

Tahini-Buckwheat Tabbouleh

Don't let the name fool you—buckwheat is not related to wheat at all, and in fact is a gluten-free grain (it's actually a member of the rhubarb family). This good-carb, good-fat, plant-protein-rich Tahini-Buckwheat Tabbouleh packs an amazing antioxidant punch with vitamins A and C and manganese. This recipe is also a good source of plant-based iron and the energy-boosting B vitamins thiamin, riboflavin, and niacin.

MAKES 6 SERVINGS

2 cups water

1 cup hulled buckwheat, rinsed

⅓ cup freshly squeezed lemon juice

¼ cup sesame tahini

2 tablespoons extra-virgin olive oil

3 garlic cloves, minced

1 teaspoon ground cumin

1 cup Italian parsley, minced

1 cucumber, seeded and cubed

1 cup sun-dried tomatoes, chopped fine

¼ cup fresh mint, minced

In a 2-quart stockpot, heat the water to boiling.

Add the buckwheat, reduce to a simmer, and cook uncovered for approximately 20 minutes, or until the buckwheat is tender and all water is absorbed.

Add the buckwheat to a mixing bowl, fluff, and allow to cool.

In a large bowl, whisk together the lemon juice, tahini, oil, garlic, and cumin. If the tahini will not mix to a smooth consistency, use a handheld immersion blender or add 2 tablespoons of warm water.

Pour the dressing over the buckwheat and toss well.

Add the parsley, cucumber, sun-dried tomatoes, and mint and toss well until all ingredients are combined.

Serve warm or chilled, with a salad and Middle Eastern White Beans (page 154).

Per serving: 238 calories, 11 g total fat (2 g saturated), 0 mg cholesterol, 208 mg sodium, 642 mg potassium, 31 g carbohydrates (4 g sugar), 6 g fiber, 8 g protein

TIP: Add ½ teaspoon of cayenne pepper for extra zing and an anti-inflammatory boost.

DINNER

Middle Eastern White Beans

These Middle Eastern white beans have got phase I detox-supporting minerals, including magnesium, copper, iron, and zinc, along with phase II folate for methylation support. There's also anti-inflammatory turmeric, coriander, and cumin, plus 11 percent of your daily bone-building calcium needs and 7 grams of fat-blasting fiber.

MAKES 6 SERVINGS

6 cups white beans

1 teaspoon ground cumin

1 teaspoon ground coriander

1 teaspoon turmeric

$\frac{1}{4}$ cup extra-virgin olive oil

2 shallots, chopped

1 garlic clove, chopped

$\frac{1}{4}$ cup freshly squeezed lemon juice

$\frac{1}{4}$ cup water

$\frac{1}{4}$ teaspoon sea salt

Use white beans cooked according to the directions on page 147 or use canned beans. Drain and rinse the beans, then drain again.

Heat a sauté pan over medium heat. Add the cumin, coriander, and turmeric to the hot sauté pan and sauté for 30 to 60 seconds, or until the spices are fragrant, stirring constantly to avoid burning.

Add the olive oil, shallots, and garlic and sauté for 3 minutes, or until translucent.

Add the beans, lemon juice, and water and cook for 4 to 5 minutes, stirring frequently, or until the beans are heated through. Season with salt, and serve.

Per serving: 244 calories, 10 g total fat (1 g saturated), 0 mg cholesterol, 106 mg sodium, 651 mg potassium, 32 g carbohydrates (0 g sugar), 7 g fiber, 10 g protein

TIP: Substitute Eden Organic BPA-free canned drained and rinsed white beans for a cooking shortcut. Buy organic spices at Frontier Natural Foods (frontiercoop.com) or Simply Organic (simplyorganic.com).

Day 4 Mind-Body Detox

PRACTICE MINDFUL EATING

Today you get to add solid food back to the menu. After 3 days of liquids, texture is a big deal. Make the most of it by practicing mindful eating. What does that mean? Instead of gobbling down your food on autopilot, take the time to really notice it, savor it, experience it, and enjoy it. Studies have demonstrated that this is an effective tool in promoting weight loss and controlling diabetes. The more slowly you eat, the more likely you are to feel fully satisfied with your meal without having to overeat.

Before you even scoop a bite onto your fork, notice the colors, aromas, textures, and shapes of every little component of the dish you're about to dig into—how they all work together to create a multisensory experience for your nourishment on every level. Take a small forkful, bring it up to your nose, and inhale deeply. What do you smell? Hold the fork up to your eyes: What do you see? When you put the food in your mouth, take a moment to touch it with your tongue. What do you feel?

Next, chew the food slowly, allowing the flavors to develop over time. Put the fork down between bites. Close your eyes. Tune out everything else except for the experience of chewing and tasting your food. No multitasking, no talking, watching TV, or checking your e-mail, no distractions of any sort. Swallow, then wait for 30 seconds before taking another bite to allow for a sensation of satiety to arise.

It may be impossible to eat every meal this way, especially when you're eating with family, in restaurants, or at the office. But simply enjoying one meal a day in a mindful fashion can transform the way you experience and think about food.

Get a Jump on Day 5

If you want to make them ahead, you can prepare and assemble Lentil-Cashew–Stuffed Peppers (follow the recipe on page 158 through step six) and store them in the baking pan in the refrigerator. When it's time for dinner, just pop the whole thing in the oven to bake as directed.

Day 5 Menu

BEVERAGE: Detox Tea (Dandelion, Chicory, or Burdock Root)

BREAKFAST: Coconut Yogurt, Berry, and Hemp Heart Parfait

MIDMORNING SNACK: Nut Milk from 3-Day Turbo Cleanse, Your Choice

LUNCH: Lentil-Cashew-Stuffed Peppers

MIDAFTERNOON SNACK: Your Choice (see page 139)

DINNER: Roasted Lemon-Garlic Artichokes with Mediterranean Kidney Beans and Salad

BREAKFAST

Coconut Yogurt, Berry, and Hemp Heart Parfait

This colorful parfait really brightens up your morning, while the hemp hearts add heartiness and contain the powerful phytochemicals ellagic acid and resveratrol, which reduce inflammation, inhibit oxidation of LDL ("lousy" cholesterol), protect nerve cells, and prevent insulin resistance. Berries have a lot less sugar by weight than many other fruits, and what sugars are there are released relatively slowly due to the 10 grams of fiber.

MAKES 1 SERVING

⅓ cup strawberries

⅓ cup raspberries

⅓ cup blackberries

⅓ cup blueberries

8 ounces plain coconut yogurt

2 tablespoons shelled hemp hearts

Pinch of ground cinnamon, optional

Pinch of ground nutmeg, optional

In a small bowl, mix the berries together.

In the bottom of a serving bowl, layer ⅓ cup of the berries. Top with ⅓ cup yogurt, another ⅓ cup berries, ⅓ cup yogurt, another ⅓ cup berries, ⅓ cup yogurt, and the last ⅓ cup berries.

Sprinkle the hemp hearts on top of the finished parfait. Sprinkle with the cinnamon and nutmeg (if using).

Per serving: 250 calories, 14 g total fat (6 g saturated), 0 mg cholesterol, 20 mg sodium, 281 mg potassium, 24 g carbohydrates (12 g sugar), 10 g fiber, 9 g protein

TIP: Berries can be expensive; use any combination here. You can also use thawed frozen berries—just be aware that the texture will change. Remember to rinse frozen produce just as you do fresh. Coconut milk yogurt is a great nondairy alternative for people who are cow milk protein or lactose intolerant. Several brands are available, but we especially like the product made by So Delicious; find a store near you at sodeliciousdairyfree.com.

LUNCH

Lentil-Cashew–Stuffed Peppers

This recipe puts the C in cashew—with 576 percent of your daily vitamin C requirement met, you're sure to ward off colds and infection. And we'll also give this recipe an A for its 198 percent vitamin A content: Carotenoids, lutein, zeaxanthin, lycopene, and beta-carotene act as antioxidants and have anticancer activity. Kale, onion, and curry boost the detox power, and the super antioxidants ellagic acid and resveratrol (found in the raisins) quell free-radical activity—all in a mouthwatering, proteinaceous, peppery delight!

MAKES 4 SERVINGS

1 tablespoon curry powder

1 cup Raw Cashew Milk (page 120)

2 tablespoons extra-virgin olive oil

1 medium yellow onion, chopped

1 cup curly kale leaves, roughly chopped

¾ cup diced tomato

⅓ cup unsulphured raisins

½ cup cashews, roughly chopped

2 cups cooked brown lentils (see "All about Lentils," page 142)

Sea salt, to taste

4 red, yellow, and/or orange bell peppers, cut in half lengthwise, cored, and seeded

Preheat the oven to 350°F. In a small bowl, whisk the curry powder into the cashew milk. Set aside.

In a 7" skillet, heat the oil over medium heat. Add the onion and cook for about 3 minutes, or until soft and translucent.

Add the kale, tomato, and raisins and sauté for 4 to 5 minutes, or until the kale leaves begin to wilt.

Reduce the heat to low and add the chopped cashews and cashew milk mixture to the skillet. Stir until the kale and raisins are evenly coated and allow to cook for about 5 minutes.

Remove from the heat, combine with the cooked lentils, and season with sea salt to taste.

Stuff the pepper halves with the lentil-cashew mixture, arrange in a 13" x 9" oiled baking pan, and bake for about 45 minutes, or until the peppers are tender and the lentil mixture is heated through.

Per serving: 298 calories, 17 g total fat (3 g saturated), 0 mg cholesterol, 54 mg sodium, 883 mg potassium, 37 g carbohydrates (10 g sugar), 6 g fiber, 9 g protein

TIP: Since bell peppers are number seven on the Environmental Working Group's Dirty Dozen list of the most polluted produce, it's important to go with organic whenever you can. Frontier Natural Products (frontiercoop.com) and Simply Organic (simplyorganic.com) sell organic nonirradiated curry powder.

Get a Jump on Day 6

Soups, stews, and compotes are great make-ahead dishes. You can make the Granny Smith Apple Compote (page 164) and the Savory Mushroom Soup (page 166) ahead of time and store them in the refrigerator. Just reheat before serving.

DINNER

Roasted Lemon-Garlic Artichokes

Artichokes aren't everyday fare for most of us—so they can make a memorable dinner centerpiece. Peeling the leaves and using your teeth to scrape the soft artichoke flesh puts the fun in functional for this fabulous vegetable. The inulin in artichoke not only detoxifies xenobiotic toxins but is an indigestible prebiotic that stimulates the growth of good bacteria in the gut and has anticancer activity, too. The citrus pectin and bioflavonoids in the lemon boost the detox power, while the rosemary adds antimicrobial activity. If you're counting calories, you can eliminate the oil—this recipe will still taste great.

MAKES 2 SERVINGS

2 artichokes

4 tablespoons extra-virgin olive oil

8 garlic cloves, sliced (not minced)

2 sprigs rosemary, leaves removed

1 large lemon, cut in 4 thick slices

Lemon wedges, optional

Sea salt, optional

Preheat the oven to 350°F.

Cut the very bottom tip of the stem off the artichokes, leaving most of the stem on, and cut the artichokes in half lengthwise from the stem down.

In a 13" x 9" baking pan, drizzle each artichoke stem and half, interior "flesh" side facing up, with 1 tablespoon of the oil. Insert garlic slices into the artichoke interiors and top with rosemary leaves and a lemon slice.

Flip the artichokes over, lemon facing down. Cover the pan with foil and bake for 45 minutes.

Serve 2 artichoke halves with lemon wedges (if using) and sea salt (if using). Add a salad and 1 cup of Mediterranean Kidney Beans (opposite) for a protein boost.

Per serving: 320 calories, 27 g total fat (4 g saturated), 0 mg cholesterol, 123 mg sodium, 585 mg potassium, 22 g carbohydrates (0 g sugar), 10 g fiber, 5 g protein

TIP: Artichokes can intimidate even adventurous home chefs. To overcome this fear, see Ocean Mist Farms All About Artichokes "How to Prepare and Cook Artichokes" videos at oceanmist.com.

DINNER

Mediterranean Kidney Beans

If this Mediterranean Kidney Beans dish came in a cereal box, it would boast "an excellent or great source of 11 vitamins and minerals." But here's the thing: This dish is not "enriched" or "fortified"—the nutrients are naturally occurring. It also contains 60 percent of your Daily Value of fiber and the protein equivalent of 2 ounces of fish or 2 eggs. Forget "seal of approval"—this simple dish should really be sealed with a kiss.

MAKES 4 SERVINGS

4 cups red kidney beans
2 celery stalks, chopped
1 scallion, chopped
1 carrot, chopped
2 tablespoons extra-virgin olive oil
2 tablespoons freshly squeezed lemon juice
2 tablespoons red wine vinegar
1 teaspoon lemon zest
$\frac{1}{4}$ teaspoon sea salt

Cook the beans according to the directions on page 147 or use canned beans. Drain and rinse the beans, then drain again.

In a large mixing bowl, combine the beans, celery, scallion, and carrot.

In a small mixing bowl, whisk together the olive oil, lemon juice, vinegar, lemon zest, and salt.

Pour the dressing over the bean and vegetable mixture and combine well. Serve at room temperature or chilled.

Per serving: 293 calories, 8 g total fat (1 g saturated), 0 mg cholesterol, 440 mg sodium, 835 mg potassium, 44 g carbohydrates (1 g sugar), 18 g fiber, 14 g protein

TIP: For a no-cook shortcut, substitute drained and rinsed Eden Organic BPA-free canned beans. Add a yellow bell pepper to lend a peppery taste, extra crunch, and some eye-popping color.

Day 5 Mind-Body Detox

MAKE YOURSELF A MANTRA

The ancient yogis tell us that mantras are powerful, able to evoke the force of the gods themselves. I don't know about that, but I do know that bringing the mind back to a phrase over and over again can be a powerful way to focus attention, calm the nervous system, and reduce stress. You can use a typical Sanskrit mantra, like "Om" (said to be the sound of creation), or "So hum" (the sound of the breath), or "Shanti, shanti, shanti" (peace, peace, peace). Or you can choose a sacred word or phrase affiliated with your own religious tradition. The Aramaic "Maranatha" (oh Lord, come) from the Christian tradition, "Shalom" (peace) from the Jewish tradition, and "Namo Butsaya" (I bow to the Buddha) from the Buddhist tradition are three such examples. There are countless others.

Better yet, create your own mantra with the specific purpose of supporting your own health and spiritual wellness. This could be anything, though I suggest that you use the journaling exercise on page 91 to choose something that will specifically invite more joy into your life and help you find the strength and willpower to succeed in your detox efforts. Then make a bold statement—not that you are going to do something, but that you have already done it! "I am well," "I am powerful," "I am peaceful," "I am able."

Or just boil it down to the most essential mantra of them all, simply: "I am."

When you are feeling stressed or shaky, or beset by craving or doubt, take a deep breath and repeat your mantra. You may have to do this several times a day; you may have to do it hundreds of times a day at first! But every time you do it, you are affirming your own power to be in control of your mind and emotions, as well as the decisions you make about what to do and what to eat.

Day 6 Menu

BEVERAGE: Detox Tea (Dandelion, Chicory, or Burdock Root)

BREAKFAST: Polenta with Granny Smith Apple Compote

MIDMORNING SNACK: Nut Milk from 3-Day Turbo Cleanse, Your Choice

LUNCH: Savory Mushroom Soup

MIDAFTERNOON SNACK: Your Choice (see page 139)

DINNER: Rosemary Celeriac and Root Vegetables with Southwestern Black-Bean Mash and Salad

BREAKFAST

Polenta with Granny Smith Apple Compote

The apple (and citrus) pectin binds heavy metals, toxins, and radioactive compounds, and the pumpkin pie spices—cinnamon, ginger, nutmeg, cloves—and cardamom have blood-sugar-lowering, anti-inflammatory, and antimicrobial properties. This delicious breakfast feels a bit like an indulgence, but it's an investment in your health.

APPLE COMPOTE

MAKES 4 SERVINGS

$\frac{1}{2}$ cup organic unfiltered apple juice

$\frac{1}{2}$ lemon, peel on, cut in 2 wedges

1 teaspoon pumpkin pie spice

6 cardamom pods

4 large Granny Smith apples, peeled, cored, and cubed

POLENTA

MAKES 2 SERVINGS

$1\frac{1}{2}$ cups water

$\frac{1}{4}$ teaspoon sea salt

$\frac{1}{2}$ cup polenta

$\frac{1}{4}$ cup Raw Cashew Milk, optional (page 120)

To make the compote: In a 1-quart saucepan, combine the apple juice, lemon wedges (squeeze them first to release juice into the mixture), pumpkin pie spice, and cardamom and bring to a rolling boil.

Add the apples and return the heat to a simmer, stirring occasionally, for 10 to 15 minutes, or until the apples are tender and the liquid begins to thicken.

Remove the cardamom pods and lemon wedges from the apple mixture. Mash the apples with a potato masher to the desired consistency (partial mashed works best).

To make the polenta: While the apples are simmering, bring the water and salt to a boil. Add the polenta and reduce the heat. Cook on a low simmer for 5 minutes, stirring occasionally. Remove from the heat and cover until the apple compote is done.

Top 1 serving of polenta with ¾ cup apple compote. Drizzle the cashew milk on top (if desired).

Per serving: 230 calories, 1 g total fat (0 g saturated), 0 mg cholesterol, 2 mg sodium, 62 mg potassium, 55 g carbohydrates (17 g sugar), 7 g fiber, 3 g protein

TIP: Substitute pears or peaches for this compote if you like—choose whatever looks freshest and best at your grocery store.

LUNCH

Savory Mushroom Soup

This recipe should be called Make-Everything-Better Bisque, because that's what it does! The beta-glucans it contains lower cholesterol, improve immunity, and fight cancer—a delicious, savory soup that really embodies the concept of food as medicine.

MAKES 6 SERVINGS

$\frac{1}{4}$ cup extra-virgin olive oil

1 large yellow onion, chopped

8 ounces baby portobello mushrooms, sliced, stems on

8 ounces white mushrooms, sliced, stems on

4 ounces shiitake mushrooms, destemmed, sliced

$\frac{1}{4}$ cup tamari

1 tablespoon freshly squeezed lemon juice

2 teaspoons fresh thyme leaves + 2 teaspoons for garnish, optional

2 teaspoons paprika

$\frac{1}{2}$ teaspoon freshly ground black pepper

$\frac{1}{4}$ cup gluten-free flour (see recipe tip)

2 cups low-sodium vegetable broth, divided

3 cups unsweetened soy or almond milk

In a 2-quart saucepan, heat the oil on medium-high heat. Add the onion and sauté until translucent or almost caramelized.

Add the mushrooms, stirring to coat with oil, and cook for 2 to 3 minutes. Add 1 to 2 tablespoons of water as needed (adding 1 tablespoon at a time) if the onion and mushrooms are sticking to the pan.

Add the tamari, lemon juice, thyme, paprika, and black pepper and allow the mushrooms to cook down for 5 to 7 minutes.

Stir in the flour, quickly and evenly. As a paste forms, pour in 1 cup of the vegetable broth and allow the mixture to come to a simmer. Do not allow it to come to a boil, as the flour and oil will separate. Add a second cup of broth and return to a simmer.

Repeat the process with the soy or almond milk, adding 1 cup at a time and returning to a simmer—not a boil—each time.

When all the liquid is added, allow the soup to simmer for 10 to 15 minutes and remove from the heat. If desired, use a handheld immersion blender to blend some of the mushrooms to a puree consistency. Garnish with fresh thyme (if using).

Per serving: 270 calories, 20 g total fat (3 g saturated), 0 mg cholesterol, 800 mg sodium, 513 mg potassium, 20 g carbohydrates (7 g sugar), 3 g fiber, 5 g protein

TIP: Bob's Red Mill All Purpose Gluten Free Flour (bobsredmill.com) or Williams-Sonoma's Cup4Cup Gluten Free Flour (williams-sonoma.com) work best in this recipe. As for the vegetable broth, you can make your own or find good ready-made broth from Kitchen Basics, Imagine Soups, Pacific, Trader Joe's, and/or Whole Foods 365 brands.

DINNER

Rosemary Celeriac and Root Vegetables

You can't get more grounded in health than this sweet, roasted root-vegetable recipe. The health-protecting antioxidant carotenoids (sweet potatoes), flavonoids (celeriac and apple), allyl sulfides (garlic), rosemarinic acid (rosemary), and thymol (thyme) make this a tasty phytochemical feast.

MAKES 6 SERVINGS

1 medium celeriac bulb, chopped in 2" cubes

2 medium sweet potatoes, skin on, halved, quartered, and cut in thick wedges

2 parsnips, peeled and chopped in 2" cubes

2 large red apples, peels on, cored, and cut in thick wedges

4 garlic cloves, crushed

$\frac{1}{4}$ cup extra-virgin olive oil

1 tablespoon fresh rosemary leaves

1 tablespoon fresh thyme leaves

1 teaspoon sea salt

$\frac{1}{2}$ teaspoon freshly ground black pepper

Preheat the oven to 450°F.

In a large bowl, toss the celeriac, sweet potatoes, parsnips, apples, and garlic with the olive oil and coat thoroughly.

Grind the rosemary and thyme together with the salt and pepper in a mortar and pestle (or bowl), add to the vegetables and apples, and toss to coat thoroughly.

Transfer to a 13" x 9" baking pan lined with parchment paper to prevent sticking.

Roast for 35 to 40 minutes, or until fork-tender, stirring about halfway through.

Remove from the oven and serve alongside Southwestern Black-Bean Mash and a salad.

Per serving: 223 calories, 10 g total fat (1 g saturated), 0 mg cholesterol, 418 mg sodium, 475 mg potassium, 34 g carbohydrates (8 g sugar), 6 g fiber, 3 g protein

DINNER

Southwestern Black-Bean Mash

This is a humble little bean dish that does a lot: It squelches free radicals (vitamin C, zinc, manganese, antioxidants, and thiols), blasts fat (50 percent of your daily fiber!), fights cancer (carotenoids, quercetin, allicin), boosts brain power (folate, B_1, B_6), detoxifies (sulfur compounds, amino acids, and cilantro), and provides the same protein power as 2 ounces of fish or eggs. Tastes great, too.

MAKES 4 SERVINGS

4 cups black beans
2 tablespoons extra-virgin olive oil
$\frac{1}{2}$ medium onion, chopped
2 garlic cloves, chopped
1 jalapeño pepper, minced
1 large tomato, chopped

$\frac{1}{4}$ cup chopped fresh cilantro leaves, divided
$\frac{1}{4}$ cup freshly squeezed lime juice
$\frac{1}{4}$ cup water
$\frac{1}{4}$ teaspoon sea salt

Cook the black beans according to the directions on page 147 or use canned beans. Drain and rinse the beans, then drain again.

In a saucepan, heat the olive oil over medium-high heat. Sauté the onion and garlic, stirring frequently to avoid burning, for 2 minutes, or until translucent.

Add the jalapeño and tomato and sauté for 3 to 4 minutes, or until the water from the tomato cooks off and the tomato skins begin to soften.

Add the black beans, half of the cilantro, the lime juice, and the water. Bring the liquid to a boil, then reduce to a simmer. Cook for 6 to 8 minutes, or until the beans are heated through, stirring often. Remove from the heat. Transfer to a food processor and pulse until smooth.

Garnish each serving with $\frac{1}{4}$ of the remaining cilantro leaves.

Per serving: 308 calories, 8 g total fat (1 g saturated), 125 mg cholesterol, 7 mg sodium, 770 mg potassium, 46 g carbohydrates (0 g sugar), 16 g fiber, 16 g protein

TIP: **Wear plastic gloves when handling the jalepeño pepper.** Puree it up to make a dip for fresh veggies or gluten-free crackers. Feel free to amp up the spice—add more jalapeño or a dash of cayenne pepper.

Day 6 Mind-Body Detox

DO A RANDOM ACT OF KINDNESS

I've already talked about the power of connection—it keeps us from wallowing in the toxic emotions of loneliness, despair, anger, and depression. But connection doesn't necessarily always have to be deep to be effective. In fact, you can connect in a meaningful way with people you don't even know!

Today try practicing a random act of kindness (or RAOK, as the Web would have it). Opportunities are everywhere, and they cost very little in terms of time or money. Helping an elderly lady across the street is a classic example. Here are some others: Open the door for someone else. Let a harried mother cut in line at the grocery store. Spring for a cup of coffee for the guy behind you at Starbucks (you're there for a green tea, right?). Give a quarter to that kindly-looking panhandler you usually pass by. Slip an encouraging note to a stressed-out co-worker. Pick up some trash on the street. Allow others to merge in front of you on the interstate (or in line for the train). Pay a compliment to a total stranger.

Of course, you can go big and do more formal volunteer work, too. I fully encourage that as a way to create ongoing relationships and do real service within your community. But these little RAOKs remind you that you are connected to *everyone* you meet—and that you have an opportunity to serve literally hundreds of times every day. You don't have to make a special occasion out of it. When you take the time and effort to put forth positive energy, I believe you will be repaid manifold . . . maybe not literally, but certainly in terms of personal well-being. After all, with every little random act of kindness you do, you remind yourself that you are a compassionate, loving, and connected human being. And certainly a slightly less toxic one.

Get a Jump on Day 7

Prepare the Carrot-Rhubarb Soup (page 173); store it in a glass bowl or stainless steel pot in the refrigerator. Reheat before serving.

Day 7 Menu

BEVERAGE: Detox Tea (Dandelion, Chicory, or Burdock Root)

BREAKFAST: Savory Green Tea-Buckwheat Cereal

MIDMORNING SNACK: Nut Milk from 3-Day Turbo Cleanse, Your Choice

LUNCH: Carrot-Rhubarb Soup

MIDAFTERNOON SNACK: Your Choice (see page 139)

DINNER: Three-Bean Kale Sauté with Brown Rice and Salad

BREAKFAST

Savory Green Tea–Buckwheat Cereal

Buckwheat is a wheat- and gluten-free grain (there is no "wheat" in it at all). The matcha green tea powder not only packs a savory punch and cancer-fighting and cholesterol-lowering green tea polyphenols, it also provides approximately 2,600 free-radical-scavenging antioxidant units per teaspoon. There's a reason they call it gunpowder tea—it starts your day with a nutritional bang! So much so that if you know you're supersensitive to caffeine, you may want to scale back the matcha powder a bit . . . or even eliminate it.

MAKES 2 SERVINGS

1 teaspoon matcha green tea powder

$\frac{1}{4}$ teaspoon sea salt

$2\frac{1}{4}$ cups unsweetened soy or nut milk

$\frac{3}{4}$ cup cream of buckwheat cereal

In a 1-quart saucepan, whisk the tea powder and salt into the soy or nut milk and bring to a boil.

Add the cream of buckwheat cereal, turn the heat down, cover, and simmer on low for 10 minutes.

Remove from the heat and serve immediately.

Per serving: 222 calories, 3 g total fat (0 g saturated), 0 mg cholesterol, 493 mg sodium, 213 mg potassium, 47 g carbohydrates (0 g sugar), 3 g fiber, 10 g protein

TIP: Try Bob's Red Mill Organic Creamy Buckwheat (bobsredmill.com) or Pocono Cream of Buckwheat (poconofoods.com). Republic of Tea (republicoftea.com) sells organic matcha green tea powder. Ito En is another good source for matcha and other green tea supplies—though they're not necessarily organic (itoen.com).

LUNCH

Carrot-Rhubarb Soup

Chicken soup may be for the soul, but this soup's allyl sulfides (shallots), gingerol (ginger), curcumin (turmeric), bioactive lipids (cumin), and limonene (orange zest) blast its detox and anti-inflammatory power to the heavens.

MAKES 6 SERVINGS

2 tablespoons extra-virgin olive oil

4 shallots, minced

1 tablespoon grated fresh ginger

2 pounds carrots, peeled and cut in 1" pieces

6 green cardamom pods, lightly crushed

1 quart low-sodium vegetable broth

1 pound rhubarb stems, cut in 1" pieces

1 orange, juice and pulp

2 cups unsweetened coconut milk

2 teaspoons orange zest

1 teaspoon ground black cumin

1 teaspoon turmeric

6 teaspoons chopped fresh chives or 3 teaspoons honey, optional

In a 2-quart saucepan, heat the olive oil over medium heat. Sauté the shallots for about 3 minutes, or until soft and translucent.

Add the ginger and sauté for 1 minute.

Add the carrots, cardamom, and broth and cook for 15 minutes, until fork-tender.

Add the rhubarb, orange juice, and orange pulp, cover, and cook for an additional 15 minutes, or until the rhubarb is soft.

Remove and discard the cardamom pods and transfer the soup to a food processor or blender. Puree the soup until smooth.

Add the coconut milk, orange zest, cumin, and turmeric and process/blend briefly.

Serve topped with 1 teaspoon of chives or drizzled with ½ teaspoon of honey (if using).

Per serving: 160 calories, 7 g total fat (2 g saturated), 0 mg cholesterol, 198 mg sodium, 723 mg potassium, 24 g carbohydrates (11 g sugar), 7 g fiber, 3 g protein

TIP: Try the unsweetened coconut milk made by So Delicious (find a store at sodeliciousdairyfree.com). Substitute frozen rhubarb if necessary; just defrost first and add a little more broth or milk.

DINNER

Three-Bean Kale Sauté with Brown Rice

When you eat this you should be wearing a big cape with an S on it because you're getting super detoxifying and cancer-fighting action in one super delicious and nutritious dish. It has a whopping 191 percent of your daily vitamin A requirement, 123 percent of your daily vitamin C, 60 percent of your daily fiber, 29 percent of your daily iron, and 16 percent of your daily calcium.

MAKES 4 SERVINGS

1 cup black beans

1 cup red kidney beans

1 cup white beans

4 tablespoons extra-virgin olive oil, divided

¼ teaspoon sea salt

¼ teaspoon black pepper

1 teaspoon crushed red-pepper flakes

4 garlic cloves, smashed

½ cup low-sodium vegetable broth

1 pound kale, stems and leaves coarsely chopped

2 tablespoons red wine vinegar

4 cups cooked brown rice, prepared according to directions

Cook the beans according to the directions on page 147 or use canned beans. Drain and rinse the beans, then drain again.

In a mixing bowl, combine the beans with 2 tablespoons of the oil, the salt, pepper, and red-pepper flakes and toss thoroughly.

In a large sauté pan, heat the remaining 2 tablespoons oil over medium-high heat. Add the garlic and cook until soft but not browned.

Turn the heat up to high, add the broth and kale, and stir to combine. Cover and cook for 3 to 4 minutes.

Add the beans, stir, and cook covered for an additional 3 to 4 minutes, or until the liquid is evaporated.

Day 7 Mind-Body Detox

WALK ON THE DARK SIDE

Though it's not "officially" accounted for in the plan, I encourage you to indulge your sweet tooth by having a piece of dark chocolate. Chocolate's scientific name is *Theobroma coca*, which literally means "food of the gods." That's not just because of the flavor, though many would argue that it is divine—dark chocolate contains plenty of powerful antioxidant polyphenols (more than blueberries, blackberries, artichokes, or cherries) and the mood-boosting chemical phenylethanolamine. Recent studies have demonstrated that the stuff can also lower blood pressure and bad cholesterol and reduce the risk of developing cardiovascular disease. It may even offset age-related cognitive decline. It really is a health food!

You'll need to read labels. Most commercial bars labeled milk chocolate contain only about 10 percent cocoa, and those labeled dark only about 20 percent. To reap the benefits without the baggage (the excessive calories that come with added sugars), choose a dark bar that is at least 70 percent cocoa. Most studies were done on chocolate that contained at least 80 percent cocoa, so if you're going for real health benefits, err on the dark side. If you can find a bar in the 75 to 85 percent cocoa range—and tolerate it, for it may be a bit more bitter than what you are used to—this is optimal. My favorite brands are Green and Black, Theo Chocolates, Newman's Organic, and Endangered Species.

Take your time with your chocolate—don't eat the whole bar, just eat a square or two, and eat it slowly. Enjoy it. And remember: It's your own little taste of heaven.

Remove from the heat, toss with the vinegar, top each serving with ½ cup brown rice, and serve immediately, accompanied by a salad.

Per serving: 454 calories, 16 g total fat (3 g saturated), 0 mg cholesterol, 316 mg sodium, 714 mg potassium, 65 g carbohydrates (0 g sugar), 15 g fiber, 17 g protein

TIP: This dish is great served warm or cold. After the 7-Day In-Depth Detox is over, you can make this dish again and serve it warm and topped with a poached egg for a protein-packed power breakfast. It also pairs well with wild salmon.

Check In with Yourself

Congratulations—you've finished the **7-Day In-Depth Detox**. Now it's time to check in with yourself and see how you're feeling. We'll follow the same process we used just after the 3-Day Turbo Cleanse.

First, flip back to Chapter 2 and retake both the Medical Symptom Questionnaire (page 35) and the Environmental Factors Questionnaire (page 42). You should see even more improvement on both scales, as you have taken another big step toward a less toxic lifestyle.

Second, get out your journal. Review what you wrote when you started this plan (see page 91) and what you wrote down just 4 days ago. See what was making you feel bad then . . . and what was making you feel good. See how you felt about your successes and your frustrations.

Then make a new inventory. How are you feeling now? What's your energy level? Do you see subjective changes in your mood? In the way you look or feel or think? How has doing the 7-Day In-Depth Detox changed your perspective? What did you learn in the process? Write down any mental or emotional challenges or frustrations you encountered during the last 4 days. Record all your triumphs and your struggles. Write down whether you accomplished what you set out to do—and how you felt about it. Make a record of everything.

When you're done, take a good last look. Add your own thoughts to the results of the Medical Symptom Questionnaire and the Environmental Factors Questionnaire. Then close your eyes and assess your situation. Do you need and want to go even deeper?

If so, get ready to start the 21-Day Clean and Lean Diet. . . .

Get a Jump on Day 8

The Red Pepper–Cashew spread (page 192) you'll be eating on Day 8 is easy to make ahead and stores well. In fact, you might want to double the recipe and keep some extra on hand for easy snacks—spread it on vegetable slices or gluten-free crackers. Need more nut milk? Make a batch tonight.

the 21-day clean and lean diet

Days 8 to 21—Going the distance to cleanse your mind and body, gain great new eating habits, and lose weight in a sustainable way

Ah, day 8—it's an exciting time. You've completed the 3-Day Turbo Cleanse, the 7-Day In-Depth Detox . . . you're feeling fantastic. Now you're ready to make the transition back to "real life." You might be daydreaming about juicy cheeseburgers and fries (if that was what you were into before you started the Detox Prescription)—but this is a bad plan. Worse now, even, than it was before. Why wreck your cleaned-up body and newly optimized digestion by returning to bad habits? "Retox" might sound like a lot of fun, but trust me—it will feel absolutely horrible.

Instead of relapsing (or "re" anything), now is your chance to embrace a way of living and eating that is detoxifying, health-optimizing, and sustainable. For the next 14 days, we'll guide you through our 21-Day Clean and Lean Diet, which provides an intelligent transition from the total phytochemical immersion of the 3 days of drinking juices and nut milks to "real life."

Here, we slowly return to what was likely your pre-detox normal: More grains make it onto the menu now, as well as soy, eggs, some dairy, and some fish. The menu was carefully created to do a few smart things. The 21-Day Clean and Lean Diet is:

BOTANICALLY DIVERSE: Part of what makes this plan uniquely healing is its sheer variety. Buckwheat, parsnips, endive, black rice, mustard greens, and chia seeds may not be in your usual repertoire, but they are incredibly healthy and delicious foods. Here, Mary Beth has used them in recipes that are both delicious and accessible. By the end of these 2 weeks, you will have made many new food friends. I realize you may not continue to cook this way forever—the reality is that we all gravitate to 5 or 10 favorite dishes that we make over and over again. But hopefully you will realize that you can rely on the familiar while still making room for what is fresh and best—cycling new greens, grains, berries, mushrooms, squashes, and seasonal fruits onto the menu. This will give you maximum botanical diversity, resulting in the widest exposure to beneficial nutrients, a limited repetition of naturally occurring toxins, and ultimately, a lowering of all-cause mortality.

COLORFUL: We talked in Chapter 3 about the benefits of the rainbow diet . . . the colors themselves are what contain the powerful chemical constituents of the foods. Antioxidant flavonoids and anthocyanins are what make foods red, blue, and purple. Eye-protective lutein and zeaxanthin are found in green and yellow foods. Vitamin A–rich carotenoids color yellow and orange fruits and veggies. Liver-protective, cancer-fighting isothioncyanates power green cruciferous foods. And white foods like garlic and onion contain the tumor-fighting compound allicin and detoxifying sulfur compounds. Every day is designed to put a rainbow on your plate—not just for the aesthetic appeal (though honestly, that is mighty) but for the incredible healing power of it.

WHEAT AND GLUTEN FREE: You'll get grains once or twice daily now, but you won't get wheat. That's because I truly believe that what passes for wheat these days is more likely to cause more harm than good for too many people. (See page 83 for more information.) Instead, you'll expand your palate—without compromising your health—by focusing on good grains such as those mentioned above, plus protein-rich quinoa, flavorful black and wild rice, luxurious polenta, and more. In my experience, wheat is problematic for about 50 percent of the patient population. So for the next 2 weeks, keep all wheat off the menu and see how you feel. When and if you decide to reintroduce it after the 21-Day Clean and Lean Diet, watch carefully—your body will tell you if it is a problem for you.

GLOBALLY INFLUENCED: When asked to pick the "world's healthiest cuisine," I find it impossible to pick just one. Japanese, Indian, and Mediterranean diets all have a lot going for them, frankly. So we've allowed them all to impact our plan. We use a liberal amount of anti-inflammatory spices—such as turmeric, cinnamon, cayenne pepper, cardamom, and cumin—just as any good Indian chef would do. In our cooking, we stick to extra-virgin olive oil, as they do in the Mediterranean, and cleave to herbs, greens, beans, and grains. And as in Japan, we keep meals small, frequent, and focused on plants—with only an occasional serving of soy and seafood. Overall, it's a sensational, sensible mix of world fusion flavors.

GEARED TOWARD WEIGHT LOSS: There's no doubt that the 21-Day Clean and Lean Diet can help you lose weight, for three reasons. First, it clears your body of toxins like PCBs, which have been linked to weight gain in recent studies. Second, because it is rich in whole foods, the diet provides lots of greens and natural fiber selected specifically to promote the health of the gut by supporting the immune system and positively impacting the natural balance of intestinal flora. Eating this way, you'll naturally develop more good bacteria—aka probiotics—which have been associated with weight loss. And third, this plan is by nature low in calories—somewhere in the neighborhood of 1,200 to 1,500 a day in the basic plan, which includes three meals, a salad with dressing, two snacks, and one juice or nut milk. Chances are this is significantly less than what you were taking in before you started down the detox path! (The USDA estimates that the average American eats about 2,700 calories a day.) Most of us will lose weight eating in this range of calories, and lose it the way that is by far the most healthful—slowly and steadily. Calorie counts are provided for everything, however, so that you can customize your own experience and dial the weight loss up or down. If you feel you can afford a few more calories and don't care so much about weight loss, add an extra snack and/or nut milk or juice every day, or maybe one of our optional desserts. This plan is easily managed in a way that works for weight maintenance. And though it will take some doing, it can even work for weight gain—just adjust proteins, nut milks, and healthy fats when making your snack choices.

HIGH CONSCIOUSNESS, LOW IMPACT: Eggs and fish are included on this menu. We urge you to shop consciously for the foods that will be best for your body—and, coincidentally, for the planet.

With eggs, it's pretty simple: Always buy organic and cage free. Eggs get a bad rap: They do have cholesterol in the yolks, but studies refute a relationship to heart disease. They also contain choline for brain, mood, and methylation; biotin for hair, skin, and nails; iron; carotenoids lutein and zeaxanthin for eyesight; and vitamin D in the yolk—one of the few food sources of it.

Fish can be a terrific source of lean protein and vital omega-3 fatty acids, but sourcing can be complex. It's worth doing a little research to find out where your fishmonger got today's catch. Conditions and recommendations regarding seafood are volatile, to say the least—but it's worthwhile to check in with your purveyor in person. One rule of thumb: Smaller is safer when it comes to toxic load, because toxins such as mercury accumulate in the flesh and are concentrated up the food chain. We have included three fish recipes in the 3 weeks of the plan and encourage you to read more about the healthiest (and most sustainable) fish in the box on the opposite page.

VERSATILE: Within the basic principles of the plan—that the food be whole, natural, colorful, organic, and diverse—you can mix it up in the way that pleases and suits you best. Yes, it's called the Detox Prescription. Yes, we're dosing it out to you, three meals a day. Just follow the menu plan, prepare the recipes as they are presented, and you have an incredible healthy, detox-optimized, and coincidentally delicious way of living and eating that will last a lifetime. But the truth is, you don't *have* to follow the plan to the letter. There may be ingredients or recipes you are allergic to or you just don't like. (I'm very sensitive to both shrimp and peanuts—though both healthy foods are represented in this plan.) There may be recipes you don't have time for or interest in. That's perfectly fine. Read through these pages, and find something else that *does* work for you. You can have breakfast for lunch, or lunch for dinner. You can repeat a favorite dish anytime. You can double up batches to make two dinners, lunches, or breakfasts at a time (our soup, pâté, and grain dishes work well for making multiple meals).

For your midmorning snack, you are now free to choose among your favorite juices, smoothies, and nut milks from the 3-Day Turbo Cleanse. If

Fishing Around

The Detox Prescription includes a limited amount of fish—and we encourage you to experiment. Haven't tried Arctic char before? Now is the time. Fish is by far the healthiest of animal products—containing lean protein, minimal or no saturated fats, and healthy omega-3 fats, among many other nutrients.

It's always best to buy what is fresh, clean, and of highest quality—and the best way to find out about that is to talk to the fish vendor directly. Find a good seafood shop, or a grocery store that takes fish seriously and offers an extensive selection, and talk to the guys or gals behind the counter. You will probably find that they love their work, often passionately, and welcome the opportunity to help educate a newbie. They can offer shopping and sustainability tips and can often tell you how to best cook a fish (or offer their strong opinions).

As with everything else, diversity is always good, not only because it helps broaden the nutritional profile, but because it also reduces the chances of overexposure to toxins—unfortunately a reality in a world like ours, with increasingly polluted oceans, lakes, and rivers. Mercury, arsenic, and PCBs are particular concerns—especially for pregnant women. It is not possible to lay down hard-and-fast rules, such as always go with wild caught and avoid farmed, or vice versa. One dictum I do use is: Any fish that swims in the ocean that you can cook head-to-tail in a pan is generally healthy and relatively safe—toxins travel upstream with predatory fish (bigger ones have a larger amount). But of course, things aren't that simple. And though I'd like to hand you a fixed list of what's safe and what's not, that list is changing so frequently and so fast, it's impossible to do.

What I can tell you is that you can keep up with the latest on the seafood shopping guides available from the Environmental Defense Fund (edf.org) and Monterey Bay Aquarium (montereybayaquarium.org). These are the resources I use and trust, and recommend to my patients and to you. It is worth doing the research to keep yourself and your family safe and healthy.

Salmon is almost always a good pick, and a good choice for a protein (and healthy fat) addition to any meal. Canned or smoked can be healthy choices, too, especially if you buy from a company that offers sustainable, wild (usually Pacific) salmon in BPA-free packaging. Good brands include Vital Choice (vitalchoice.com), Rain Coast Trading (raincoasttrading.com), Wild Planet (wildplanet.com), 365 (Whole Foods), and Trader Joe's.

you choose to go with juices or smoothies and need to carry them with you to work, take a little extra care to keep them sealed and cool so that the natural plant enzymes don't degrade. Better yet, do what I do and carry the raw ingredients in a NutriBullet container and blend at work! (I know this isn't possible for everyone, but it's great if you can swing it.) Of course, you can go out for a raw juice or smoothie, too—just make sure you're getting it from a source that's using real fruits and vegetables (not sweetened concentrates or artificial colors or flavors, and preferably organic, especially within the "Dirty Dozen"). No fast-food frappés!

For your midafternoon snack, it's back to the snack list (see page 139), only now you can feel free to introduce dairy if you like—choose fat-free Greek yogurt or low-fat goat cheese. But be conscious about it, paying close attention to quality as well as quantity. Get organic dairy only, and be certain that it does not contain recombinant bovine growth hormone. Personally, I love organic goat cheese—I eat it with crackers, with soup, and with fresh veggies—or even with a spoon. Both of these options are very filling, high-protein, low-fat foods. Be aware that (especially cow-based) dairy is a bit harder to digest—which is why we didn't eat it during the first 7 days of the Detox Prescription—and that some people are allergic or sensitive to it. Pay close attention to how you feel when you add it back into the diet.

Remember that you should consider your activity level when choosing snacks to make sure that your protein needs are met. The daily RDA for protein for an average-size woman is 46 grams and 56 grams for men, but you may need more if you are especially active—and during this part of the Detox Prescription, you really should start exercising vigorously and aiming to break a sweat five or more times a week (see page 202). One way to usefully and easily calculate your protein needs is to multiply your body weight by 0.4. So a 200-pound guy would need around 80 grams of protein; a 120-pound woman would need 48 grams. Here, the basic meal plan averages about 50 to 60 grams a day—you can easily move that number into your range by choosing protein-rich snacks and nut milks.

Now that you're in it for a longer haul, you can also have an occasional dessert. Let me be clear once again: I don't like sugar—it's probably what's behind much of the American heart disease and diabetes epidemics and can be toxic for many. But I understand that some people have a sweet tooth or like a reward from time to time for taking good care of themselves. For the sake of your health, if you are going to eat dessert, have it in moderation—and only have the really good stuff: We give you a few examples here.

Moderation, when it comes to dessert, means once or twice a week. If you can, make it fruit only and enjoy its natural inherent sweetness. In "Just Desserts" (page 186) we offer two incredible recipes that add flavor complexity to apples and peaches without adding sugar so you can reward your taste buds without setting yourself up for the dysfunctional cycle of sugar craving. Two more recipes are indulgent and minimally sweetened confections—for occasional use only! Rawsome Chocolate Truffles are full of fiber, nuts, and antioxidant-rich cacao. And Moo-Less Avocado-Chocolate Mousse boasts an incredible dose of healthy fats and phytonutrients that almost balances out the sugar load. You can also add in a "breakfast" yogurt (preferably coconut or soy) parfait or goat cheese with fruit for an after-dinner treat.

As you reintroduce some foods that were off the menu for a while—like soy, eggs, and dairy—you'll have an opportunity to notice how your body reacts to them and watch for any potential food allergy. The Detox Prescription was not designed as an official elimination diet—in which you would bring back foods one at a time in a more deliberate way. But nevertheless, when you reintroduce each food, observe how you feel from head to toe.

For 24 hours after you eat, say, dairy or soy, watch for changes in your mood or energy level. See whether you develop postnasal drip, headaches, or shortness of breath. Do you have stomach pain or bloating, constipation or diarrhea, or notice bits of undigested food or oil in your stool? Do your joints or muscles ache? All of these signs and symptoms can be caused by food reactions (allergies or sensitivities; see Chapter 8). If you suspect a link, edit the food back out of your diet and see if the symptoms subside. If they do, you have your answer and can plan your meals accordingly.

Every little piece of information you get about how food makes you feel contributes to a better life. When you are able to tap into your body's true responses, you'll no longer be fooled by the surface-level sensations peddled by the food-industrial complex. When you eat with awareness and mindfulness, you'll begin to understand and feel that those cheeseburgers and fries you were fantasizing about are toxic to your system—they are dragging you down in the most literal sense. And in the near future you may even find yourself daydreaming about kale smoothies and quinoa instead.

21-DAY CLEAN AND LEAN DIET MENU, WEEK 2

	Day 8	Day 9	Day 10
Beverage	Detox Tea (Dandelion, Chicory, or Burdock Root)	Detox Tea (Dandelion, Chicory, or Burdock Root)	Detox Tea (Dandelion, Chicory, or Burdock Root)
Breakfast	Kick-Butt Coconut Oatmeal	Parsnip and Pear Puree	Vanilla Quinoa with Raspberry Compote
Midmorning Snack	Smoothie, Juice, or Nut Milk from 3-Day Menu	Smoothie, Juice, or Nut Milk from 3-Day Menu	Smoothie, Juice, or Nut Milk from 3-Day Menu
Lunch	Red Pepper–Cashew Endive with Grape Salad	Hummus and Veggie Rainbow Tortilla	Stuffed Black Bean–Cabbage Rolls
Midafternoon Snack	Snack from "Grab and Go Snacks" (page 139)	Snack from "Grab and Go Snacks" (page 139)	Snack from "Grab and Go Snacks" (page 139)
Dinner	Curried Lentils with Sweet Potato and Chard and Salad	Wild Arctic Char and Roasted Radicchio and Salad	Rosemary Portobello Mushrooms with Tahini Green Beans and Salad

Day 11	Day 12	Day 13	Day 14
Detox Tea (Dandelion, Chicory, or Burdock Root)	Detox Tea (Dandelion, Chicory, or Burdock Root)	Detox Tea (Dandelion, Chicory, or Burdock Root)	Detox Tea (Dandelion, Chicory, or Burdock Root)
Zucchini and Sweet Potato Frittata	Polenta with Apple Compote and Vanilla Cashew Cream	Baked Acorn Squash with Apples and Walnuts	Buckwheat-Banana-Walnut-Cereal
Smoothie, Juice, or Nut Milk from 3-Day Menu	Smoothie, Juice, or Nut Milk from 3-Day Menu	Smoothie, Juice, or Nut Milk from 3-Day Menu	Smoothie, Juice, or Nut Milk from 3-Day Menu
Chickpea and Arugula–Stuffed Avocado	Roasted Root Vegetables and Salad	"Creamy" Garlic Soup with Spinach	"Creamy" Avocado- Broccoli Soup
Snack from "Grab and Go Snacks" (page 139)	Snack from "Grab and Go Snacks" (page 139)	Snack from "Grab and Go Snacks" (page 139)	Snack from "Grab and Go Snacks" (page 139)
Peanut Satay Tofu Stir-Fry with Broccoli and Salad	Spicy White Bean and Spinach Soup and Salad	Caramelized Sea Scallops with Bok Choy and Salad	Black Bean and Spinach Tortilla and Salad

Just Desserts

Dessert is not my favorite course . . . at least from a health perspective. That's because sugary foods cause inflammation, which we now know is the culprit behind so many diseases—not just the obvious diabetes, but also heart disease (yes, cholesterol's a problem, but it's inflammation of the arterial walls that sets it loose to cause heart attacks). And they all too often set up swings of sugar and insulin and brain chemistry changes that make people continually want more.

In many ways, dessert is toxic to the body—certainly, that's true for me. I don't have much of a sweet tooth, but the last time I really indulged in dessert, a thick slice of chocolate cake on my wife's birthday, I was comatose on the floor for about 45 minutes afterward. It literally knocked me down. When you eat sugar all the time, your insulin receptors become desensitized to it, and you don't feel the crash-and-burn as acutely. But when you get off sugar and stay off for a while, you'll be able to feel how negatively it's affecting you, as I did. Then you'll see why it's worth avoiding the stuff!

All that said, if you find yourself needing a sweet fix, first consider keeping it simple with a luscious piece of organic fresh fruit—really, there is nothing more magnificent on heaven or Earth than a peak-season peach or a truly ripe fig. Barring that, choose a dessert that that is rich in phytonutrients, anti-inflammatory spices, fiber, and essential fatty acids, as all four of these simple recipes are. These aren't included in the daily menu, as they are meant to be only occasional indulgence. I consider each one a net gain for personal health in terms of nutrition, but they are also additional calories and sugar grams. Whether you have them or not is a personal decision—if and when you do, I encourage you to go slowly and savor every bite. (If you need tips on how to eat mindfully, see our advice on page 155.)

RAWSOME CHOCOLATE TRUFFLES

These are a natural, raw, awesome dessert—hence the name. As a bonus, nuts have cholesterol-lowering properties, cacao has blood-pressure-lowering flavonoids, and the dates contain antioxidants, carotenoids, and phenolics.

MAKES 12 TO 16 TRUFFLES

2 tablespoons raw pumpkin seeds, coarsely chopped

2 tablespoons unsweetened coconut flakes

$\frac{1}{4}$ teaspoon coarse sea salt

1 cup walnuts

$\frac{1}{2}$ cup raw cacao powder or $\frac{3}{4}$ cup unsweetened cocoa powder

1 cup dates, pitted

2 tablespoons coconut oil, melted

2 teaspoons maple syrup

In a small mixing bowl, combine the pumpkin seeds, coconut flakes, and sea salt. Set aside.

In a food processor, process the nuts to a crumb or "meal" consistency. Add the cacao or cocoa powder, dates, coconut oil, and maple syrup and process until the mixture resembles a smooth, wet cookie dough.

Dampen your hands slightly, scoop out dough, and roll into truffle-size balls (resisting the urge to lick your fingers). Roll the balls in the pumpkin seed mixture. Place on parchment paper, on a plate, or in mini-muffin liners and refrigerate or freeze for 30 minutes (if you can wait that long).

Per serving: 125 calories, 8 g total fat (3 g saturated), 0 mg cholesterol, 47 mg sodium, 131 mg potassium, 13 g carbohydrates (9 g sugar), 2 g fiber, 2 g protein

TIP: Find organic cacao powder at Navitas Naturals (navitasnaturals.com) or Essential Living Foods (essentiallivingfoods.com). You can refrigerate truffles for up to a week or freeze them for up to a month.

JUST PEACHY

This simple, succulent dessert is ready in a flash and is just peachy, with vitamins A and C, free-radical-quenching antioxidants, carotenoids, cancer-fighting and detoxifying quercetin, and limonene.

MAKES 4 SERVINGS

1 tablespoon extra-virgin olive oil

4 peaches, skin on, halved and pitted

4 teaspoons lime juice

1 teaspoon ground cinnamon, nutmeg, or cumin

1 cup plain coconut or Greek yogurt, optional

Preheat the oven broiler.

Lightly brush a 13" x 9" baking dish with the oil.

Place the peaches in the baking dish, cut half facing up. Drizzle the peaches with the lime juice and spices.

Broil 4" to 5" from the heat, or until the peaches are golden brown and fork-tender. Remove from the heat and serve warm. Serve alone or topped with yogurt (if using).

Per serving: 70 calories, 0 g total fat, 0 mg cholesterol, 0 mg sodium, 322 mg potassium, 18 g carbohydrates (15 g sugar), 3 g fiber, 1 g protein

TIP: Freeze plain coconut or Greek yogurt before preparing this recipe for a creamy peach à la mode!

(continued)

Just Desserts—*Continued*

NUTTY BAKED APPLES

We call these Nutty Baked Apples because everyone goes nuts for them. With detoxifying, heavy-metal-binding apple pectin, antiwrinkle alpha hydroxy malic acid, 4 grams of fiber (rare in a dessert!), good fats, and phytonutrients, it's okay to go nutty. Eat with or without the yogurt.

MAKES 4 SERVINGS

4 small apples

8 tablespoons chopped walnuts or pecans

2 Medjool dates or dried figs, finely chopped

1 teaspoon orange zest

1 teaspoon ground cinnamon or pumpkin pie spice

$\frac{1}{2}$ teaspoon ground ginger

4 teaspoons extra-virgin olive oil, coconut oil, or Earth Balance dairy- and soy-free spread

$\frac{1}{4}$–$\frac{1}{2}$ cup water

1 cup plain coconut or Greek yogurt, optional

Preheat the oven to 375°F and brush an 8" x 8" baking dish with oil.

With a paring knife or apple corer, core the apples to just above the bottom of the apple, leaving a small amount of apple core on the bottom. Slice a small slice off the bottom of the apple if needed to allow it to sit flat in the baking dish.

In a small mixing bowl, combine the nuts, dates or figs, orange zest, cinnamon or pumpkin pie spice, ginger, and oil or spread.

Place the apples in the baking dish and stuff with the nut and fruit mixture.

Add $\frac{1}{4}$ cup water to the bottom of the baking dish. Bake for 30 to 40 minutes, checking after 20 minutes and adding $\frac{1}{4}$ cup water to the dish as needed. Remove from the oven when the apples are fork-tender but not mushy. Serve alone or topped with plain coconut or Greek yogurt (if using).

Per serving: 172 calories, 10 g total fat (2 g saturated), 0 mg cholesterol, 1 mg sodium, 200 mg potassium, 21 g carbohydrates (14 g sugar), 4 g fiber, 2 g protein

TIP: Freeze plain coconut or Greek yogurt before preparing this recipe to eat it à la mode!

MOO-LESS AVOCADO-CHOCOLATE MOUSSE

This dairy-free chocolate mousse will fool even your foodie friends! They won't believe that this gourmet vegan delight lowers cholesterol, fights belly fat, and delivers a whopping 9 grams of fiber per serving. (As an added bonus, the orange peel supports detox, too.)

MAKES 3 SERVINGS

2 ripe large avocados, pitted and scooped

$\frac{1}{3}$ cup honey

$\frac{1}{3}$ cup unsweetened cocoa powder

2 teaspoons vanilla extract

4 teaspoons orange zest, divided

$\frac{2}{3}$–1 cup coconut milk

OPTIONAL TOPPINGS

$\frac{1}{2}$ cup sliced strawberries, raspberries, or blueberries

$\frac{1}{4}$ cup organic unsweetened toasted coconut flakes or chopped nuts

In a food processor, blend the avocado for about 30 seconds, or until smooth.

Add the honey, cocoa powder, vanilla extract, and 1 teaspoon of the orange zest (reserve the remainder of the zest) and process until mixed through. With a rubber spatula, scrape down the sides of the food processor as needed.

Add $\frac{2}{3}$ cup coconut milk (reserve the remainder) and process until smooth, scraping down the sides of the food processor as needed. If the mousse is too thick, add the remainder of the coconut milk to desired consistency (the mousse will continue to thicken when chilled).

Spoon into 3 small ramekins, top each serving with 1 teaspoon of orange zest, and chill in the refrigerator for 2 hours, or in the freezer for half an hour. Serve alone or with toppings (if using).

Per serving: 267 calories, 15 g total fat (3 g saturated, 2 g polyunsaturated, 9 g monounsaturated), 0 mg cholesterol, 15 mg sodium, 575 mg potassium, 36 g carbohydrates (25 g sugar), 9 g fiber, 3 g protein

TIP: Look for Trader Joe's, So Delicious, and Bliss brands of dairy-free coconut milk. To make a chocolate-mint variation that would make a Girl Scout weep, substitute organic peppermint extract for vanilla and leave out the orange. You can substitute agave syrup or raw coconut nectar for the honey, if desired.

Day 8 Menu

BEVERAGE: Detox Tea (Dandelion, Chicory, or Burdock Root)

BREAKFAST: Kick-Butt Coconut Oatmeal

MIDMORNING SNACK: Smoothie, Juice, or Nut Milk

LUNCH: Red Pepper-Cashew Endive with Grape Salad

MIDAFTERNOON SNACK: Your Choice (see page 139)

DINNER: Curried Lentils with Sweet Potato and Chard and Salad

BREAKFAST

Kick-Butt Coconut Oatmeal

This powerhouse oatmeal starts your day with 50 percent of your daily requirement for vitamin B$_{12}$, 30 percent of your vitamin D, 20 percent of your iron, and 12 percent of your calcium. It's rounded out with the protein equivalent of an egg and about 20 percent of your daily fiber—all with a coconut-vanilla creamy goodness.

MAKES 2 SERVINGS

2 cups coconut milk (see tip below)
$\frac{1}{2}$ vanilla bean, split, seeds scraped and reserved, or 1 teaspoon vanilla extract
$\frac{1}{2}$ teaspoon pumpkin pie spice
1 cup gluten-free rolled oats
Honey, optional
Toasted unsweetened coconut flakes, optional

In a 1-quart saucepan, bring the coconut milk, scraped vanilla seeds or extract, and pumpkin pie spice to a boil.

Add the oats, reduce the heat, and cook uncovered for 15 to 20 minutes, to desired consistency.

Remove from the heat, drizzle the top with honey (if using), and top with the toasted coconut flakes (if using).

Per serving: 241 calories, 9 g total fat (6 g saturated), 0 mg cholesterol, 15 mg sodium, 5 mg potassium, 33 g carbohydrates (1 g sugar), 5 g fiber, 7 g protein

TIP: Try Trader Joe's light coconut milk for a creamy consistency or So Delicious coconut milk for a thinner and lighter taste. If you don't like coconut, omit the coconut flakes and coconut milk and substitute rice, nut, or soy milk instead for Kick-Butt Oatmeal. For a nutty variation with a higher protein content, add 2 tablespoons almond butter, substitute almond milk for coconut milk and omit the coconut flakes, and top with toasted sliced almonds.

LUNCH

Red Pepper–Cashew Endive with Grape Salad

This punchy, proteinaceous spread is packed with carotenoids, flavonoids, sulfur compounds, and phenols—plus a whopping 210 percent of your daily vitamin C—making it a detox delight. Plus the tart sumac spice makes your taste buds really sing.

MAKES 6 SERVINGS

RED PEPPER-CASHEW ENDIVE

2 cups raw cashews

2 roasted red peppers (see tip below)

$\frac{1}{2}$ cup water

2 garlic cloves

3 tablespoons lemon juice

3 tablespoons tahini

1 teaspoon sumac powder (see tip below)

$\frac{1}{2}$ teaspoon sea salt

18 endive leaves

GRAPE SALAD

6 cups seedless green grapes, halved

1$\frac{1}{2}$ cups fresh mint, chopped

To make the endive: Place the cashews, peppers, water, garlic, lemon juice, tahini, sumac powder, and salt in a food processor or blender and mix until smooth.

Place 3 tablespoons of red pepper–cashew spread on each endive leaf.

To make the salad: Toss together the green grapes and mint.

Serve 3 endive leaves with 1 cup grape salad.

Per serving, endive spread: 325 calories, 25 g total fat (5 g saturated), 0 mg cholesterol, 211 mg sodium, 399 mg potassium, 21 g carbohydrates (3 g sugar), 3 g fiber, 9 g protein

Per serving, salad: 62 calories, 0 g total fat, 0 mg cholesterol, 0 mg sodium, 176 mg potassium, 16 g carbohydrates (15 g sugar), 1 g fiber, 0 g protein

TIP: If not roasting your own, try Mezzetta Organics jarred Fire-Roasted Red Bell Peppers (mezzetta.com). Buy sumac at a Middle Eastern grocery store, or online at thespicehouse.com. Or, substitute $\frac{1}{2}$ teaspoon lemon zest and $\frac{1}{4}$ teaspoon paprika.

DINNER

Curried Lentils with Sweet Potato and Chard

The carotenoid-rich sweet potato lends a slight sweetness that complements the spicy gingery, jalapeño-y, curry flavor. The curry powder, onion, and garlic provide a triple detox whammy, and the ginger and jalapeño make this an inflamer-tamer, too.

MAKES 4 SERVINGS

3 tablespoons extra-virgin olive oil

1 small yellow onion, diced

2 garlic cloves, minced

1 slice (2") fresh ginger, peeled and minced

1 small red jalapeño pepper (1"–2"), deseeded and minced

1 tablespoon curry powder

1 cup dried lentils

4 cups low-sodium vegetable broth, divided

1 cup So Delicious unsweetened coconut milk

2 cups sweet potatoes, peeled and cubed

2 cups Swiss chard, stems removed, leaves coarsely chopped

In a 3-quart saucepan, heat the oil. Add the onion and sauté until soft but not brown.

Add the garlic, ginger, jalapeño pepper, and curry powder and sauté for 1 to 2 minutes, stirring to prevent the spices from burning.

Add the lentils and 2 cups of the vegetable broth, reserving the remainder for later use. Bring to a boil, then reduce the heat and gently simmer, covered, for 10 to 15 minutes.

(continued)

Add the remaining broth, coconut milk, and sweet potatoes. Return to a gentle simmer and cook, covered, for 15 to 20 minutes, or until the sweet potatoes are fork-tender.

Remove from the heat, add the Swiss chard, stir, and cover for 5 minutes to allow the chard to soften. Serve in soup bowls.

Per serving: 278 calories, 12 g total fat (3 g saturated), 0 mg cholesterol, 311 mg sodium, 869 mg potassium, 36 g carbohydrates (3 g sugar), 10 g fiber, 8 g protein

TIP: Wear plastic gloves when handling the jalepeño pepper. Simply Organic or Frontier Natural Products sell nonirradiated organic curry powder. Use Trader Joe's light coconut milk for a creamier consistency.

Get a Jump on Day 9

Tomorrow's Parsnip and Pear Puree (page 197) is easy to make ahead of time. Just simmer the parsnips, sauté the pears, and throw it all into a food processor or blender. It's delicious hot or cold. Double the recipe for a simple, healthy snack.

Day 8 Mind-Body Detox

WALKING MEDITATION

When I suggest meditation to my patients, they often respond with an automatic "No way!" They think they just can't do it. That's because they envision some kind of ultimate Zen situation in which they're supposed to sit in an uncomfortable position for hours with an absolutely blank mind, no thoughts whatsoever.

Obviously that's not possible—or appealing—for most of us. And it doesn't have to be—there are many forms of meditation. One type that's particularly accessible to Westerners is walking meditation, since it fits perfectly with our on-the-go aesthetic.

Find a relatively quiet room or walking path where you can walk undisturbed (it doesn't have to be silent, just free from obstacles—a clear hallway or park path will do). Allow your arms to hang freely at your sides, shoulders relaxed and held back (none of the hunching we too often walk around with), head centered over the neck, and gaze soft and focused on the ground about 2 feet ahead. With your left foot planted firmly on the ground, roll the right foot onto the toe, pause, then lift the right foot. Plant the heel of the right foot about 6 inches in front of the left foot as you roll down onto the sole of the right foot and up onto the left toes. Pause again. Then with your right foot planted firmly on the ground, lift the left foot. Plant the heel of the left foot about 6 inches in front of the right as you roll down onto the sole of the left foot and up onto the right toes. Pause again. Then repeat this action for 10 to 20 steps or more.

This is not exercise—you are deliberately moving slowly with the intention of feeling every micromovement. Feel every little corner of your feet coming into contact with the earth—as though you were walking on the beach. (If you can do this exercise with bare feet, so much the better!) The eyes and ears are open. Don't try to tune out sights and sounds around you, rather register them in service to your walk. If your mind wanders, bring it back to the sensations of the feet lifting, rolling, and stepping again and again. If you get distracted by something pretty or loud, simply notice whether or not that impacts your walk, and return to your walk.

When you are done, I recommend that you stop and close your eyes for a few breaths and feel your feet. They may feel simply amazing! After all, they're not used to so much attention. You are truly grounded now.

Day 9 Menu

BEVERAGE: Detox Tea (Dandelion, Chicory, or Burdock Root)

BREAKFAST: Parsnip and Pear Puree

MIDMORNING SNACK: Smoothie, Juice, or Nut Milk

LUNCH: Hummus and Veggie Rainbow Tortilla

MIDAFTERNOON SNACK: Your Choice (see page 139)

DINNER: Wild Arctic Char and Roasted Radicchio and Salad

BREAKFAST

Parsnip and Pear Puree

This parsnip-pear puree has a whopping 43 percent of your daily vitamin C to support phase I glutathione, so do your liver a great big detox favor and eat up.

MAKES 4 SERVINGS

4 large parsnips, peeled and chopped

2 tablespoons extra-virgin olive oil

2 large pears, peeled and chopped

$\frac{1}{2}$ cup organic unfiltered apple juice

$\frac{1}{2}$ teaspoon allspice

$\frac{1}{4}$ teaspoon ground nutmeg

$\frac{1}{4}$ teaspoon sea salt

$\frac{1}{4}$–$\frac{1}{3}$ cup nut milk, homemade or store bought

Pinch of cinnamon, optional

1 teaspoon coconut cream concentrate, or Vanilla Cashew Cream (page 219), optional

In a 1-quart saucepan, place the parsnips in water to cover. Bring to a boil, then reduce the heat and simmer, uncovered, for 15 to 20 minutes, or until the parsnips are fork-tender. Remove from the heat and drain.

While the parsnips are simmering, heat the oil in another 1-quart saucepan and sauté the pears for 4 to 5 minutes. Add the apple juice, allspice, nutmeg, and salt and simmer, uncovered, for about 15 minutes, stirring often.

Transfer the parsnips, pears with any remaining apple juice, and nut milk to a food processor and pulse until desired consistency—chopped or pureed.

Top with cinnamon and coconut cream concentrate or Vanilla Cashew Cream (if using).

Per serving: 243 calories, 8 g total fat (1 g saturated), 0 mg cholesterol, 179 mg sodium, 775 mg potassium, 45 g carbohydrates (16 g sugar), 9 g fiber, 3 g protein

TIP: Coconut cream concentrate is different from coconut milk or coconut oil. It's basically 100 percent coconut "meat" ground very fine, giving it a creamy consistency due to its high (mainly healthy) fat content, much like other nut butters. Tropical Traditions sells organic coconut cream concentrate (tropicaltraditions.com).

The Sweet Deal

Actually, *there is no sweet deal.* Agave nectar has enjoyed a halo effect recently because of claims that it is low on the glycemic index. But it turns out that's only because it's high in fructose, which is just as problematic for the body as sucrose, or table sugar, because fructose can unleash processes that lead to liver toxicity and other metabolic diseases. In my opinion, beyond what comes naturally packaged in fruits and vegetables, there is no such thing as a "good" sugar, despite the best efforts of health food manufacturers to convince you otherwise.

That said, I do understand that it does take a teaspoon of the sweet stuff here and there to make the medicine of detoxification go down easy—and we allow for that in some of our juice and smoothie recipes. It's always optional, and I suggest you minimize it. Mary Beth recommends that if you must use it, then treat it as you do any other category of food and aim for optimal botanical diversity—that is to say, keep three or four varieties on hand and rotate them frequently. Here are some options.

Natural Sweeteners

AGAVE NECTAR AND SYRUP

Harvested from Mexican Agave cactus, the same plant whose sap is a source of tequila, agave nectar resembles honey but is less thick and dissolves easier in liquids. Evidence-based studies of agave's glycemic index and blood sugar effects in humans and long-term risks and benefits of agave consumption are lacking, despite agave proponents' claims.

BROWN RICE SYRUP

Brown rice syrup is produced commercially by breaking down brown rice flour or starch with enzymes. The resulting syrup is filtered and excess water evaporated to thicken it. A recent study revealed high levels of arsenic in organic brown rice syrup, so don't overdo this one.

COCONUT SUGAR, POWDER, AND NECTAR

Coconut sweeteners are harvested from the blossoms of the coconut tree. The sugar, powder, and syrup have a subtle, brown sugar–like taste with a slight hint of caramel. Studies of coconut sugar's glycemic index and blood sugar effects in humans are lacking.

HONEY

The world's oldest sweetener is rich in history, symbolism, and allure. It is made by bees using nectar from many flower varieties, such as clover, wildflower, alfalfa, orange blossom, tupelo, chestnut, or manuka. Interestingly, honey does contain some antibacterial compounds and has been studied for use in burns and sore throats. But it's not medicine and is not a good source of nutrition.

JERUSALEM ARTICHOKE SWEETENER

Jerusalem artichoke syrup is made from Jerusalem artichokes, using acid or enyzmes to break down the starch and extract the fructose that lends the sweetening power. It has an earthy, sweet flavor, similar to agave; is blander than honey, maple syrup, or molasses; and it contains trace amounts of inulin fiber, a prebiotic.

MAPLE SYRUP

This boiled-down sap of maple tree is less refined than other sweeteners. Use it for its distinctive, caramel-like flavor. Though it is not considered a good source of minerals, it does contain some manganese, zinc, iron, and calcium in trace amounts. Also contains antioxidant phenols. Classified by grades (A and B) and by colors (light amber, medium amber, dark amber). Grade B and darker colors have a richer maple taste and are typically used in baking.

MOLASSES

Molasses is made from sugarcane or sugar beets. The juice of the crushed leaves is boiled, which crystallizes the sugar, and then boiled for a second time, and finally a third time for the traditional blackstrap molasses, which has a very hearty, robust, almost smoky taste and is used most often in baking. It contains trace amounts of calcium, magnesium, potassium, and iron. Tastes great drizzled sparingly on vegetables, fruits, greens, and grains. Buy unsulphured.

RAW CANE SUGAR

This crystallized evaporated cane juice with a caramel taste is still mostly cane sugar.

YACON SYRUP AND POWDER

From the tuberous yacon plant of the Andes mountains, this traditional sweetener is used in Peru, Bolivia, and Brazil and contains fructooligosaccharides (FOS), which act as a prebiotic.

LUNCH

Hummus and Veggie Rainbow Tortilla

When sliced, the tortilla's interior is a beautiful display of red, orange, yellow, green, and blue-purple (ROYGBV!). With 95 percent of your daily vitamin A, D-glucaric acid in the tomato, sulfur in the cabbage, vitamin B_6 for methylation and sulfation, and quercetin in the lemon, this rainbow tortilla looks beautiful, tastes great, and is a detoxer's dream come true.

MAKES 1 SERVING

1 gluten-free brown rice tortilla

$\frac{1}{3}$ cup organic store-bought hummus

$\frac{1}{2}$ tomato, sliced

$\frac{1}{2}$ carrot, shredded

$\frac{1}{2}$ cup arugula

$\frac{1}{4}$ cup purple cabbage, shredded

$\frac{1}{4}$–$\frac{1}{2}$ lemon, optional

1–2 sprigs fresh thyme, leaves removed, optional

Warm the tortilla in a sauté pan for 2 to 3 minutes, or until soft.

Remove from the pan and spread the hummus on the tortilla while still warm.

Layer the tomatoes, shredded carrot, arugula, and cabbage on top. Squeeze the lemon (if using) and thyme leaves (if using) on top.

Roll the tortilla into a wrap, slice it in the middle on a diagonal, and serve immediately.

Per serving: 306 calories, 11 g total fat (1 g saturated), 0 mg cholesterol, 509 mg sodium, 549 mg potassium, 45 g carbohydrates (3 g sugar), 9 g fiber, 10 g protein

TIP: Try Tribe Organic hummus (tribehummus.com) or Desert Pepper Trading Company White Bean Dip (desertpepper.com) in this recipe. Food for Life makes a good gluten-free brown-rice tortilla; find a store at foodforlife.com.

DINNER

Wild Arctic Char and Roasted Radicchio

The orange zest's quercetin and radicchio's copper and magnesium support phase I detox, and the amino acids in the Arctic char support phase II.

MAKES 4 SERVINGS

2 heads radicchio, halved lengthwise
8 tablespoons extra-virgin olive oil
1 teaspoon sea salt, divided
1 teaspoon ground peppercorn
   blend, divided
2 teaspoons fennel seeds

4 teaspoons orange zest
$\frac{1}{4}$ teaspoon ground cayenne pepper
4 Arctic char fillets (6 ounces each)
1 lime, juiced
$\frac{1}{4}$ cup unsulphured molasses

Arrange 1 rack on the upper part of the oven and 1 rack on the lower part of the oven. Preheat the oven to 400°F. Brush 2 rimmed baking sheets with oil.

Coat the radicchio halves with 2 tablespoons oil, sprinkle with $\frac{1}{2}$ teaspoon of the sea salt and peppercorns, and place flat side down on the baking sheets. Roast for 12 to 15 minutes, turning once halfway through, or until the leaves are slightly wilted and charred. While the radicchio roasts, prepare the fish for roasting.

With a mortar and pestle, grind the fennel seeds, orange zest, remaining sea salt, remaining peppercorns, and cayenne pepper.

Brush the skin of the fish fillets with the remaining 2 tablespoons oil and the lime juice, place skin side down, and sprinkle the tops of the fillets with the crushed seed-zest-spice blend.

Place the fish on the upper rack of the oven and roast for 10 to 12 minutes, or until the fish flakes easily with a fork, basting with the baking sheet juices halfway through. When almost done, broil for 2 minutes, or until browned on top.

Remove the fish and radicchio from the oven. Plate 1 fillet and 1 radicchio quarter per plate. Drizzle molasses on the radicchio before serving.

Per serving: 572 calories, 35 g total fat (5 g saturated), 36 mg cholesterol, 707 mg sodium, 1,200 mg potassium, 20 g carbohydrates (12 g sugar), 2 g fiber, 43 g protein

TIP: According to Monterey Bay Seafood Watch, Arctic char is a "Best Choice."

Day 9 Mind-Body Detox

GET SWEATY

If you haven't been breaking much of a sweat up until now, just do it. Sweating helps release toxins through the skin and has been shown to accelerate release of toxins from the internal fat cells.

In European circles, no detox plan is complete without good old-fashioned sweat therapy. You can do it one of two ways. There, the use of saunas is nearly ubiquitous. If you have access to one, do get in it three to five times a week, starting with 10 minutes at a time and working your way up to at least 20 minutes. If you have access to an infrared sauna, even better—it will heat you from the inside out, whereas a traditional sauna works from the outside in. Some people might find it a little easier to tolerate longer turns in an infrared—up to 30 minutes at a time (the maximum I recommend). Either option is a good one—especially if you use your sauna as a sacred space to unwind tension from your body and mind.

If you can't sauna, don't worry—you can get your sweat on with exercise. Amp up your Sun Salutations (page 124), walking routine (page 216), or other exercise efforts so that you hit the sweaty aerobic zone. (That's moderate intensity, defined as 50 to 70 percent of your maximum heart rate—for most people somewhere between 120 and 150 beats per minute.) Exercise raises your core body temperature and makes you sweat just as a sauna does, and offers additional heart-healthy benefits, too.

Get a Jump on Day 10

Stuffed Black Bean–Cabbage Rolls (page 205) are a classic comfort food dinner—even more comforting if you've made them ahead and all you have to do is pull them out of the refrigerator and pop them in the oven. Follow the recipe through step seven, and store until dinnertime, if you like.

Day 10 Menu

BEVERAGE: Detox Tea (Dandelion, Chicory, or Burdock Root)

BREAKFAST: Vanilla Quinoa with Raspberry Compote

MIDMORNING SNACK: Smoothie, Juice, or Nut Milk

LUNCH: Stuffed Black Bean-Cabbage Rolls

MIDAFTERNOON SNACK: Your Choice (see page 139)

DINNER: Rosemary-Portobello Mushrooms with Tahini Green Beans and Salad

BREAKFAST

Vanilla Quinoa with Raspberry Compote

With 90 percent of your daily riboflavin—for mood support, energy production, and phase I of detox support—this quinoa will put some get up in your morning. And the 8 grams of fiber it contains will also get you "going."

MAKES 4 SERVINGS

2 cups water

1 vanilla bean, split, seeds scraped and reserved, or 2 teaspoons vanilla extract

1 cup quinoa

2 cups raspberries

$\frac{1}{2}$ teaspoon cinnamon + extra for sprinkling

2 tablespoons maple syrup or honey

$\frac{1}{3}$ cup pecans, or any other nut, coarsely chopped

1 cup raw nut milk, optional (see recipes, Chapter 5)

In a 1-quart saucepan, combine water, vanilla bean seeds, and quinoa. Bring to a boil over high heat.

Reduce the heat to a gentle simmer and cook, covered, for approximately 12 minutes, or until most of the liquid is absorbed.

While the quinoa is simmering, mash the raspberries, cinnamon, and maple syrup or honey together with a fork to a semimashed consistency.

Optional: While the quinoa is simmering, roast the pecans over medium-high heat in a dry sauté pan for 3 minutes, stirring often until fragrant but not burnt.

When the water is absorbed, turn off the heat and add the raspberry mash to the top of the quinoa. Let stand, covered, for 5 minutes.

Stir in the nut milk (if using) and top with the pecans and sprinkle with cinnamon.

Per serving: 297 calories, 10 g total fat (1 g saturated), 0 mg cholesterol, 2 mg sodium, 156 mg potassium, 46 g carbohydrates (8 g sugar), 8 g fiber, 8 g protein

TIP: Blueberries and blackberries are great alternatives to the raspberries. Frozen berries can work, too, and may be a more affordable alternative.

LUNCH

Stuffed Black Bean–Cabbage Rolls

A crucifer to remember! This hearty stuffed cabbage is chock-full of free-radical-scavenging vitamin C, manganese, and carotenoids and pumped up with folate, vitamin B_6, and riboflavin, methylation supporters. Add the jalapeño's luteolin, magnesium, and quercetin for toxin biotransformation and you (and your taste buds) will be transformed.

MAKES 8 SERVINGS

2 cups cooked brown rice

3 teaspoon sea salt, divided

¼ cup extra-virgin olive oil

1 head of cabbage, cored

1 medium onion, diced

4 garlic cloves, crushed

1 yellow pepper, diced

1 red pepper, diced

1 orange pepper, diced

1 small red jalapeño pepper (1"–2"), deseeded and minced

1 can (16 ounces) black beans, drained and rinsed

1 bottle (32 ounces) organic crushed or diced tomatoes

¼ cup Italian leaf parsley, minced

1 teaspoon ground black pepper

1 lemon, juiced

1 cup Daiya mozzarella-style vegan "cheese" shreds, optional

Preheat the oven to 350°F.

Prepare the rice according to package directions.

Fill a 6-quart stockpot, large enough to submerge the cabbage head, with water. Add 2 teaspoons of the salt to the water and bring to a boil.

(continued)

While the water is coming to a boil, heat the oil in a large sauté pan over medium-high heat. Add the onion and sauté until translucent. Add the garlic and peppers and sauté until soft. Remove from the heat.

In a large mixing bowl, add the brown rice, black beans, onion and peppers mixture, 1 cup of the diced tomatoes, parsley, the remaining 1 teaspoon salt, and pepper, and combine well.

Gently submerge the cabbage head in boiling water for 2 to 3 minutes, just long enough for the outer leaves to soften. Remove the cabbage head with tongs, allow to cool for 1 minute, and remove 2 to 3 large outer softened leaves. Resubmerge the cabbage in the water, remove, and repeat the process until you have removed 8 large softened leaves.

Spread the cabbage leaves out and place about ¾ cup of the filling in the center of each leaf. Roll up like a burrito.

Take the cooled cabbage head, cut 4 to 6 leaves in half, and line the bottom of a large (ideally 3-quart) baking dish. (You can also use two smaller baking dishes.) Place the stuffed cabbage leaves, seam side down, on top of the cut cabbage leaves.

Mix the lemon juice and the remaining diced tomatoes, pour over the cabbage leaves, and bake, covered with foil, for 45 to 50 minutes.

Optional: When almost done, increase the oven heat to 450°F, sprinkle the mozzarella-style shreds, and broil for 5 minutes, or until the "cheese" is bubbly and browned.

Remove from the heat and serve.

Per serving: 267 calories, 8 g total fat (1 g saturated), 0 mg cholesterol, 523 mg sodium, 743 mg potassium, 42 g carbohydrates (4 g sugar), 10 g fiber, 8 g protein

TIP: Wear plastic gloves when handling the jalepeño pepper. Eden Organic sells canned beans with BPA-free liners and organic bottled diced tomatoes. Jovial and Bionaturae sell organic strained and diced tomatoes as well as paste; both can be purchased online at tropicaltraditions.com. Daiya vegan cheese shreds are free of dairy, soy, gluten, eggs, rice, peanuts, and tree nuts, except coconut oil (find a store at daiyafoods.com).

DINNER

Rosemary-Portobello Mushrooms

The copper, niacin, riboflavin, and selenium in these medicinal mushrooms support phase I detox and methylation and quench free radicals. Plus, the rosemary adds immune-supportive antimicrobial activity. The "meaty" texture of portobello will really satisfy any carnivorous cravings you've been harboring.

MAKES 4 SERVINGS

$\frac{1}{4}$ cup extra-virgin olive oil

$\frac{1}{4}$ cup balsamic vinegar

4 sprigs fresh thyme, leaves removed

2 sprigs fresh rosemary, leaves removed

$\frac{1}{4}$ teaspoon sea salt

$\frac{1}{4}$ teaspoon ground peppercorns

4 large portobello mushrooms

Preheat the oven to 375°F.

In a bowl, whisk together the oil, vinegar, thyme, rosemary, salt, and peppercorns.

Brush the mixture on the portobello mushroom tops and bottoms, place on a rimmed baking sheet, and roast for 10 to 12 minutes, or until browned.

Per serving: 159 calories, 14 g total fat (2 g saturated), 0 mg cholesterol, 157 mg sodium, 502 mg potassium, 8 g carbohydrates (4 g sugar), 2 g fiber, 3 g protein

TIP: To boost the protein power of this meal, serve with 1 cup of Mediterranean Kidney Beans (page 161).

Get a Jump on Day 11

Tomorrow's dinner features a fabulous satay sauce. Make it tonight if you want. Consider doubling the recipe—you can thin it with a little bit with water for a tasty salad dressing. You can also go ahead and roast the sweet potato for tomorrow's frittata.

DINNER

Tahini Green Beans

In this recipe, more than 12 micronutrients are excellent (>20 percent of your daily requirement) or good (10 to 19 percent of your daily requirement) sources, including phosphorus, vitamin C, manganese, vitamin A, thiamin, folate, vitamin E, calcium, iron, riboflavin, magnesium, and copper. These Tahini Green Beans give multivitamins a run for their money!

MAKES 4 SERVINGS

1 pound green beans, ends trimmed
2 tablespoons extra-virgin olive oil
2 garlic cloves, minced
1 teaspoon red-pepper flakes
8 tablespoons Lemon-Tahini Dressing (page 145)
2 teaspoons sea salt, optional
1 teaspoon lemon zest, optional

Fill a 2-quart stockpot with water and optional salt (if using) and bring to a boil.

Blanch the green beans for about 2 minutes, or until bright green.

Drain immediately and shock in a bowl of ice water to stop the green beans from cooking.

Heat the oil in a large sauté pan. Add the garlic and red pepper and sauté for about 30 seconds, or until fragrant but not browned.

Add the green beans and sauté for about 5 minutes, stirring often to prevent sticking.

Remove from the heat, toss with the dressing, salt (if using), and lemon zest (if using) and serve immediately.

Per serving: 320 calories, 19 g total fat (3 g saturated), 0 mg cholesterol, 183 mg sodium, 330 mg potassium, 12 g carbohydrates (1 g sugar), 5 g fiber, 3 g protein

TIP: Double the red-pepper flakes in this recipe to boost the anti-inflammatory and analgesic activity.

Day 10 Mind-Body Detox

BE A WARRIOR

Combat an afternoon slump by cultivating a little of your own warrior energy. We all have it, and yoga offers a simple technique for getting in touch with it. This simple flow can be done anytime, anywhere—no special clothes or yoga mat is needed, just a little space and a willingness to be fierce. These are variations on the yoga postures known as Warrior Pose One and Warrior Pose Two—there's no need to go as fully and deeply into the poses as you would in a yoga class. Here, we're aiming to capture the essence and energy of the postures, rather than the full stretch. Here's how to do the simple Warrior Flow:

Standing Salute: Stand tall with your feet together, chin slightly tucked, crown of the head reaching toward the ceiling. Bring your hands together at your heart, and take a few deep breaths. On an inhalation, sweep your arms out to the sides and overhead, bringing your palms to touch. Hook the thumbs behind the hands to lock the palms together in a prayer position. Keep the head neutral and the gaze forward.

Warrior One: Exhale and step your right foot back about 3 feet. The right leg should be extended, the left leg bent, moving toward a 90-degree angle. Keep the arms overhead and the head lifted and neck neutral. As you inhale again, square the hips forward, open the chest, drop a little more deeply into the left leg, and look slightly up as you come into a fuller expression of Warrior Pose One (aka *Virabhadrasana* One). Exhale and drop your arms down to chest level, with your locked hands pointing directly forward from the heart. Maintain the same position in the feet and hips.

Warrior Two: On an inhalation, swing your right arm and right hip open to the right in line with the left arm and left shoulder. Keep both arms parallel to the floor, the left pointing straight in front of you and the right pointing to the rear. The right leg should be extended, the left leg bent. This is Warrior Pose Two (*Virabhadrasana* Two). Exhale and swivel your hips forward again as you swing the right arm to meet the left. Clasp the hands again in prayer pose, arms extending forward from the heart as before.

Standing Salute: Inhale, raise the arms overhead, and step forward. Exhale and lower your hands to your heart center. This is one repetition. Repeat the entire sequence on the other side, this time leading with the left leg.

Day 11 Menu

BEVERAGE: Detox Tea (Dandelion, Chicory, or Burdock Root)

BREAKFAST: Zucchini and Sweet Potato Frittata

MIDMORNING SNACK: Smoothie, Juice, or Nut Milk

LUNCH: Chickpea and Arugula-Stuffed Avocado

MIDAFTERNOON SNACK: Your Choice (see page 139)

DINNER: Peanut Satay Tofu Stir-Fry with Broccoli and Salad

BREAKFAST

Zucchini and Sweet Potato Frittata

This frittata has only 4 grams of saturated fat and almost four times more good fats (monounsaturated and polyunsaturated fats) than that. And anyway, the phytonutrient-dense vegetables and spices outmuscle the animal food in this recipe. Amino acids, carotenoids, free-radical-scavenging antioxidants vitamins A, C, E, and the mineral manganese, along with methylation supporters vitamins B_2, B_6, and B_{12} make this a real detox food. And as a bonus, it's a beautiful dish that would steal the show at the most elegant brunch.

MAKES 6 SERVINGS

6 tablespoons extra-virgin olive oil, divided

2 tablespoons molasses + 1 tablespoon, optional for garnish

1 teaspoon salt, divided

2 sprigs fresh thyme, leaves removed

2 medium sweet potatoes, peeled and cubed

12 cherry tomatoes, quartered

1 small onion, chopped

2 medium zucchini, sliced lengthwise, seeded and grated

$\frac{1}{4}$ cup basil leaves, coarsely chopped

1 teaspoon red-pepper flakes

6 extra-large eggs

1 cup Daiya vegan Cheddar- or Pepperjack-style shreds, optional

Arrange 1 rack on the upper part of the oven and 1 rack on the lower part of the oven. Preheat the oven to 375°F.

Lightly oil 2 baking sheets.

In a small mixing bowl, whisk 4 tablespoons of the olive oil with the molasses, $\frac{1}{2}$ teaspoon of the salt, and the thyme.

In a large mixing bowl, toss the sweet potato cubes with $\frac{1}{2}$ of the oil mixture. Spread in a single layer on a baking sheet. Roast for 25 to 30 minutes, or until tender.

(continued)

In another mixing bowl, toss the cherry tomato quarters and onion with the remaining oil mixture. Lay in a single layer on the second baking sheet. Roast for 15 to 20 minutes, or until browned.

Remove the sweet potatoes, tomatoes, and onion from the oven when done. Increase the oven heat to 450°F for the final finishing of the frittata.

Transfer the sweet potatoes to a large mixing bowl and add the roasted tomatoes and onion, draining and discarding any juice before adding. Add the grated zucchini, basil, red-pepper flakes, and the remaining ½ teaspoon salt to the bowl. Combine.

Spread all the ingredients in a well-oiled, large, oven-safe skillet. Lightly beat the eggs and pour into the skillet. Cook over medium heat for 8 to 10 minutes, or until the eggs begin to set.

Add the Cheddar- or Pepperjack-style shreds, if using. Transfer the skillet to the oven for 5 minutes, or until the frittata is lightly browned and completely set on top.

Invert the frittata on a plate and slice with a pizza wheel into 6 servings. Drizzle each frittata wedge with molasses (if using).

Per serving: 280 calories, 20 g total fat (4 g saturated), 215 mg cholesterol, 488 mg sodium, 678 mg potassium, 19 g carbohydrates (9 g sugar), 3 g fiber, 9 g protein

TIP: This frittata freezes well. Just thaw it overnight and gently rewarm it just before serving.

LUNCH

Chickpea and Arugula–Stuffed Avocado

This recipe can't be beat for its utter simplicity—or nutrient density. It's an A–Zinc powerhouse, with 14 micronutrients providing either good (10 to 20 percent) or excellent (>20 percent) sources of your daily requirements! With all the free-radical-scavenging antioxidants and anti-inflammatory compounds, it's no wonder the avocado is rumored to be an antiaging superfood.

MAKES 1 SERVING

$\frac{1}{2}$ cup chickpeas

1 cup arugula

6 cherry tomatoes, quartered

2 tablespoons lemon juice

1 tablespoon apple cider or balsamic vinegar

$\frac{1}{8}$ teaspoon sea salt

$\frac{1}{4}$ teaspoon black pepper, coarsely ground

1 avocado, halved lengthwise and pit removed

In a small mixing bowl, combine the chickpeas, arugula, tomatoes, lemon juice, vinegar, salt, and pepper.

Fill the avocado halves with the salad and allow the salad to overflow the avocado halves.

Serve immediately.

Per serving: 463 calories, 28 g total fat (4 g saturated), 0 mg cholesterol, 666 mg sodium, 1,420 mg potassium, 50 g carbohydrates (5 g sugar), 19 g fiber, 11 g protein

TIP: Cook your own chickpeas (see page 147), or use Eden Organic BPA-free canned chickpeas. Add 3 ounces of wild salmon to boost the omega-3-rich anti-inflammatory and protein power of this recipe.

DINNER

Peanut Satay Tofu Stir-Fry with Broccoli

This dish is an excellent (20 percent of RDA) source of 17 vitamins and minerals! Ask not what this super crucifer, high-omega-3, capsaicin-, gingerol-, carotenoid-, flavonoid-, and sulfur-compound-rich dish does—rather, what *doesn't* it do?

MAKES 4 SERVINGS

1 pound firm tofu

¼ cup grapeseed oil, divided

1 large red bell pepper, deseeded and cut in thin strips

2 carrots, quartered and cut lengthwise in thin strips

4 garlic cloves, minced

1 slice (1") fresh ginger, peeled and minced

1 small red jalapeño pepper (1"–2") , deseeded and minced

1 pound broccoli florets

⅓ cup water

1 tablespoon wheat-free non-GMO tamari

½ cup Peanut Satay Sauce (opposite page)

Drain the tofu, press between paper towels to drain the excess liquid, and cut into 1"-long pieces.

In a large sauté pan, heat 2 tablespoons of the oil on medium-high heat and stir-fry the tofu until lightly golden. Remove from the heat and drain on a bed of paper towels. Set aside.

Add the remaining oil to the pan. Sauté the bell pepper and carrots for about 5 minutes, or until the vegetables begin to soften. Add the garlic, ginger, and jalapeño and stir-fry for 1 minute, being careful not to brown the garlic.

Add the broccoli and stir-fry for 1 to 2 minutes, then add the water. Stir until the water is almost evaporated, then stir in the tamari, Peanut Satay Sauce, and tofu, coating the vegetables and tofu. Stir-fry for 4 to 5 minutes, or until fragrant and hot.

Per serving: 367 calories, 31 g total fat (4 g saturated), 0 mg cholesterol, 456 mg sodium, 917 mg potassium, 22 g carbohydrates (4 g sugar), 9 g fiber, 22 g protein

Peanut Satay Sauce

MAKES 16 SERVINGS (2 TABLESPOONS EACH)

1 cup organic crunchy peanut butter

2 ounces apple cider vinegar

2 tablespoons sesame oil

1 tablespoon tamari

3 Medjool dates, pitted

2 garlic cloves, pressed with a garlic press or finely minced

1 piece (1") fresh ginger, peeled and pressed with a garlic press or finely minced

1 small red jalapeño pepper (about 2" long), deseeded and finely minced

2–4 ounces hot water

In a food processor, blend the peanut butter, vinegar, oil, tamari, dates, garlic, ginger, and pepper.

Add water in 1-tablespoon increments to thin to desired consistency.

Refrigerate, for up to 1 week, in a glass Mason jar or shaker bottle and shake well before using.

Per serving: 117 calories, 10 g total fat (2 g saturated), 0 mg cholesterol, 142 mg sodium, 140 mg potassium, 5 g carbohydrates (3 g sugar), 2 g fiber, 4 g protein

TIP: Wear plastic gloves when handling the jalapeño pepper. Look for wheat-free, non-GMO tamari, such as that made by San-J (san-j.com). Santa Cruz, MaraNatha, and Arrowhead Mills sell organic crunchy peanut butter. This raw Peanut Satay Sauce also makes a nice accompaniment to tofu, vegetables, shrimp, and even egg dishes.

Day 11 Mind-Body Detox

STEP IT UP

Movement is a critical part of a nontoxic, health-oriented lifestyle, but it can be hard for busy people to carve out chunks of time. I know, I've been there. For those patients who can't find even 15 minutes in their day to go out for a walk, I recommend investing in a good pedometer and counting steps rather than minutes.

The average sedentary American takes between 2,000 and 3,000 steps every day—that's not very many, about the equivalent of walking a mile. By contrast, the health community is big on promoting 10,000 steps a day—and if you take them, you'll be burning an additional 2,500 to 3,000 calories a week, which is significant if weight control is an issue for you.

Moreover, a recent Stanford University study found that just owning a pedometer makes you move more—to the tune of about 2,000 steps a day. It is, in itself, an incredible motivator. The best news of all is that you can get a good one for about $25, or even less—and if you have a smartphone, you can download an app that lets you count not only steps but miles and calories, too.

So clip on a pedometer, then walk around the block, around the office, and around the house. Walk to lunch and back again, to the grocery store, to the neighbor's house. Park the car a little farther away than you otherwise might. You'll be surprised at all the little opportunities you can find when you go looking for them, and how rewarding it can be to watch them all add up.

Get a Jump on Day 12

Tomorrow's lunch is Roasted Root Vegetables (page 220); these are easy to make ahead—just pop them in the oven and go about your evening's business. Store them in the refrigerator overnight and eat them cold or at room temperature. Put your cashews for the cashew cream in the refrigerator to soak overnight.

Day 12 Menu

BEVERAGE: Detox Tea (Dandelion, Chicory, or Burdock Root)

BREAKFAST: Polenta with Apple Compote and Vanilla Cashew Cream

MIDMORNING SNACK: Smoothie, Juice, or Nut Milk

LUNCH: Roasted Root Vegetables and Salad

MIDAFTERNOON SNACK: Your Choice (see page 139)

DINNER: Spicy White Bean and Spinach Soup and Salad

BREAKFAST

Polenta with Apple Compote

Apple (and citrus) pectin binds heavy metals, toxins, and radioactive compounds, and the pumpkin pie spices—cinnamon, ginger, nutmeg, cloves—have blood-sugar-lowering, anti-inflammatory, antimicrobial, and detox properties. It's no wonder some applesauce each day keeps the doctor away.

MAKES 2 SERVINGS

½ cup organic unfiltered apple juice

½ lemon, peel on, cut in 2 wedges

1 teaspoon pumpkin pie spice

6 cardamom pods

4 large Granny Smith apples, peeled, cored, and cubed

1½ cups water

¼ teaspoon sea salt

½ cup polenta

¼ cup Raw Cashew Milk (page 120), optional

1–2 tablespoons Vanilla Cashew Cream (opposite page), optional

In a 1-quart saucepan, add the apple juice, squeezed lemon wedges, pumpkin pie spice, and cardamom and bring to a rolling boil.

Add the apples and return the heat to a simmer, stirring occasionally, for 10 to 15 minutes, or until the apples are tender and the liquid begins to thicken.

While the apples are simmering, bring the water and salt to a boil in a separate pan. Add the polenta and reduce the heat. Cook on low and simmer for 5 minutes, stirring occasionally, until slightly thickened but not overly thick (thin with water as needed to desired consistency). Remove from the heat and cover.

Remove the cardamom pods and lemon wedges from the compote. Mash with a potato masher to desired consistency (partial mashed tastes best).

Top 1 serving of polenta with ¾ cup apple compote. Drizzle on Raw Cashew Milk or Vanilla Cashew Cream (if using).

Per serving: 230 calories, 1 g total fat (0 g saturated), 0 mg cholesterol, 2 mg sodium, 62 mg potassium, 55 g carbohydrates (17 g sugar), 7 g fiber, 3 g protein

TIP: You can substitute pears or peaches for the apples in this compote. Frontier Natural Products (frontiercoop.com) and Simply Organic sell organic pumpkin pie spice (simplyorganic.com).

Vanilla Cashew Cream (REQUIRES SOAKING)

This vegan Vanilla Cashew Cream is versatile and healthy. With a high proportion of unsaturated fats, vitamin E, phytosterols, flavonoids, resveratrol, and anthocyanidins, this is one "cream" that's great for your heart.

MAKES APPROXIMATELY 2 CUPS

2 cups whole raw unsalted cashews, rinsed well

$\frac{1}{2}$–1 cup water

$\frac{1}{4}$ cup honey

1 vanilla bean, split, and seeds scraped and reserved, or 2 teaspoons vanilla extract

Place the cashews in a cup or bowl with just enough cold water to cover them. Cover and refrigerate for 3 to 4 hours, or overnight.

Remove the cashews from the refrigerator and drain the water.

Place in a blender or food processor with $\frac{1}{2}$ cup water. Blend on high speed until the nuts are blended. Stop and scrape down the sides of the blender. Continue to drizzle in water in 1-ounce increments to reach desired thickness (very thick cream, semithick cream, or thin cream sauce) and smoothness, turning off the blender and scraping down the sides as needed between water additions. Once smooth, blend in the honey and vanilla bean seeds or vanilla extract.

Refrigerate in an airtight container for up to 1 week.

Per serving: 114 calories, 8 g total fat (2 g saturated), 0 mg cholesterol, 3 mg sodium, 100 mg potassium, 10 g carbohydrates (5 g sugar), 1 g fiber, 3 g protein

TIP: A handheld blender can be used to blend the cashews in a bowl. Dried dates, apricots, or figs can be used to make a creamy fruit-cashew dip. Add lemon, nutritional yeast, tahini, and spices to make a Mediterranean cashew cream.

LUNCH

Roasted Root Vegetables

If the Peanut Satay Tofu Stir-Fry with Broccoli is the King of All Micronutrient Dishes, then say hello to the Queen. This is a very good source of 15 vitamins and minerals. Detoxifier, inflammation tamer, cancer fighter, heart healthy—this is a Warrior Queen, protecting you from head to toe.

MAKES APPROXIMATELY 6 SERVINGS (2 CUPS EACH)

½ cup extra-virgin olive oil

2 sprigs fresh rosemary, leaves removed

2 sprigs fresh thyme, leaves removed

1 tablespoon curry powder

1 teaspoon sea salt

1 teaspoon coarsely ground mixed peppercorns

1 whole head of garlic cloves, unpeeled

8 large carrots, peeled and cut in 1" pieces

4 large parsnips, peeled and cut in 1" pieces

2 medium turnips, peeled and cubed

2 medium sweet potatoes, peeled and cubed

2 large beets, peeled and cubed

1 large onion, peeled and halved

6 lemon wedges, optional

12 teaspoons nutritional yeast, optional

Preheat the oven to 400°F.

In a small mixing bowl, mix the oil, rosemary, thyme, curry powder, salt, and peppercorns.

Place the garlic cloves, carrots, parsnips, turnips, sweet potatoes, beets, and onion in a large baking dish with the onion halves flat side down.

Pour the oil mixture over the vegetables, tossing to coat thoroughly.

Roast for 40 to 45 minutes, stirring occasionally, or until tender and golden brown.

Transfer the vegetables to a platter. Squeeze the garlic cloves from the peel.

Serve warm over salad with 1 freshly squeezed lemon wedge (if using) and 2 teaspoons nutritional yeast (if using) sprinkled on top.

Per serving: 380 calories, 23 g total fat (3 g saturated), 0 mg cholesterol, 500 mg sodium, 978 mg potassium, 42 g carbohydrates (14 g sugar), 10 g fiber, 5 g protein

TIP: Fortified nutritional yeast adds a nutty, cheesy flavor and provides vitamin B_{12}—a key nutrient that is often lacking in vegetarian and vegan dishes. Bragg (bragg.com), Red Star (redstaryeast.com), and Now Foods (nowfoods.com) all make nutritional yeast flakes. If you know or think that you are yeast sensitive, skip this. To boost the protein power of this meal, prepare and serve with 1 cup Southwestern Black-Bean Mash (page 169).

DINNER

Spicy White Bean and Spinach Soup

Good for your vision (83 percent of daily vitamin A), red blood cells (37 percent of daily iron), bones (16 percent of daily calcium), and muscles (30 percent daily magnesium), plus free-radical-quenching antioxidants and anti-inflammatory gingerol and capsaicin—this is a bowl that will cure whatever ails you. The spices make it a great choice for treating winter colds.

MAKES 6 SERVINGS

2 tablespoons extra-virgin olive oil

3 garlic cloves, pressed or finely chopped

1 medium onion, diced

2 cups diced tomatoes

½ cup diced carrots

¼ cup diced celery

2 slices (1" each) fresh ginger, peeled and pressed (or 1 teaspoon ground)

2 teaspoons paprika

2 teaspoons ground cumin

1 teaspoon cayenne pepper

1 teaspoon sea salt

2 cans (15 ounces each) Eden Organic cannellini beans (with liquid)

1 cup water

4 cups spinach, shredded

In a 3-quart saucepan, heat the oil over medium-high heat. Sauté the garlic and onion for 2 to 3 minutes.

Add the tomatoes, carrots, celery, ginger, paprika, cumin, pepper, and salt and sauté for 4 to 5 minutes, stirring often.

Add the beans and water, stir thoroughly, and reduce the heat to simmer, uncovered, for 25 minutes.

Add the spinach, simmer 5 minutes to wilt, and remove from the heat.

Per serving: 277 calories, 6 g total fat (1 g saturated), 0 mg cholesterol, 429 mg sodium, 1,172 mg potassium, 45 g carbohydrates (1 g sugar), 11 g fiber, 14 g protein

TIP: Eden Organic Cannellini Beans are BPA free. If you used to be a real cheese lover, you can sprinkle on some Parma Vegan Parmesan or Parma Chipotle Cayenne (eatparma.com); Daiya Cheddar-style or Daiya mozzarella-style "shreds" (daiyafoods.com); or B_{12}-fortified nutritional yeast for a comfort-food familiarity.

Day 12 Mind-Body Detox

GET ON A ROLL

The benefits of massage are manifold and well documented: It is a proven strategy for reducing stress. However, it can also be a costly one—not everyone has the time and money to invest in this kind of hands-on healing. Luckily, high-density foam rollers—such as those made by Gaiam (gaiam.com), Trigger Point Performance Therapy (tptherapy.com), Perform Better (performbetter.com), and GoFit (gofit.net)—are the next best thing.

Long used by physical therapists, rollers have made their way into gyms—and now into living rooms—across the country. These simple tools provide sturdy support for you to roll away your own physical stress. All you need to do is lie atop them and roll yourself back and forth, using your own body weight to provide pressure. Roll your back, hips, buttocks, thighs, IT bands, and neck—anywhere your body stores tension. (For more isolated or hard-to-reach areas of tension—say, up under the shoulder blades—try rolling around on a tennis ball or a softer massage ball.) You can roll yourself lengthwise or crossways; you can lie still atop the roller with it positioned along your spine and simply stretch (one of my favorites). It may be a little uncomfortable at first if you're especially wound up, but as you learn to relax into the massage, it will begin to feel addictively good. And that's fine—this is an appointment you can afford to make, and keep, every single day.

Get a Jump on Day 13

Bake your acorn squash for tomorrow's surprisingly sweet breakfast. If you'd like, you can make the "Creamy" Garlic Soup with Spinach (page 226) ahead of time and store it in the refrigerator. Just rewarm it on the stovetop before serving.

Day 13 Menu

BEVERAGE: Detox Tea (Dandelion, Burdock, or Chicory Root)

BREAKFAST: Baked Acorn Squash with Apples and Walnuts

MIDMORNING SNACK: Smoothie, Juice, or Nut Milk

LUNCH: "Creamy" Garlic Soup with Spinach

MIDAFTERNOON SNACK: Your Choice (see page 139)

DINNER: Caramelized Sea Scallops with Bok Choy and Salad

BREAKFAST

Baked Acorn Squash with Apples and Walnuts

This recipe is a nutritionist's dream. It features free-radical-scavenging antioxidants (vitamin C and manganese), detox phase I supporters (copper and magnesium), and detox phase II supporters (vitamin B_6, D-glucaric acid, and quercetin).

MAKES 8 SERVINGS

2 tablespoons grapeseed oil, coconut oil, or extra-virgin olive oil

2 acorn squash, halved and deseeded

1 cup unsulphured raisins

1 cup walnuts, chopped

2 apples, cored and cut in $\frac{1}{2}$" cubes

1 tablespoon freshly squeezed lemon juice

2 tablespoons maple syrup

$\frac{1}{2}$ teaspoon sea salt

$\frac{1}{4}$ teaspoon ground nutmeg

$\frac{1}{4}$ teaspoon ground cloves

Preheat the oven to 375°F.

Brush the oil on the outer skin and interior pulp of the acorn squash. Place the acorns cut side down on a baking sheet and bake for 45 minutes, or until fork-tender. (Bake an additional 10 minutes if needed.)

While the squash bakes, combine the raisins, walnuts, apples, lemon juice, syrup, salt, nutmeg, and cloves in a small mixing bowl.

Turn the squash halves cut side up, stuff with the fruit and nut mixture, and return to the oven for 10 to 15 minutes, or until the mixture is heated through and the top browns. Remove from the oven and cut the acorn halves in half.

Per serving: 267 calories, 14 g total fat (1 g saturated), 0 mg cholesterol, 152 mg sodium, 651 mg potassium, 39 g carbohydrates (20 g sugar), 5 g fiber, 4 g protein

TIP: A stuffed acorn half also makes a great dinner, especially when accompanied by a mesclun salad or a savory bowl of red miso broth.

LUNCH

"Creamy" Garlic Soup with Spinach

This "Creamy" Garlic Soup with Spinach will keep you vampire free (garlic), scurvy free (125 percent of your daily vitamin C), cold free (it's terrific for immunity), and will lower both your blood pressure and cholesterol. And with the allicin and ajoene in the garlic, and the DIM, I3C, glucosinolates, and isothiocyanates in the cauliflower, this is a big bowl of cancer prevention, too.

MAKES 6 SERVINGS

6 cups wild rice

3 bulbs garlic

4 tablespoons extra-virgin olive oil, divided

4 shallots, chopped

1 head of cauliflower, cored and chopped

1 cup celery, chopped

6 cups low-sodium vegetable broth

1 teaspoon ground turmeric

1 teaspoon cayenne pepper + $\frac{1}{2}$ teaspoon for garnish, optional

2 cups baby spinach, shredded in 1" pieces

Prepare the rice according to package directions.

Preheat the oven to 400°F.

Peel away the outer excess layers of the garlic skin but leave the skin on the cloves. Cut $\frac{1}{4}$" to $\frac{1}{2}$" off the tops of the bulbs, exposing the clove tops. Drizzle 2 teaspoons oil onto each bulb, coating the cloves well, and wrap each bulb in aluminum foil.

On a baking sheet or in a muffin tin, bake the bulbs for 30 to 40 minutes, checking to see if the bulbs feel soft when pressed. (They will be tender when they are done.) Remove from the oven and cool.

Once the garlic is cooled, take 2 bulbs and squeeze each clove into a small bowl.

Heat the remaining 2 tablespoons oil in a 3-quart saucepan over medium-high heat. Add the shallots and sauté for 3 to 4 minutes, or until lightly browned.

Add the roasted garlic from the bowl (reserving 1 garlic bulb for garnish or a spread), cauliflower, celery, broth, turmeric, and cayenne pepper to the saucepan and bring to a boil. Reduce the heat and simmer for 20 minutes, or until the cauliflower is fork-mashable.

Transfer the soup to a food processor and puree until smooth. Stir the spinach in by hand and cover for 5 minutes to allow the spinach to wilt. Serve immediately, topped with 1 or 2 garlic cloves, a drizzle of olive oil, and a pinch of cayenne pepper (if using).

Serve accompanied by a cup of cooked wild rice.

Per serving: 172 calories, 10 g total fat (1 g saturated), 0 mg cholesterol, 195 mg sodium, 618 mg potassium, 20 g carbohydrates (2 g sugar), 5 g fiber, 5 g protein

TIP: Make your own vegetable broth, or buy a good one from Pacific, Imagine Foods, Trader Joe's, or Whole Foods 365. Chew a little parsley as a breath freshener after this odorific soup.

DINNER

Caramelized Sea Scallops with Bok Choy

Not only is this a great match of textures and flavors, this dish has incredible health-boosting properties. Vitamins, minerals, amino acids, antioxidants, antibacterials, micronutrients, and phytonutrients galore support detoxification, immunity, mood, and more. It's no wonder that with dishes such as this the Japanese enjoy such incredible longevity.

MAKES 2 SERVINGS

12 sea scallops, washed and patted dry

$\frac{1}{4}$ teaspoon ground ginger

$\frac{1}{4}$ teaspoon cayenne pepper

$\frac{1}{4}$ teaspoon curry powder

$\frac{1}{4}$ teaspoon sea salt

3 tablespoons extra-virgin olive oil

$\frac{1}{4}$ cup freshly squeezed lemon juice

1 teaspoon lemon zest

2 tablespoons honey

2 stalks chives, snipped in 1" pieces

$\frac{1}{2}$ cup low-sodium vegetable broth

3 garlic cloves, coarsely chopped

6 baby bok choy

1 tablespoon sesame oil

Wash the scallops and pat dry with a paper towel.

In a small mixing bowl, mix the ginger, pepper, curry powder, and salt together. Season both sides of the scallops with the mixture.

Heat the oil in a large stainless steel sauté pan over medium-high heat. Place the scallops in the sauté pan, sides not touching (otherwise the scallops will steam, not caramelize). Cook, without moving the scallops, for 3 to 4 minutes, or until the bottoms of the scallops start to pull away from the pan and are a deep golden brown. Turn over, using tongs, and repeat on the second side. Transfer the scallops to a serving dish.

Add the lemon juice, lemon zest, and honey to the pan, whisking quickly for 1 minute, then pour over the plated scallops and top with the chives.

Add the vegetable broth and garlic to the sauté pan and return to medium-high heat, whisking any remaining caramelized scallop pieces from the bottom of the pan. Add the baby bok choy and simmer uncovered, turning occasionally, for about 8 minutes, or until the bok choy is tender, adding the sesame oil for the last 1 to 2 minutes of cooking.

Serve 6 scallops with 3 pieces of baby bok choy.

Per serving: 548 calories, 29 g total fat (4 g saturated), 60 mg cholesterol, 674 mg sodium, 945 mg potassium, 39 g carbohydrates (19 g sugar), 9 g fiber, 38 g protein

TIP: Pacific, Imagine Foods, Trader Joe's, and Whole Foods 365 brands all sell organic, gluten-free, low-sodium vegetable broth.

Get a Jump on Day 14

If you want to get a start on tomorrow's lunch, blanch the broccoli and celery from the "Creamy" Avocado-Broccoli Soup (follow the recipe on page 233, step one) and store in the refrigerator. When it's time for lunch, just get out the blender and go!

Day 13 Mind-Body Detox

KISS WORKOUT

The benefits of exercise are unparalleled—it improves heart health, diabetes, brain function, bone density . . . pretty much everything. If you're not already doing it, it is probably the most powerful step toward wellness you could possibly take (unless you're smoking—in which case, quitting is). If you've already got a routine, keep up the good work. If not, try my keep-it-super-simple (KISS) workout—the three-step bottom line for good health. Do it at least three times a week. Here's how:

1. **TAKE A BRISK WALK.** This is a no-brainer (see page 91 for more information on why you should do it). Walk briskly for a half hour. Aim to get your heart rate up to about 70 percent of its maximum capacity (calculate that by subtracting your age from 220, then multiplying by 0.70). Ballpark it at about 120 beats per minute, or about 20 beats in a 10-second count. You should be able to carry on a conversation, but only just.

2. **DO 20 PUSHUPS.** Classic pushups provide upper-body strength. You can do them with straight legs, on your knees, or against the wall—place your hands under your shoulders, bend your elbows back toward your hips, lower your body to the floor or wall, then extend your elbows and push your body away again. That's one rep. Don't worry if you can't do 20 full reps at first; start with just one or two if that's all you can do, and add one or two more each day. Don't stress, just get stronger.

3. **DO 60 CRUNCHES.** To build core strength, do this gentler and safer variation on the situp. Lie on your back with your legs bent and feet on the ground. Put your hands behind your head to support it. Tuck your chin slightly, contract your abdominal muscles, and curl your body up so that your shoulder blades just lift off the floor. Hold for a moment, then lower back down. That's one rep. You can do your 60 in three sets of 20—work up to the full number if need be. (*Note:* Keep your lower back on the floor and don't pull up on your neck—this is especially important if you have back problems.)

Day 14 Menu

BEVERAGE: Detox Tea (Dandelion, Burdock, or Chicory Root)

BREAKFAST: Buckwheat-Banana-Walnut Cereal

MIDMORNING SNACK: Smoothie, Juice, or Nut Milk

LUNCH: "Creamy" Avocado-Broccoli Soup

MIDAFTERNOON SNACK: Your Choice (see page 139)

DINNER: Black Bean and Spinach Tortilla and Salad

BREAKFAST

Buckwheat-Banana-Walnut Cereal

This hearty Buckwheat-Banana-Walnut Cereal will fully power you through the morning—no slump. With 10 grams of fiber to lower your net carbs, 13 grams of protein, 100 percent of your daily manganese, 51 percent of your daily magnesium (no headaches or muscle aches), 49 percent of your vitamin E, 43 percent of your calcium (who needs milk?), plus vitamin B$_6$, niacin, riboflavin, and thiamin for mood support, and cinnamon to lower your blood sugar, this recipe should replace your doctor's prescription pad.

MAKES 3 SERVINGS

2½ cups soy or nut milk (any nut milk recipe from 3-Day Turbo Cleanse)
1 stick cinnamon
1 cup buckwheat groats, rinsed
1 large banana, sliced
6 tablespoons walnuts, chopped

In a 1-quart saucepan over medium-high heat, add the soy or nut milk and cinnamon and bring to a boil, stirring frequently to avoid scorching on bottom.

Add the buckwheat, reduce the heat to a simmer, and cook for 30 minutes, or until the buckwheat is tender and all liquid is absorbed. Optional: If you like a thinner cereal, add more soy or nut milk as desired.

Remove and discard the cinnamon stick. Top each serving with ⅓ of the sliced bananas and 2 tablespoons of walnuts.

Per serving: 456 calories, 24 g total fat (2 g saturated), 0 mg cholesterol, 152 mg sodium, 719 mg potassium, 57 g carbohydrates (6 g sugar), 10 g fiber, 13 g protein

TIP: Look for a non-GMO soy milk, such as EdenSoy by Eden Foods (edenfoods.com). For a quicker morning cereal, you can use cream of buckwheat, prepared according to package directions.

LUNCH

"Creamy" Avocado-Broccoli Soup

Avocado gives this soup a creamy consistency. It's chock-full of B vitamins for mood support, cognition, neurological health, and phase II methylation support. With detox-inducing and cancer-fighting cruciferous phytochemicals to boot, "Creamy" Avocado-Broccoli Soup is the bomb.

MAKES 4 SERVINGS

1 large bunch broccoli florets and stems, chopped

2 stalks celery, chopped

1 large cucumber, peeled and deseeded

$\frac{1}{4}$ cup basil leaves, shredded

1 garlic clove, minced

1 slice (1") fresh ginger, peeled and chopped

1 teaspoon fresh thyme leaves

1 teaspoon fresh oregano, chopped

1 lemon, juiced

$\frac{1}{2}$ teaspoon lemon zest

$\frac{1}{4}$ teaspoon sea salt

2 avocados, halved and pitted, one half reserved

$\frac{1}{4}$ cup pine nuts, toasted

$\frac{1}{2}$ teaspoon cayenne pepper

2–3 cups water

In a 3-quart saucepan, bring salted water to a boil and blanch the broccoli and celery for 2 to 3 minutes. Drain immediately.

In a blender, add all the ingredients except 1 avocado half, the pine nuts, cayenne, and water.

Blend on high speed for 1 to 2 minutes. Turn the blender off and scrape the sides with a spatula as needed. Add the water, $\frac{1}{2}$ cup at a time, thinning to desired consistency.

(continued)

Transfer to serving bowls.

Toast the pine nuts in a dry sauté pan on medium-high heat for 30 to 60 seconds, stirring continually to avoid burning.

Slice the remaining avocado half and cut into cubes. Top the soup with avocado cubes, toasted pine nuts, and a pinch of pepper.

Per serving: 264 calories, 20 g total fat (2 g saturated), 0 mg cholesterol, 232 mg sodium, 1,210 mg potassium, 21 g carbohydrates (2 g sugar), 12 g fiber, 8 g protein

TIP: This soup is great hot or cold: Just use boiling water to make a warm soup and cold water for a cold soup.

DINNER

Black Bean and Spinach Tortilla

This dish could be renamed detoxitilla! It's high in thiamin, riboflavin, folate, and vitamin B_6, with D-glucaric acid and quercetin for glucuronidation, sulfur for sulfation, and free-radical-scavenging antioxidants A, C, and E.

MAKES 1 SERVING

1 tablespoon extra-virgin olive oil

2 tablespoons chopped onion

$\frac{1}{2}$ cup black beans, drained and rinsed

$\frac{1}{4}$ cup organic salsa, divided

2 corn tortillas

1 handful of spinach

1 teaspoon lemon or lime juice

$\frac{1}{2}$ avocado, pitted

Pinch of sea salt

In a small sauté pan, heat the oil over medium-high heat.

Sauté the onion, black beans, and 1 tablespoon of the salsa in the oil for 2 to 3 minutes. Transfer to a small bowl.

Place 1 tortilla in the sauté pan, top the tortilla with the onion-bean-salsa mixture, and add the spinach on top. Place the second tortilla on top and press down firmly. Cook for 2 to 3 minutes, checking the color underneath the bottom tortilla for browning. When the spinach is wilted and the bottom of the tortilla is golden brown, gently flip and cook an additional 2 to 3 minutes, or until golden brown.

Transfer to a plate. Slice with a pizza wheel.

Drizzle the lemon or lime juice into an avocado half, sprinkle with sea salt, and add the remaining salsa to the avocado. Serve the avocado alongside the tortilla.

Per serving: 564 calories, 31 g total fat (5 g saturated), 0 mg cholesterol, 251 mg sodium, 1,035 mg potassium, 62 g carbohydrates (6 g sugar), 22 g fiber, 15 g protein

Day 14 Mind-Body Detox

FIND A NEW SWEETENER

If you find yourself missing your old sugar habit, take a little time to consider deeply this question: What makes your life sweeter? Chances are, it's not just sugar. Think about all the little things that make you smile, or laugh, or bring you a feeling of lightness and ease. These are your own personal sweeteners, and you should keep them handy and use them liberally.

If you're not sure what those things are, make a list. Think about colors, music, animals, flowers, fragrances, words, actions, places, and things. A single red rose might sweeten your life better than a pound of chocolate ever could. A whiff of tangerine essential oil might be more elevating in the morning than a chocolate-frosted doughnut. A saucy samba might pick you up out of your afternoon slump more effectively than your usual afternoon candy bar. A snuggle with a child or a cat can satisfy a nighttime craving for sweetness.

The key is to really notice these other forms of sweetness and let them satiate you. The next time you find yourself reaching for a toxic sugary food, take your list out instead. Then reach for something truly nourishing to body and soul.

Get a Jump on Day 15

Tomorrow morning's Chia Porridge (page 243) is best if you make it the night before and let it soak overnight in the refrigerator. All you have to do then at breakfast is pull it out and let it sit at room temperature for 10 to 15 minutes in the morning before topping with blueberries. You can also prepare the Lentil-Walnut Pâté (page 244) for tomorrow's lunch. This dish is a savory, sophisticated flavor hit, so you might want to make some extra to share with hungry co-workers.

Check In with Yourself

You've got another week behind you. That's great work! You're almost there. Celebrate by taking time to check in with yourself and see how you're feeling.

Flip back to Chapter 2 and retake both the Medical Symptom Questionnaire (page 35) and the Environmental Factors Questionnaire (page 42). You should see marked improvements on both scales from last week.

Second, get out your journal. Review what you wrote when you started this plan (see page 91) and what you wrote down just last week. See what was making you feel bad then . . . and what was making you feel good. See how you felt about your successes and your frustrations. See how you've progressed (or not).

Then make a new inventory. How are you feeling now? What's your energy level? Do you see subjective changes in your feeling of wellness? In the way you look or feel or think? Do you feel happier or more level? Are you finding that the diet plan comes easily to you, or are you struggling with it? Are you learning about new foods? New cooking techniques? Are you enjoying yourself?

Use your journal as a safe space to put your feelings. Record all of your highs and lows. You've got a week left to go, so go ahead and do a little visualization. Using your experience from the last week, what would you wish for yourself for the next 7 days? How do you see it all coming together? What results are you hoping for? Write it all in your journal.

Then close your eyes and visualize yourself at the end of the Detox Prescription—a little happier, healthier, and leaner than you were when you started.

Keep on going. You can do it.

Tips for Eating on the Move

If you're in a time crunch—you are traveling or you need to grab something quick at the office—or dining out, you don't have to give up on your plan. Take Mary Beth's advice for making good on-the-go decisions.

Quick and Easy Foods

Here are some good quick meal options. Grab, spread, roll, toss—or some combination—and go. Choose from the following (and choose organic when you can):

- Gluten-free tortilla
- Brown rice cakes
- Gluten-free bread
- Vegetable spreads
- Chopped vegetables
- Cultured vegetables (like kimchi or sauerkraut)
- Leafy greens
- Avocado
- Julienned sun-dried tomatoes
- BPA-free canned organic beans
- Bean spreads
- Nuts and seeds
- Nut and seed butters
- Chopped fruits
- 100% fruit butters
- Unsulphured dried fruits
- Natural salad dressings
- Natural salsas
- Natural tapenades
- Natural chutneys
- Dried seaweeds
- Vegan cheeses
- Dairy-free yogurts
- Organic vegetarian soups (Kitchen Basics, Imagine Soups, Pacific, Trader Joe's, and Whole Foods 365 brands)
- Hard-boiled eggs (after week 1)
- Greek yogurt (after week 1)
- Fresh juice from juice bar
- Fresh dairy-free smoothie from juice bar
- Store-bought nut milks

ADD THOSE UP

Get creative in how you combine any and all of the above: Spread black bean dip, fruit salsa, and vegan cheese on a gluten-free tortilla and you have a New Wave Detoxitilla; chop hard-boiled eggs and a couple of celery sticks, mix with curry powder, dried raisins, a few cashews, and a bit of Greek yogurt for a Quick Curried Egg Salad; make a Brown Rice Super Stacker by layering hummus, avocado, sun-dried tomatoes, and sunflower seeds on a brown rice cake, and drizzling with a bit of yogurt. If all else fails, an Almond Butter and Fruit Butter on gluten free toast (an enlightened take on the classic PB&J) can be healthy, filling, and fast.

Out to Eat

When you are in a restaurant, don't panic. Breathe deeply, close your eyes, and recite Mary Beth's detox mantra: "Grains, greens, veggies, beans, fruits, seeds, nuts, and weeds." Now open your eyes, and look at the menu. These foods are probably on there somewhere. The trick is picking them out skillfully and eliminating all the toxic trappings (like wheat-based breads and fatty cheese) that often come with them. Enjoy a salad, construct a veggie plate, and remember that side dishes and appetizers can easily become entrees when you add them up. Also, most decent restaurants will be happy to work with your special needs—don't hesitate to explain that you'd like to stick with fresh plant-based, wheat-free foods and olive oils. You can even tell them you're a vegan—trust me, they've heard it before.

If you do feel the need for a protein-based entree, tofu and free-range chicken breast make good choices, as does grilled fish—especially if you know it's a clean catch. What's the best way to be sure? Consult the Seafood Selector at the Environmental Defense Fund's Web site, edf.org, or download the excellent Seafood Watch app from Monterey Bay Aquarium for up-to-date info.

Even if you're not able to do the best job, don't worry—having one less-than-perfect meal at a restaurant won't "retox" you. Just return to the diet ASAP.

On the Road

Many of the foods listed on the Fast and Easy Foods menu are available just about anywhere—from convenience stores to airports to hotel lobbies. But you can play it safe by carrying some of your favorites on the road with you—just store them in BPA-free plastic containers or freezer bags, and tuck them into suitcases or carry-ons. Dried fruits and trail mix are traveling must-haves! Also good for travelers:

Buckwheat or quinoa flakes (just add hot water for a healthy breakfast)

Gluten-free crackers

Shelf-stable boxed rice, nut, or soy milk

Organic 100% juice boxes

Gluten-free whole-foods nutrition bars (Kind, Pure, Bumble Bar, Raw Revolution)

Any of the protein powders (see page 102)

Any of the Rainbow Superfood Boosters (see page 103)

Meal replacement powders or bars (see page 305)

21-DAY CLEAN AND LEAN DIET MENU, WEEK 3

	Day 15	Day 16	Day 17
Beverage	Detox Tea (Dandelion, Chicory, or Burdock Root)	Detox Tea (Dandelion, Chicory, or Burdock Root)	Detox Tea (Dandelion, Chicory, or Burdock Root)
Breakfast	Chia Seed Porridge with Blueberries	Pumpkin-Oat Pancakes	Poached Egg–Avocado Tortilla
Midmorning Snack	Smoothie, Juice, or Nut Milk from 3-Day Menu	Smoothie, Juice, or Nut Milk from 3-Day Menu	Smoothie, Juice, or Nut Milk from 3-Day Menu
Lunch	Lentil-Walnut Pâté	Kale, Pecan, and Dried Cherry Salad with Rosemary Quinoa	Roasted Veggie and Hummus Romaine Wraps
Midafternoon Snack	Snack from "Grab and Go Snacks" (page 139)	Snack from "Grab and Go Snacks" (page 139)	Snack from "Grab and Go Snacks" (page 139)
Dinner	Broiled Wild Salmon with Cauliflower "Rice" and Salad	Tomato and Kidney Bean Soup with Maple-Sesame Oranges and Salad	Roasted Spaghetti Squash and Tomatoes and Salad

Day 18	Day 19	Day 20	Day 21
Detox Tea (Dandelion, Chicory, or Burdock Root)	Detox Tea (Dandelion, Chicory, or Burdock Root)	Detox Tea (Dandelion, Chicory, or Burdock Root)	Detox Tea (Dandelion, Chicory, or Burdock Root)
Tofu-Veggie Scramble with Gluten-Free Toast	Orange-Pecan-Millet Cereal	Twice-Baked Fruit-and-Nut-Stuffed Sweet Potatoes	Black Rice Porridge with Blueberries and Toasted Walnuts
Smoothie, Juice, or Nut Milk from 3-Day Menu	Smoothie, Juice, or Nut Milk from 3-Day Menu	Smoothie, Juice, or Nut Milk from 3-Day Menu	Smoothie, Juice, or Nut Milk from 3-Day Menu
Roasted Brussels Sprouts and Hazelnuts with Miso Soup	Tuna Niçoise and White Bean Salad	Green Gazpacho with Chive-Cayenne Oil and Tortilla Toasts	Red Quinoa–Avocado Salad
Snack from "Grab and Go Snacks" (page 139)	Snack from "Grab and Go Snacks" (page 139)	Snack from "Grab and Go Snacks" (page 139)	Snack from "Grab and Go Snacks" (page 139)
Quinoa with Asian Mushrooms and Black Truffle Oil and Salad	Spinach-Tofu Soup with Gluten-Free Garlic Crostini	Chickpea Burger with Tahini Dressing and Red Cabbage Slaw	Curried Mustard Greens with Lentils and Eggs and Salad

Day 15 Menu

BEVERAGE: Detox Tea (Dandelion, Burdock, or Chicory Root)

BREAKFAST: Chia Seed Porridge with Blueberries

MIDMORNING SNACK: Smoothie, Juice, or Nut Milk

LUNCH: Lentil-Walnut Pâté

MIDAFTERNOON SNACK: Your Choice (see page 139)

DINNER: Broiled Wild Salmon with Cauliflower "Rice" and Salad

BREAKFAST

Chia Seed Porridge with Blueberries

(BEST SOAKED OVERNIGHT)

Chia and chai are anagrams—and this chia porridge happens to taste great with chai spice. This dish builds bones, with a whopping 24 percent calcium when prepared with raw nut milk or 54 percent calcium when prepared with commercially purchased fortified organic nut milk. Let's not forget the fantastic fiber—17 grams of the stuff—to help keep you full, stabilize blood sugar and insulin levels, and promote fat-burning, not fat storage. Power breakfast indeed.

MAKES 2 SERVINGS

6 level tablespoons chia seeds

$1\frac{1}{3}$ cups nut milk

1 teaspoon herbal chai blend, optional

Nut milk or water, optional to thin porridge

$\frac{2}{3}$ cup blueberries

2 teaspoons maple syrup

In a small mixing bowl, mix the chia seeds, nut milk, and herbal chai blend (if using). Let the mixture sit refrigerated or at room temperature for at least 45 minutes (best if prepared in advance and soaked in refrigerator overnight) while it doubles in volume and becomes gelatinous.

Transfer to a serving bowl. If the chia has clumped, break up the clumps with a fork or spoon. Thin with additional nut milk or water, as needed, to desired consistency.

Top each serving of porridge with $\frac{1}{3}$ cup of blueberries and drizzle on 1 teaspoon of maple syrup.

Per serving: 250 calories, 11 g total fat (0 g saturated), 0 mg cholesterol, 123 mg sodium, 355 mg potassium, 28 g carbohydrates (9 g sugar), 17 g fiber, 10 g protein

TIP: Frontier Natural Products sells Indian Spice Tea (Herbal Chai) blend. Add a protein powder for a protein boost. Tastes great topped with apple butter, too.

LUNCH

Lentil-Walnut Pâté

This yummy pâté supports the liver as it detoxes your body, with phase I detox micronutrients (magnesium and iron), phase II detox methylation supporters (folate and vitamin B$_6$), free-radical-quenching antioxidants (vitamin C and manganese), quercetin and sulfur compounds (onion and garlic), and the glutathione inducers curcumin (turmeric) and carnosol (rosemary).

MAKES 6 SERVINGS

1 cup walnuts

4 tablespoons extra-virgin olive oil, divided

1 small onion, chopped

2 garlic cloves, chopped

1 teaspoon ground turmeric

1 tablespoon fresh rosemary leaves, roughly chopped

2 cups cooked red lentils

1 lemon, juice squeezed and reserved

½ teaspoon sea salt

6 endive leaves

In a small, dry sauté pan, toast the walnuts over medium-high heat for 3 to 4 minutes, or until lightly browned and fragrant, stirring frequently to avoid burning. Transfer to a food processor when done.

In a medium sauté pan, heat 2 tablespoons oil (reserving the remaining 2 tablespoons oil for later use) over medium-high heat, add the onion and garlic and sauté for 3 to 4 minutes, or until softened but not browned. Add the turmeric and rosemary and sauté for 1 to 2 minutes more. Transfer to a food processor when done.

Add the lentils, lemon juice, remaining olive oil, and sea salt to the food processor. Process the mixture to desired consistency—slightly chunky or smooth.

Spread ⅓ cup Lentil-Walnut Pâté on each endive leaf and serve with a cup of vegetable or miso broth (see page 264).

Per serving: 259 calories, 23 g total fat (3 g saturated), 0 mg cholesterol, 196 mg sodium, 258 mg potassium, 12 g carbohydrates (1 g sugar), 5 g fiber, 6 g protein

DINNER

Broiled Wild Salmon

With 2,000 milligrams of omega-3 fatty acids, Broiled Wild Salmon is a super inflammation tamer. Plus, because it also has 76 percent of your daily selenium, 37 percent of your daily C, bioflavonoids, and quercetin (lemon juice and peel), it's also an antioxidant delight. The 29 grams of protein here just round out an already well-rounded dish.

MAKES 4 SERVINGS

2 tablespoons extra-virgin olive oil, divided

2 teaspoons lemon peel

1 teaspoon coarsely ground black pepper

½ teaspoon sea salt

¼ teaspoon ground cayenne pepper

1 lemon, juiced

4 wild salmon fillets (4 ounces each)

Preheat the oven broiler. Brush a small baking sheet with 1 tablespoon of the oil.

With a mortar and pestle, mix the lemon peel, black pepper, salt, and cayenne pepper.

Mix the remaining 1 tablespoon oil with the lemon juice. Brush over the salmon fillets. Rub the lemon peel–spice mixture into the salmon flesh.

Broil the salmon for 6 to 8 minutes, depending upon thickness, or until easily flaked with a fork.

Per serving: 243 calories, 13 g total fat (2 g saturated), 0 mg cholesterol, 646 mg sodium, 761 mg potassium, 4 g carbohydrates (0 g sugar), 2 g fiber, 29 g protein

TIP: To add a little sweet and savory to the spicy cayenne pepper, add 1 tablespoon maple syrup and 1 tablespoon red miso paste to the lemon juice–olive oil mixture.

DINNER

Cauliflower "Rice"

The cruciferous cauliflower takes on the starring, low-carb, super-detoxifying role of rice in this appearance. Carotenoids, free-radical-quenching antioxidants (A, C, E, manganese), anti-inflammatory gingerol and capsaicin (ginger and cayenne pepper), quercetin and sulfur (onion and garlic), and methylation- and mood-supporting B vitamins make Cauliflower "Rice" a star in the nutrition firmament.

MAKES 6 SERVINGS

1 head of cauliflower, cored and leaves removed

$\frac{1}{4}$ cup extra-virgin olive oil, divided

1 medium onion, chopped

3 garlic cloves, chopped

1 red bell pepper, cut in $\frac{1}{2}$" cubes

1 yellow bell pepper, cut in $\frac{1}{2}$" cubes

2 carrots, cut in $\frac{1}{2}$" cubes

2 cups kale, shredded in small pieces

1 tablespoon wheat-free tamari

1 piece (1") fresh ginger, peeled and grated or pressed

1 teaspoon cayenne pepper

2 tablespoons sesame or peanut oil

In a food processor, process $\frac{1}{4}$ head of cauliflower into small, rice-size pieces. Transfer to a large mixing bowl and repeat with each remaining $\frac{1}{4}$ head of cauliflower.

In a large sauté pan or wok, heat 2 tablespoons of the olive oil over medium-high heat. Add the onion and garlic and sauté for 2 to 3 minutes, stirring often, being careful not to burn.

Add the bell peppers and carrots and sauté for 4 to 5 minutes, or until the vegetables are softened but not mushy. Remove from the heat and transfer to a mixing bowl.

Heat the remaining olive oil in the same sauté pan or wok and add the cauliflower, tossing and stirring for 5 to 6 minutes, to make sure the cauliflower toasts and water cooks out.

Return the cooked vegetables to the pan with the cauliflower. Add the kale, tamari, ginger, and cayenne pepper, combining thoroughly. Reduce to medium heat and sauté for 2 to 3 minutes to heat through.

Add the sesame or peanut oil, sauté for 1 to 2 minutes, remove from the heat, and serve.

Per serving: 203 calories, 14 g total fat (2 g saturated), 0 mg cholesterol, 236 mg sodium, 752 mg potassium, 18 g carbohydrates (2 g sugar), 6 g fiber, 5 g protein

TIP: Adding 2 scrambled cage-free organic eggs (whites only if you prefer less fat) to this dish would add 14 grams of protein power—add eggs after combining the kale, tamari, and ginger. Push the cauliflower rice to the outer sides of the sauté pan, make a small well in the middle of the pan, and stir in the scrambled eggs. Cook until soft, then combine with the cauliflower rice, add sesame or peanut oil, sauté for 1 to 2 minutes, and serve.

Day 15 Mind-Body Detox

TURN OFF YOUR HEAD BEFORE BED

Time for bed, but you can't turn off your head? Try the meditative technique known as *tratak*, or candle gazing. It's a nice way to transition from your bright busy day into the darkness and stillness necessary for restorative, detoxifying sleep. Here's how to do it:

Get yourself ready for bed. Make sure your room is cool and dark and that your sleeping space is clear and uncluttered. Then find a spot on the floor near your bed where you can sit comfortably in an upright position, propping your hips with cushions if need be.

Place a lighted candle on the floor in front of you, about 2 feet away from where you are sitting. Then dim or turn off all the other lights in the room.

Sit quietly and gaze at the candle, allowing your focus to soften and your peripheral vision to fall away altogether. Focus on the center of the flame, where it is slightly darker. Then move your focus to the edges of the flame. Finally, let your vision encompass the entire flame. Watch carefully as it dances in the unseen drafts in the room. Let your mind become fully absorbed—almost hypnotized—by the motion of this single flame. If your attention wanders, just return it to the flame. Don't try to stare without blinking—just let your looking be natural, an extension of your attention. If you need to move or cough, that's okay. Just keep watching the flame.

After 10 or 20 minutes, you can blow out the candle and go directly to bed. Or you can turn on some low lighting and do some restful evening activity.

Get a Jump on Day 16

Go ahead and make Pumpkin-Oat Pancakes (page 250) for tomorrow's breakfast; in the morning, you can pop them in the toaster to warm and crisp them! If you like, you can also prepare the Rosemary Quinoa (page 251).

Day 16 Menu

BEVERAGE: Detox Tea (Dandelion, Burdock, or Chicory Root)

BREAKFAST: Pumpkin-Oat Pancakes

MIDMORNING SNACK: Smoothie, Juice, or Nut Milk

LUNCH: Kale, Pecan, and Dried Cherry Salad with Rosemary Quinoa

MIDAFTERNOON SNACK: Your Choice (see page 139)

DINNER: Tomato and Kidney Bean Soup with Maple-Sesame Oranges and Salad

BREAKFAST

Pumpkin-Oat Pancakes

These Pumpkin-Oat Pancakes should get an A+ rating, not only because they are so delicious, but because they contain 96 percent of your daily vitamin A and are supercharged with carotenoids. Add the blood-sugar-lowering (cinnamon and fiber), antimicrobial (clove), anti-inflammatory (ginger), cholesterol-lowering (ginger), and analgesic (nutmeg) activity of the pumpkin pie spice, and these pancakes truly are food as medicine. Simple to make, too.

MAKES 12 TO 16 PANCAKES (2 PANCAKES PER SERVING)

3 teaspoons EnerG egg replacer + 4 tablespoons water (or 2 eggs)
1½-cups gluten-free rolled oats
1 cup vanilla coconut yogurt
½ cup organic canned pumpkin
1½ teaspoons aluminum-free baking powder
2 teaspoons pumpkin pie spice
1 teaspoon ground cinnamon

Mix the egg replacer and water together.

In a food processor, add the oats, yogurt, pumpkin, baking powder, pumpkin pie spice, and egg replacer mixture and process until smooth.

Heat a large oiled skillet over medium-high heat. Pour the batter into the skillet. When air bubbles cover the surface of the pancakes, flip and cook through.

Sprinkle the pancakes with a pinch of cinnamon before serving.

Per serving: 163 calories, 4 g total fat (1 g saturated), 0 mg cholesterol, 32 mg sodium, 258 mg potassium, 31 g carbohydrates (5 g sugar), 6 g fiber, 5 g protein

TIP: EnerG makes a starch-based thickening egg-replacement powder that is free of wheat, dairy, soy, nuts, sodium, and—you guessed it—eggs. Shop online at ener-g.com. To boost the protein power of this recipe (an additional 8 grams per serving), substitute organic Greek yogurt for the coconut yogurt and 2 egg whites for the egg replacer.

LUNCH

Kale, Pecan, and Dried Cherry Salad with Rosemary Quinoa

Get your detox on with this supercharged Kale, Pecan, and Dried Cherry Salad topped with warm Rosemary Quinoa. Quinoa is the most protein rich of all the grains. And this cruciferous combo containing the phenolic carnosol in the rosemary and the orange and lemon bioflavonoids in the Citrus Dressing make it a zesty detox trifecta.

QUINOA MAKES 3 SERVINGS (1 CUP EACH)

QUINOA

1 cup quinoa

2 teaspoons extra-virgin olive oil

2 cups water

1 garlic clove, mashed

1 teaspoon rosemary, chopped

$\frac{1}{4}$ teaspoon sea salt

SALAD MAKES 1 SERVING

SALAD

2 cups shredded kale

1 ounce pecans (20 pecan halves)

2 tablespoons unsweetened dried tart cherries, chopped

DRESSING MAKES 10 SERVINGS (2 TABLESPOONS EACH)

DRESSING

$\frac{1}{2}$ cup extra-virgin olive oil

4 lemons, squeezed/juiced (about $\frac{1}{2}$ cup lemon juice)

1 orange, squeezed/juiced (about $\frac{1}{4}$ cup orange juice)

1 teaspoon finely grated lemon zest

1 teaspoon finely grated orange zest

$\frac{1}{2}$ teaspoon freshly ground black pepper

$\frac{1}{4}$ teaspoon sea salt

(continued)

TO MAKE THE QUINOA: Rinse the quinoa in a fine-mesh strainer to reduce bitterness, and drain.

In a 2-quart saucepan, heat the olive oil over medium-high heat.

Add the drained quinoa to the oil, stirring until the water evaporates and the quinoa is lightly toasted to a golden color.

Add the water, garlic, rosemary, and salt to the saucepan and bring to a boil. Lower the heat to medium-low for a gentle simmer, cover, and cook for 15 minutes.

After 15 minutes, remove the quinoa from the heat and let stand for 5 minutes, covered. Fluff the quinoa with a fork and serve warm, 1 cup topped on the Kale, Pecan, and Dried Cherry Salad.

TO MAKE THE SALAD AND DRESSING: While the quinoa is cooking, mix the salad ingredients in a bowl.

Add the dressing ingredients to a shaker container or glass Mason jar.

Seal the container or jar and shake vigorously until blended.

Toss the salad with 2 tablespoons of dressing and refrigerate the remaining dressing for future use.

Per serving: 689 calories, 39 g total fat (4 g saturated), 0 mg cholesterol, 320 mg sodium, 828 mg potassium, 75 g carbohydrates (18 g sugar), 16 g fiber, 13 g protein

TIP: Grate more lemon and orange zest than you need, and save some peels and pectin-rich pith, too. Refrigerate leftover dressing for later use on salads, grains, and/or veggies—or add it to a little warm water to make a citrus detox tea.

DINNER

Tomato and Kidney Bean Soup with Maple-Sesame Oranges

This soup's got it all—the phytonutrient carotenoids, flavonoids, D-glucaric acid, quercetin, thiols, plus it's an excellent source of vitamin A, vitamin C, folate, and manganese and a good source of copper, iron, phosphorus, B_1, B_2, B_6, magnesium, and vitamin E. On top of all that, the spicy cayenne pepper kick and an amazing 12 grams of fiber rev your metabolism and signal your body to burn fat.

MAKES 4 SERVINGS

¼ cup extra-virgin olive oil

1 medium onion, chopped

3 garlic cloves

4 cups chopped tomatoes

2 teaspoons fresh thyme leaves

2 bay leaves

1 teaspoon cayenne pepper

3 cups low-sodium vegetable broth

2 cups canned red kidney beans, with juice, divided

¼ cup fresh basil, shredded

1 teaspoon white sesame seeds

1 teaspoon black sesame seeds

2 oranges, peeled and sectioned

2 teaspoons maple syrup

In a 3-quart saucepan, heat the oil over medium-high heat. Add the onion and garlic and sauté until translucent.

Add the tomatoes, thyme, bay leaves, and cayenne pepper and sauté until the tomatoes have reduced in size and are soft and mushy.

(continued)

Add the broth and 1 cup of the beans and simmer, uncovered, for 15 to 20 minutes. Remove the bay leaves when done simmering.

Use a handheld immersion blender or transfer to a blender and blend until desired consistency—partially chunky or smooth. Add the remaining kidney beans, return to a simmer, and simmer, uncovered, for 10 minutes.

During the final 2 minutes of cooking, add the shredded basil.

Toast the sesame seeds in a small dry skillet for 2 to 3 minutes, or until lightly browned and fragrant, stirring frequently to avoid burning. In a small mixing bowl, combine the orange sections, maple syrup, and toasted sesame seeds. Serve the soup accompanied by orange salad for a tart, savory, and sweet meal ending.

Per serving, soup: 294 calories, 15 g total fat (2 g saturated), 0 mg cholesterol, 559 mg sodium, 806 mg potassium, 34 g carbohydrates (2 g sugar), 12 g fiber, 9 g protein

Per serving, oranges: 120 calories, 2 g total fat (0 g saturated), 0 mg cholesterol, 1 mg sodium, 360 mg potassium, 27 g carbohydrates (21 g sugar), 5 g fiber, 2 g protein

TIP: Use Eden Organic BPA-free canned kidney beans in this recipe if you're short on time. Pacific, Imagine Foods, Trader Joe's, and Whole Foods 365 brands all sell organic gluten-free low-sodium vegetable broth.

Get a Jump on Day 17

Just relax—everything tomorrow is quick and easy, or totally hands-off cooking. But if you need more nut milk, now's a good time to make a batch.

Day 16 Mind-Body Detox

LOG YOURSELF OUT

It used to be that I recommended to my stressed-out patients that they turn off their TVs to reduce their access to bad news; now I tell them to log off of all their digital devices. Staying wired 24/7 keeps us receptive to news, both good (what we're hoping for) and bad (what we're more likely to get). We may have the best intentions to make ourselves available to family and friends, but we end up also making ourselves available to our employers, the news media, marketers, and all manner of other folks who may not have our best interests at heart. And when you look at these screens late at night, the EMFs coming from them are overly stimulating—making it harder for your brain to relax enough for you to fall asleep (insomniacs especially take note!).

These digital feeds can become a real addiction—you might not even realize how wired you really are, between your computer, mobile phone, and iPad. Checking these devices becomes habitual, receiving and returning texts automatic, updating our status a constant duty. Just stop—for an hour, for 2 hours, for an evening, for a day. The first time I did this, I did it by accident. I was traveling and lost my phone. I was in a total panic. What would I do? How would I survive? Did they even make pay phones anymore? Then it dawned on me: I was free! I could spend my time in the back of the taxi just sitting and breathing. I could be totally present for my lunch. At night, in my hotel room, I could read a book! It was incredible. I got my phone back the next day, but I'd stumbled on a powerful new practice—something I'd come back to again and again.

You might think this is impossible; it is not. The digital world will spin on without you. You might have a little anxiety that you'll be left out of the loop, what psychologists are now calling FOMO, or "fear of missing out." You won't. Messages will be left and will be waiting for you when you come back. But you will be surprised how empowered you feel by this time away from your online duties—empowered to be present with your family and friends and surroundings. I recommend you enjoy a window of digital-free time every day, maybe even a couple of times a day. Take a deep breath and remember: Real life happens in the real world. Be there for it.

Day 17 Menu

BEVERAGE: Detox Tea (Dandelion, Burdock, or Chicory Root)

BREAKFAST: Poached Egg-Avocado Tortilla

MIDMORNING SNACK: Smoothie, Juice, or Nut Milk

LUNCH: Roasted Veggie and Hummus Romaine Wraps

MIDAFTERNOON SNACK: Your Choice (see page 139)

DINNER: Roasted Spaghetti Squash and Tomatoes and Salad

BREAKFAST

Poached Egg-Avocado Tortilla

Studies reveal eggs contain the satiety (fullness) hormone PYY. Eating eggs for breakfast can suppress hunger and calorie consumption during the day.

MAKES 1 SERVING

½ avocado

2 pinches of sea salt

Juice of ¼ lime

1 teaspoon lemon juice

1 large egg

1 teaspoon extra-virgin olive oil

Pinch of cayenne pepper

1 corn tortilla

With a fork, mash the avocado in a bowl with a pinch of sea salt and the lime juice.

Fill a 1-quart saucepan with water, the lemon juice, and a pinch of sea salt and bring the water to a simmer.

Crack an egg into a small bowl or ramekin.

While gently stirring the water, add the egg to the water by tipping the egg in just above the surface of the water. Cook for 4 to 5 minutes, or until the egg white is semifirm but the yolk appears tender. Remove with a slotted spoon to a clean small bowl or ramekin.

Heat the olive oil and pinch of pepper over medium-high heat.

Warm the tortilla in the olive oil–pepper mixture on both sides for 30 seconds, and remove to a plate.

Top the tortilla with the mashed avocado and poached egg.

Per serving: 326 calories, 24 g total fat (4 g saturated), 0 mg cholesterol, 322 mg sodium, 589 mg potassium, 23 g carbohydrates (1 g sugar), 8 g fiber, 10 g protein

TIP: Add a mashed clove of garlic to the oil and cayenne pepper to boost the detox power of this recipe.

LUNCH

Roasted Veggie and Hummus Romaine Wraps

These wraps have as much protein as an egg, 8 grams of fiber, good fat, and good carbs. Methylation donors vitamin B$_6$, thiamin, and folate support energy production, mood and cognition, detoxification, and lower homocysteine levels to protect the heart. Carotenoids, vitamins A and C, and manganese quench free radicals, while capsaicin decreases inflammation and pain.

MAKES 4 SERVINGS

1 small eggplant (1 pound), cut into $\frac{1}{2}$"-thick slices

1 large red bell pepper, deseeded and cut in quarters

1 small red onion, cut in $\frac{1}{2}$"-thick slices

2 tablespoons extra-virgin olive oil, divided

1 tablespoon balsamic vinegar

$\frac{1}{4}$ teaspoon sea salt

$\frac{1}{4}$ teaspoon coarsely ground black pepper

$\frac{1}{8}$ teaspoon crushed red-pepper flakes

4 romaine lettuce leaves

1 cup store-bought organic hummus

Brush the eggplant, bell pepper, and onion with 1 tablespoon of the oil.

Heat the remaining 1 tablespoon oil in a large sauté pan over high heat. Sauté the vegetables for 3 to 4 minutes on each side, or until lightly charred, and transfer to a cutting board.

Chop the vegetables coarsely and toss with the balsamic vinegar, salt, black pepper, and red-pepper flakes.

Lay 1 romaine leaf flat, spread $\frac{1}{4}$ cup hummus in the leaf, top with $\frac{1}{4}$ of the vegetables, roll up the wrap, and cut on a diagonal.

Per serving: 212 calories, 13 g total fat (2 g saturated), 0 mg cholesterol, 388 mg sodium, 497 mg potassium, 20 g carbohydrates (0 g sugar), 8 g fiber, 7 g protein

DINNER

Roasted Spaghetti Squash and Tomatoes

You won't be missing pasta when spaghetti squash hits the plate. The tomatoes pop, the garlic pows, and the spices sizzle in this hearty, carotenoid-rich dish. Quercetin, thiols, sulfur compounds, D-glucaric acid, phase I supporters vitamin A, magnesium, copper, and iron, and phase II supporters thiamin, niacin, folate, and B$_6$ make this dish a detoxer's delight. Pasta-loving kids will embrace it.

MAKES 6 SERVINGS

1 spaghetti squash (4 pounds)

¼ cup extra-virgin olive oil, divided

2 teaspoons ground cumin

1 teaspoon coriander

12 plum tomatoes, halved with white center membrane removed

8 garlic cloves, peeled and thinly sliced

1 teaspoon sea salt

1 teaspoon coarsely ground black pepper

1 teaspoon crushed red pepper

8 sprigs thyme

¼ cup Italian flat-leaf parsley, chopped

Arrange 1 rack on the upper part of the oven and 1 rack on the lower part of the oven. Preheat the oven to 375°F.

Oil 2 rimmed baking sheets.

Cut the squash in half lengthwise, deseed, brush the inside of the squash halves with 2 tablespoons of the olive oil, and sprinkle on the cumin and coriander. Roast the squash face down on the baking sheet on the lower rack of the oven for 40 to 45 minutes.

Toss the tomatoes and garlic with the remaining 2 tablespoons olive oil. Spread the tomatoes cut side down on the second baking sheet. Sprinkle the salt, black

(continued)

pepper, and red pepper and layer the thyme on top. Roast the tomatoes on the upper rack for 25 to 30 minutes, or until the tomatoes start to shrink and wrinkle.

Remove the tomatoes, transfer to a chopping board, and drain any juices in a large mixing bowl. Chop the tomatoes coarsely and toss with the parsley in a mixing bowl.

Remove the squash from the oven. Scrape the squash flesh with a large fork, adding the strands to the mixing bowl until the squash flesh is all scraped out and only the hard flesh or rind remains. It should look just like bright yellow pasta. Toss the tomatoes and squash. Add additional olive oil as needed. Serve immediately.

Per serving: 174 calories, 10 g total fat (1 g saturated), 0 mg cholesterol, 440 mg sodium, 577 mg potassium, 22 g carbohydrates (5 g sugar), 5 g fiber, 3 g protein

TIP: Add a little Parma! vegan "cheese" for a tasty finishing touch—Original Parma!, Chipotle Cayenne Parma!, and Garlicky Green Parma! are all delicious (eatparma.com). You can also boost flavor and get a little vitamin B_{12} by sprinkling on some nutritional yeast, such as Bragg (bragg.com) or Red Star (redstaryeast.com). To increase the protein power of this meal, prepare and serve with 1 cup of Middle Eastern White Beans (page 154).

Get a Jump on Day 18

You can make your Roasted Brussels Sprouts and Hazelnuts (page 264) ahead of time, if you like. Replenish your store of Citrus Zinger Detox Dressing (page 145)—it's great served on salad alongside Quinoa with Asian Mushrooms and Black Truffle Oil (page 266).

Day 17 Mind-Body Detox

START THE PEACE PROCESS

There is no doubt that anger and resentment are toxic emotions—if you are carrying them around, you already know that. Forgiveness is the only known antidote, but that's easier said than done, especially if hurts run deep or have been carried for many years. There is no such thing as "just let go." Forgiveness is a process that you must engage with some effort, and sometimes sustain over time. Here's how you might approach it:

Tell your story. Get out your journal and write it all down: What happened, when it happened, how it happened. Who was involved, and what was said and done? Most important: How did you feel? Don't edit yourself, just try to capture the essence of the bad feeling you're holding on to.

See the other side. Next, imagine that you are the other person telling the story. What's the opposite point of view? What reasons might they have had? What conditions might have compelled them to act? What unseen forces might have been at play? This story doesn't have to be "right"—or even accurate—just plausible. Allow yourself to feel compassion for the other person, if you can.

Observe from the outside. Next, pretend you're a benevolent but disinterested third party observing the situation. Talk to yourself and the other party in the second person, naming both your negative feelings from the past and your desire for more positive feelings in the future. This exercise allows you to move out of the victim (you-did-this-to-me) stance and see the situation from a broader perspective.

Acknowledge any resistance. Envision that future time when forgiveness has already happened—you are past it, you have already moved on. Is some part of you screaming *no*? If so, why are you attached to this resentment? Will letting go of it mean redefining yourself in some essential way? If so, acknowledge that. You may have to work through it again to discover the root of your resistance. If you're truly stuck, you may need to seek counseling to get to the bottom of your attachment to the trauma.

Release your resentment. When you're ready to shed your resentment, you can mark the occasion. One way is to directly communicate with the forgiven—this can be a truly healing and liberating experience. If that's not possible, mark the occasion by writing your forgiveness on a piece of paper and either casting it into a fire or releasing it into a stream (make sure it's eco-friendly and biodegradable paper and ink, of course). Release it into the trash, if that's the best you can do. The idea is to marry a physical sense of release to your emotional intention as a way to seal the deal. You are free.

Day 18 Menu

BEVERAGE: Detox Tea (Dandelion, Burdock, or Chicory Root)

BREAKFAST: Tofu-Veggie Scramble with Gluten-Free Toast

MIDMORNING SNACK: Smoothie, Juice, or Nut Milk

LUNCH: Roasted Brussels Sprouts and Hazelnuts with Miso Soup

MIDAFTERNOON SNACK: Your Choice (see page 139)

DINNER: Quinoa with Asian Mushrooms and Black Truffle Oil and Salad

BREAKFAST

Tofu-Veggie Scramble with Gluten-Free Toast

You won't be missing scrambled eggs, because this tofu has a terrific tongue-tickling turmeric taste. It's antioxidant rich (manganese, zinc, vitamin C, and selenium) and has anti-inflammatory action (turmeric and scallions), anticancer activity (carotenoids, quercetin, sulfides), and more. Plus 57 percent of your daily calcium.

MAKES 2 SERVINGS

1 block firm tofu

2 tablespoons extra-virgin olive oil

2 scallions, chopped in 1" pieces

1 small green bell pepper, chopped in 1" pieces

2 plum tomatoes, seeded and cut in 1" pieces

$\frac{1}{2}$ teaspoon turmeric

$\frac{1}{2}$ cup shredded vegan Cheddar-style "cheese"

4 slices gluten-free bread

Extra-virgin olive oil, optional

B_{12}-fortified nutritional yeast, optional

Press the tofu block between paper towels to drain excess fluid. Crumble the tofu.

In a large sauté pan, heat the oil over medium-high heat. Sauté the scallions and pepper for 2 to 3 minutes, add the tofu, and sauté for an additional 3 to 4 minutes, or until the tofu is lightly browned.

Add the tomatoes and turmeric, stirring to combine well, and sauté for 5 to 7 minutes, or until heated through.

Remove from the heat, top with the vegan cheese, and cover for 2 to 3 minutes to allow the "cheese" to melt.

Toast the bread. Brush with olive oil (if using) and sprinkle on the yeast (if using).

Per serving: 270 calories, 19 g total fat (3 g saturated), 0 mg cholesterol, 248 mg sodium, 414 mg potassium, 26 g carbohydrates (1 g sugar), 5 g fiber, 17 g protein

TIP: For a lower-carb meal, skip the toast and serve the tofu scramble over wilted spinach or Swiss chard.

LUNCH

Roasted Brussels Sprouts and Hazelnuts with Miso Soup

Unbeknownst to many, the mustard seed is also in the cruciferous family (along with mustard greens). The kelp and kombu seaweeds are heavy-metal "chelators"—they bind metals such as copper, lead, and arsenic. Add the bioflavonoids, citrus pectin, and quercetin in the grapefruit, and you've got three detox powerhouses in this dish. Pair the sweet maple syrup with the tart grapefruit and the rich and indulgent hazelnut, and all your senses will be satisfied.

MAKES 4 SERVINGS

1 pound Brussels sprouts

$\frac{1}{4}$ cup extra-virgin olive oil

1 large red grapefruit, juice and pulp

2 tablespoons maple syrup

$\frac{1}{2}$ teaspoon sea salt

$\frac{1}{4}$ teaspoon coarsely ground black pepper

$\frac{1}{8}$ teaspoon ground mustard

1 cup hazelnuts

4 cups water

3 tablespoons white miso paste

2 teaspoons kelp and kombu flakes

1 scallion, sliced in $\frac{1}{2}$" pieces

Preheat the oven to 375°F. Oil the bottom of a 13" x 9" baking pan.

Cut the stems from the Brussels sprouts and remove any wilted or brown leaves.

In a large mixing bowl, whisk together olive oil, grapefruit juice, maple syrup, sea salt, black pepper, and mustard and toss with the Brussels sprouts. Spread the Brussels sprouts in a single layer in the baking pan, drizzling in all remaining dressing in the mixing bowl.

Roast the Brussels sprouts for 40 to 45 minutes, stirring every 10 to 15 minutes, or until fork-tender.

While the Brussels sprouts are roasting, spread the hazelnuts in a single layer on a rimmed, dry baking sheet. Roast for 8 to 10 minutes, or until lightly browned and fragrant, being careful to avoid burning.

While the hazelnuts are roasting, boil the water. Whisk in the miso paste, kelp and kombu flakes, and scallion. Cover and reduce the heat to warm.

Toss the hazelnuts and Brussels sprouts together before serving.

Accompany each serving of Roasted Brussels Sprouts and Hazelnuts with 1 cup of miso soup.

Per serving: 443 calories, 32 g total fat (3 g saturated), 0 mg cholesterol, 729 mg sodium, 846 mg potassium, 38 g carbohydrates (10 g sugar), 9 g fiber, 9 g protein

TIP: Frontier Natural Products (frontiercoop.com) and Simply Organic (simplyorganic.com) sell organic nonirradiated ground mustard. Maine Coast Sea Vegetables (seaveg.com) sells wild Atlantic kelp and kombu flakes. If you want to get results even quicker, Trader Joe's and most natural food stores sell natural miso soup packets—just add hot water, and voilà!

DINNER

Quinoa with Asian Mushrooms and Black Truffle Oil

Immune-enhancing beta-glucan, rich mushrooms, and anti-inflammatory garlic and ginger make this a must-eat dish, while the indulgent and rich truffle oil makes you forget all about meat and keeps you focused on the plant kingdom.

MAKES 4 SERVINGS

2 cups enoki mushrooms, whole (or substitute cremini mushrooms)

2 cups low-sodium vegetable broth

1 cup quinoa

3 tablespoons extra-virgin olive oil

3 garlic cloves, grated

2 teaspoons grated ginger

2 cups shiitake mushrooms, sliced thick (or substitute baby portobellos)

2 tablespoons black truffle oil

Clean the enoki mushrooms gently by swishing in a bowl of water.

In a 1-quart saucepan, add the broth and bring it to a boil. Stir in the quinoa, reduce the heat to low, cover, and simmer gently for 15 minutes, or until the quinoa is tender and translucent.

While the quinoa is cooking, heat the olive oil in a large sauté pan over medium-high heat. Add the garlic and ginger and sauté for 1 to 2 minutes, being careful not to burn.

Add the enoki and shiitake mushrooms and sauté for 4 to 5 minutes, or until the mushrooms are softened but not mushy (not more than 7 to 8 minutes).

Reduce the heat to low, stir in the truffle oil, and sauté for 1 to 2 minutes more.

Transfer the quinoa to a serving bowl. Top with the mushrooms, using a spatula to transfer the oil onto the quinoa. Toss lightly and serve immediately.

Per serving: 349 calories, 20 g total fat (2 g saturated), 0 mg cholesterol, 74 mg sodium, 235 mg potassium, 36 g carbohydrates (5 g sugar), 4 g fiber, 8 g protein

TIP: Topping each serving with a scrambled or poached egg adds 7 grams of protein per serving. A few spoonfuls of the Korean cabbage kimchi on top add some fermented and spicy sizzle to this exotic dish.

Day 18 Mind-Body Detox

PUT YOUR LEGS UP A WALL

Restorative yoga postures can be a good stand-in for sleep on days when you just haven't had enough rest. Never plan for less than 7 hours a night, but when insomnia strikes, do all you can to get your body the rest it needs to de-stress and detoxify. One of my favorite restorative poses is Legs-Up-the-Wall Pose, also known as *Viparita Karani.* Because the legs are extended over the heart, this is an inverted posture that lets the legs take a rest. It calms the mind very effectively (especially if you use props to make yourself warm and comfortable in the pose) and can relieve mild backache. Here's how to do it:

Place a yoga bolster, if you have one, or a couch cushion, or a firm pillow lengthwise along a wall. Sit on the end of the cushion and roll onto your back so that your hips come onto the cushion and your legs rotate directly over the hips and up the wall (you'll be positioned with your back perpendicular to the wall). The hips can be an inch or two away from the wall; the feet can be together or hip-distance apart, whichever feels more comfortable to you.

Roll your shoulders away from your ears and relax your arms out to your sides with the elbows bent in "cactus arms." Roll the head gently from side to side until you find that sweet spot where absolutely no tension is needed to support its weight. Then release all effort, and allow the weight of your upper body to sink into the floor. You can cover your eyes with a beanbag, if you like, or a folded washcloth.

Stay in the pose for 5 to 15 minutes; set a timer, if you like, so that you don't have to keep checking. When it's time to come out of the pose, bend your knees, roll onto your right side, push away from the wall and off the bolster. Pause for a moment in fetal position on your right side. Then push yourself up to a seated position. Take a moment to enjoy the refreshed, relaxed after-effects of Legs-Up-the-Wall Pose.

Get a Jump on Day 19

Cook the Orange-Pecan-Millet Cereal (page 269) for tomorrow's breakfast. You can also make the Spinach-Tofu Soup with Gluten-Free Garlic Crostini (page 271).

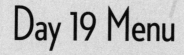

Day 19 Menu

BEVERAGE: Detox Tea (Dandelion, Burdock, or Chicory Root)

BREAKFAST: Orange-Pecan-Millet Cereal

MIDMORNING SNACK: Smoothie, Juice, or Nut Milk

LUNCH: Tuna Niçoise and White Bean Salad

MIDAFTERNOON SNACK: Your Choice (see page 139)

DINNER: Spinach-Tofu Soup with Gluten-Free Garlic Crostini

BREAKFAST

Orange-Pecan-Millet Cereal

Cardamom belongs to the ginger family and is likewise anti-inflammatory. Cinnamon lowers blood sugar; the orange bioflavonoids, quercetin, and citrus pectin support detox; and the dates provide antioxidants and carotenoids. And with 7 grams of fiber, this cereal may expand your stomach and fill you up, but it will help shrink your waistline due to its effect on reducing blood sugar and insulin's effect on abdominal fat storage.

MAKES 4 SERVINGS

1 cup millet

3 cups boiling water

2 oranges, juice and pulp

4 Medjool dates, pitted and finely chopped

1 cinnamon stick

6 green cardamom pods

Extra water as needed

1 cup pecans, coarsely chopped

In a large skillet, toast the millet over medium-high heat, stirring constantly, for 3 to 4 minutes, or until lightly browned and fragrant.

Transfer the millet to a 2-quart saucepan. Add the water, orange juice and pulp, dates, cinnamon, and cardamom and bring to a boil. Reduce the heat to a gentle simmer, cover, and simmer for 30 to 40 minutes, stirring occasionally, until the millet is tender and translucent. If the millet is getting too thick and sticking to the bottom of the saucepan, add extra water as needed.

Remove the cinnamon stick and cardamom pods. Transfer to serving bowls and top with pecans.

Per serving: 327 calories, 22 g total fat (2 g saturated), 0 mg cholesterol, 1 mg sodium, 378 mg potassium, 32 g carbohydrates (15 g sugar), 7 g fiber, 5 g protein

TIP: To up the protein of this recipe, top with ⅓ cup Greek yogurt or use nut milk for cooking water.

LUNCH

Tuna Niçoise and White Bean Salad

Full of lean protein, good fats, and low net carbs, this lunch is an excellent source of vitamin B_{12} and iron, a good source of the bone-building minerals magnesium and calcium, and has phytonutrients galore.

MAKES 2 SERVINGS

4 cups mixed greens

1 cup cherry or grape tomatoes, halved

½ cucumber, sliced and scored

10–12 organic olives, kalamata, black, or green

½ cup white beans

1 jar (6 ounces) tuna in olive oil, drained, with 1 tablespoon oil reserved

¼ cup freshly squeezed lemon juice

2 tablespoons balsamic vinegar

½ teaspoon lemon peel

¼ teaspoon ground mustard

½ teaspoon coarsely ground black pepper

1–2 tablespoons fresh thyme, chives, and/or oregano, optional

12–16 gluten-free crackers, optional

Toss the mixed greens, tomatoes, cucumber, olives, and beans together.

Whisk the olive oil reserved from the tuna, lemon juice, balsamic vinegar, lemon peel, mustard, and black pepper. Toss with the salad.

Top with the tuna and fresh herbs (if using) and serve with 6 to 8 gluten-free crackers (if using).

Per serving: 323 calories, 11 g total fat (2 g saturated), 53 mg cholesterol, 285 mg sodium, 621 mg potassium, 27 g carbohydrates (2 g sugar), 7 g fiber, 30 g protein

TIP: Tonnino tuna is sold in glass jars and is wild caught, hand packed, and dolphin safe. Other sustainable wild-caught tuna in BPA-free cans include Vital Choice (vitalchoice.com), Wild Planet, and Rain Forest Trading.

DINNER

Spinach-Tofu Soup with Gluten-Free Garlic Crostini

This soup melts in your mouth and tastes decadently creamy but has none of the pro-inflammation compounds in animal-based cream. The garlic crostini add some zing and crunch as well as anti-cancer, anti-inflammatory, and detox support. An excellent source of eight nutrients (vitamins A and C; manganese; vitamins B_1, B_2, B_3, and B_6; and selenium) and a good source of eight additional nutrients (folate, magnesium, calcium, copper, iron, phosphorus, vitamin E, and vitamin B_{12}), this is a superfood, super soup recipe!

MAKES 4 SERVINGS

FOR THE SOUP

- 10 oz frozen spinach, thawed, pressed, and drained
- $\frac{1}{4}$ cup extra virgin olive oil
- 1 medium onion, chopped
- 3 garlic cloves, chopped
- 2 carrots, chopped in $\frac{1}{4}$" cubes
- 2 celery stalks, chopped in $\frac{1}{4}$" cubes
- $\frac{1}{2}$ teaspoon crushed red pepper flakes
- 2 cups low-sodium vegetable broth
- 1 low-sodium vegetable bouillon cube or 1 teaspoon vegetable bouillon powder
- 12 oz block silken firm tofu
- 1 cup organic non-GMO unsweetened soy milk
- 1 teaspoon curry powder
- Salt and pepper, to taste

FOR THE CROSTINI

- 4 slices gluten-free bread, such as Italian, crusts removed and quartered
- 2 teaspoons olive oil
- 2 teaspoons chopped garlic
- $\frac{1}{8}$ teaspoon coarse sea salt
- $\frac{1}{4}$ teaspoon coarsely ground black pepper
- 2 teaspoons B_{12} fortified nutritional yeast

(continued)

Preheat the oven to 350°F.

TO MAKE THE SOUP: Press the spinach between paper towels and drain well.

Heat the oil in a large sauté pan over medium-high heat. Add the onion, garlic, carrots, and celery and sauté 4 to 5 minutes, stirring often to avoid burning.

Add the spinach and crushed red pepper flakes, adding more oil as necessary, and sauté 5 to 6 minutes, stirring often to avoid sticking and browning.

Add the broth and bouillon cube or powder and bring to a boil. Reduce to a simmer and cook uncovered for 15 to 20 minutes.

In a blender, combine the tofu, soy milk, and curry powder, and blend until completely smooth.

Reduce the soup to low-medium heat. Spoon in the blended tofu and soy milk mixture. Use a handheld immersion blender as needed for smooth consistency. Heat for 4 to 5 minutes until heated through. Add salt and pepper to taste.

TO MAKE THE CROSTINI: While the soup simmers, brush both sides of gluten-free bread quarters with the olive oil and garlic, and sprinkle with the salt and pepper. Arrange on a rimmed baking sheet, and bake 10 to 15 minutes, flipping the crostini once when tops are golden, after 7 to 8 minutes. When both sides are done, remove them from the oven and sprinkle with the nutritional yeast.

Serve the soup with the crostini in bowls.

Per serving (soup): 250 calories, 17 g total fat (2 g saturated), 0 mg cholesterol, 180 mg sodium, 552 mg potassium, 15 g carbohydrates (4 g sugar), 5 g fiber, 11 g protein

Per serving (crostini): 113 calories, 4 g total fat (1 g saturated), 0 mg cholesterol, 181 mg sodium, 132 mg potassium, 17 g carbohydrates (0 g sugar), 2 g fiber, 3 g protein

TIP: GoBio sells organic, gluten-free, yeast-free, MSG-free, non-GMO, additive-free vegetable broth powder in bouillon cubes and as powders in glass jars. Go-Buy-o it (all puns intended) now!

Day 19 Mind-Body Detox

TAKE A BATH

Trouble unwinding at night? Try an age-old remedy: Take a bath.

A warm bath really is incredibly relaxing for mind and body. Add Epsom salts and you get the added benefit of magnesium, which will unwind muscular tension and soothe frazzled nerves. Up the relaxing ambience further by adding a few drops of lavender essential oil. Inhale deeply—in studies, lavender has been shown to improve depression and insomnia, as well as to calm the restlessness associated with anxiety. Aromatherapy really works.

Of course, there are other ways to make your bath time a luxurious, self-indulgent, special experience—dim the lights, play special music, light a few candles, or add organic bubbles (such as Deep Steep's Lavender Chamomile Bubble Bath, deepsteep.com). You might even consider adding your significant other to the mix; though it's not as relaxing, maybe, you'll benefit from the bonus of human connection. Any way you play it, a nice long bath provides premium "me" time—unplugged, unclothed, and undistracted. All you need to do is let your stress soak away.

Get a Jump on Day 20

Prepare Twice-Baked Fruit-and-Nut-Stuffed Sweet Potatoes (page 275) for tomorrow's breakfast. You can work all the way through the recipe, and when you are done, just wrap them up in the aluminum foil you used to cook them in and store them in the refrigerator. In the morning, pop them in a warm oven while you get ready for work, and enjoy a naturally sweet, nutritious breakfast before you go. (These carry well for lunches, too.) You can also assemble the Green Gazpacho (page 276)—just be sure to store it in the refrigerator in a glass or stainless steel bowl, not aluminum, which will react with the tomato juice. Make the Red Cabbage Slaw (page 280) for tomorrow's fabulous Chickpea Burgers. You'll have a busy evening, but an easy day tomorrow.

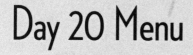

Day 20 Menu

BEVERAGE: Detox Tea (Dandelion, Burdock, or Chicory Root)

BREAKFAST: Twice-Baked Fruit-and-Nut-Stuffed Sweet Potatoes

MIDMORNING SNACK: Smoothie, Juice, or Nut Milk

LUNCH: Green Gazpacho with Chive-Cayenne Oil and Tortilla Toasts

MIDAFTERNOON SNACK: Your Choice (see page 139)

DINNER: Chickpea Burger with Tahini Dressing and Red Cabbage Slaw and Salad

BREAKFAST

Twice-Baked Fruit-and-Nut-Stuffed Sweet Potatoes

This dish is a sight for sore eyes. It contains 138 percent of daily vitamin A, 36 percent of daily vitamin C, and 13 percent of daily zinc—nutrients that decrease macular degeneration. The 8 grams of fiber here reduce the net carb content of this dish.

MAKES 4 SERVINGS

4 medium sweet potatoes

1 apple, cored and cubed

1 ounce orange juice or lemon juice

4 tablespoons unsulphured raisins

1 cup pecans, roughly chopped

2 tablespoons extra-virgin olive oil

$\frac{1}{4}$ teaspoon ground ginger

$\frac{1}{4}$ teaspoon pumpkin pie spice or cinnamon

Preheat the oven to 400°F.

Poke several holes in the sweet potatoes. Wrap in foil, place directly on the oven rack, and bake for 45 minutes, or until fork-tender.

In a small mixing bowl, combine the remaining ingredients.

When the sweet potatoes are fork-tender, remove from the oven and increase the oven temperature to 450°F.

Unwrap the foil, cut a long slit in the center, and with a fork gently mash and fluff the interior sweet potato flesh. Stuff the fruit, nut, and spice mixture into the center of each sweet potato. Loosely wrap foil around the sweet potato sides, but leave the stuffed center open. Return the sweet potatoes to the oven for 10 to 15 minutes, or until the fruit and nut stuffing is heated through and slightly browned.

Per serving: 420 calories, 29 g total fat (3 g saturated), 0 mg cholesterol, 42 mg sodium, 788 mg potassium, 41 g carbohydrates (20 g sugar), 8 g fiber, 5 g protein

TIP: Prepare a few extra potatoes and serve as a quick snack drizzled with molasses and with a dab of organic goat cheese, sliced and rewarmed for breakfast or tossed into a smoothie (like our Carotenoid Smoothie, page 122).

LUNCH

Green Gazpacho with Chive-Cayenne Oil and Tortilla Toasts

This green gazpacho is a tantalizing blend of sweet, cool, minty, spicy, and hot flavors that meet, fall in love, and then get married in your mouth. Fourteen daily vitamins and minerals, plus an almost two-to-one ratio of potassium to sodium, and the diuretic action of cucumbers makes this an inflammation tamer and a no-brainer for water retainers.

MAKES 4 SERVINGS

CHIVE-CAYENNE OIL

MAKES $\frac{1}{3}$ CUP OR 6 TABLESPOONS

$\frac{1}{3}$ cup extra-virgin olive oil

$\frac{1}{4}$ cup chives, coarsely chopped

$\frac{1}{4}$ teaspoon cayenne pepper

TORTILLA TOASTS

4 small corn tortillas

$\frac{1}{4}$ teaspoon sea salt

GREEN GAZPACHO

5 medium cucumbers, peeled, deseeded, and chopped in $\frac{1}{2}$" cubes

1 large yellow bell pepper, cut in $\frac{1}{2}$" cubes

$\frac{2}{3}$ cup scallions, chopped in $\frac{1}{2}$" pieces

1 large ripe avocado, scooped

1 cup water, plus additional as needed

3 tablespoons lemon or lime juice

2 tablespoons extra-virgin olive oil

2 garlic cloves, minced

3 tablespoons fresh mint, chopped

$\frac{1}{2}$ teaspoon sea salt

1 teaspoon ground coriander or cumin

Preheat the oven to 350°F and line a large baking sheet with parchment paper or brush with olive oil.

To make the chive-cayenne oil: In a mini-chopper, blender, or food processor, puree the oil, chives, and cayenne on high speed.

To make the tortilla toasts: Brush 1 teaspoon chive-cayenne oil on each tortilla (oil both sides), reserving the remainder of the chive-cayenne oil for garnish. Cut the tortillas into eighths with a pizza wheel. Arrange on a baking sheet and sprinkle with the sea salt. Bake the tortilla chips in the oven for approximately 10 minutes, or until crisp. Remove from the oven and reserve the tortilla chips for garnish.

To make the green gazpacho: Toss together $\frac{1}{3}$ cup each of the chopped cucumber, bell pepper, and scallions. Reserve for garnish.

Place the remaining ingredients, except the chive-cayenne oil and reserved chopped vegetables, in a large blender or food processor and blend until smooth. Add additional water, $\frac{1}{4}$ cup at a time, as needed to thin to desired consistency.

Transfer the gazpacho to 4 serving bowls. Serve topped with $\frac{1}{4}$ cup reserved cucumber, pepper, and scallion mix. Drizzle 1 teaspoon chive-cayenne oil on top. Add 8 tortilla chips.

Per serving: 364 calories, 27 g total fat (4 g saturated), 0 mg cholesterol, 453 mg sodium, 869 mg potassium, 29 g carbohydrates (5 g sugar), 8 g fiber, 5 g protein

TIP: Sprinkle 1 or 2 tablespoons nutritional yeast, such as Bragg (bragg.com) or Red Star (redstaryeast.com) on the tortillas before baking for a faux "cheesy" taste and a B_{12} boost!

DINNER

Chickpea Burger with Tahini Dressing and Red Cabbage Slaw

This hearty and flavorful chickpea burger puts meat hamburgers to shame. It's got lean protein, low net carbs, good fats, and a healthy dose of fiber. It's an excellent source of vitamins A and C, manganese, folate, and vitamin B6, and a good source of iron, phosphorus, vitamin E, copper, and thiamin, making it a winner in the burger wars.

MAKES 6 "BURGERS"

4 tablespoons extra-virgin olive oil, divided

$\frac{1}{2}$ small onion, chopped

3 garlic cloves, chopped

1 medium red bell pepper, chopped

1 teaspoon ground cumin

$\frac{1}{2}$ teaspoon cayenne pepper

1 can chickpeas (15 ounces), drained, rinsed, and patted dry

$1\frac{1}{2}$ teaspoons EnerG egg replacer + 2 tablespoons water mixed together (or 1 egg)

$\frac{1}{2}$ cup gluten-free bread crumbs (use additional as needed)

6 cups mixed greens

10–12 tablespoons Lemon-Tahini Dressing (page 145)

6 cups Red Cabbage Slaw (page 280)

Heat 2 tablespoons of the oil in a small sauté pan over medium-high heat. Add the onion, garlic, and bell pepper and sauté for 3 to 4 minutes, stirring often to avoid burning. Add the cumin and cayenne pepper and sauté for 1 to 2 minutes more. Remove from the heat and transfer to a food processor.

Add the chickpeas to a blender and process until all ingredients are combined into a thick, chunky mash. Transfer to a mixing bowl.

Add the egg replacer–water mixture (or egg) and bread crumbs to the mixing bowl and mix with your hands until everything is blended. If needed, add 2 tablespoons bread crumbs to the chickpea-vegetable mixture—the mixture should be "sticky."

Divide into 5 or 6 patties of desired size. In a large skillet or grill pan, heat the remaining 2 tablespoons olive oil over medium heat. Cook the burgers for 3 to 4 minutes, until golden, then flip and cook for 3 to 4 minutes more.

Serve each chickpea burger on a cup of mixed greens topped with 2 tablespoons Lemon-Tahini Dressing and accompanied by 1 cup Red Cabbage Slaw.

Per serving: 327 calories, 21 g total fat (3 g saturated), 0 mg cholesterol, 442 mg sodium, 265 mg potassium, 30 g carbohydrates (1 g sugar), 6 g fiber, 7 g protein

TIP: EnerG makes egg-replacement powder that is free of wheat, dairy, soy, nuts, sodium, and—you guessed it—eggs. Shop online at ener-g.com.

Red Cabbage Slaw

The ruby-colored crown jewel of the cruciferous vegetable family, Red Cabbage Slaw is a good-fat, low-carb detoxer's dream with its high content of sulfur for phase II sulfation, quercetin for glucuronidation, bioflavonoids and citrus pectin for toxin binding, and vitamins A and C, manganese, and thiols for antioxidant activity and free-radical quenching. It doesn't get better, or tastier, than that.

MAKES 8 SERVINGS

$\frac{1}{2}$ cup freshly squeezed orange juice

$\frac{1}{4}$ cup freshly squeezed lime juice

$\frac{1}{2}$ small red onion, chopped

$\frac{1}{4}$ cup fresh basil leaves, shredded

1 tablespoon apple cider vinegar

$\frac{1}{2}$ cup extra-virgin olive oil

1 teaspoon honey

1 teaspoon coriander

$\frac{1}{2}$ teaspoon orange zest

$\frac{1}{2}$ teaspoon sea salt

$\frac{1}{2}$ teaspoon coarsely ground black pepper

$\frac{1}{2}$ head red cabbage, finely shredded

With a handheld immersion blender, blend the juices, onion, basil, vinegar, oil, honey, coriander, zest, salt, and pepper.

In a mixing bowl, toss the dressing with the cabbage.

Refrigerate for at least 30 minutes before serving.

Per serving: 157 calories, 14 g total fat (2 g saturated), 0 mg cholesterol, 165 mg sodium, 233 mg potassium, 9 g carbohydrates (5 g sugar), 4 g fiber, 1 g protein

TIP: Best refrigerated overnight to allow the flavors to fully develop.

Day 20 Mind-Body Detox

MAKE EVERY DAY THANKSGIVING

Take a moment before you eat to give thanks for your food. Prayer is a powerful healing force—a tremendous body of medical literature demonstrates its effectiveness as an intervention for everything from AIDS to congestive heart failure to cancer. A new round of studies has demonstrated that it can work wonders—even when a patient has no idea he or she is being prayed for.

But I think the real benefit is for the person praying, in that prayer offers a chance to connect to something beyond and bigger than ourselves. This bigger thing might be God, it might be consciousness, it might be the universe, it might be science, it might be nature, or it might be humankind itself. What you envision is not as important as the act of envisioning it. No matter how you slice it, creation is a miracle—and there is no better time to stop and appreciate it than before you sit down to eat.

Food sustains and nourishes our bodies. It also connects us intimately to the cycles of nature, the health of the planet, and—for city folk, anyway—to the efforts of many other human beings—from the farmers to the shippers to the grocers. We have much to be thankful for with every bite . . . especially if we don't have to struggle, suffer, or fight for every meal. Pausing to offer prayerful appreciation for our food promotes a kind of mindfulness and connection that can help digestion not only on the physical level but on the spiritual level, too.

Get a Jump on Day 21

Go ahead and make tomorrow's Black Rice Porridge (page 283) and store in the fridge overnight. If you like your nuts crunchy, add them just before breakfast.

Day 21 Menu

BEVERAGE: Detox Tea (Dandelion, Burdock, or Chicory Root)

BREAKFAST: Black Rice Porridge with Blueberries and Toasted Walnuts

MIDMORNING SNACK: Smoothie, Juice, or Nut Milk (see page 139)

LUNCH: Red Quinoa-Avocado Salad

MIDAFTERNOON SNACK: Your Choice (see page 139)

DINNER: Curried Mustard Greens with Lentils and Eggs and Salad

BREAKFAST

Black Rice Porridge with Blueberries and Toasted Walnuts

People in Asian countries typically consume rice in a porridge or gruel consistency, also known as "congee." Congees can be eaten plain or may contain fish, meat, vegetables, or fruits. Individuals with digestive difficulties typically tolerate congee's well-cooked, soft, easily digestible consistency. The beauty of this dish is the blueberry-stained black rice adds an exotic-looking, totally delightful, flavonoid-rich start to your morning.

MAKES 4 SERVINGS

½ cup Thai black rice

2 cups unsweetened coconut milk (or other nut milk or soy milk if preferred)

1 cup water, plus additional as needed

2 cups blueberries

½ vanilla bean, split, seeds scraped and reserved, or 1 teaspoon vanilla extract

1 cup walnuts

In a 2-quart saucepan, bring the rice, coconut milk, and water to a boil. Reduce the heat to a gentle simmer and cook, covered, for 40 minutes, stirring occasionally.

During the last 10 minutes of cooking, check to see if additional water is needed.

During the last 5 minutes of cooking, add the blueberries and vanilla bean seeds or extract.

While the blueberries simmer, toast the walnuts in a small dry skillet over medium heat for 2 to 3 minutes, stirring constantly to avoid burning, or until golden brown and fragrant.

Serve immediately, topped with ¼ cup toasted walnuts.

Per serving: 267 calories, 19 g total fat (4 g saturated), 0 mg cholesterol, 20 mg sodium, 216 mg potassium, 22 g carbohydrates (11 g sugar), 4 g fiber, 6 g protein

TIP: Order black rice online at Tropical Traditions (tropicaltraditions.com).

LUNCH

Red Quinoa–Avocado Salad

Here, the slightly nutty, crunchy quinoa and melt-in-your-mouth avocado contrast beautifully with an explosion of minty-citrusy-honey flavor. Beyond all that tastiness, there's plenty to support detox: copper, magnesium, and iron for phase I, and folate and vitamin A for phase II. That's to say nothing of the recipe's array of phytonutrients and essential fatty acids.

MAKES 4 SERVINGS

3 cups red quinoa

2 cucumbers, sliced lengthwise and cubed

2 avocados, pitted, peeled, sliced, and cubed

½ cup fresh mint, roughly chopped

¼ cup extra-virgin olive oil

2 tablespoons freshly squeezed lemon juice

2 tablespoons balsamic vinegar

2 tablespoons honey

8 cups mixed greens

Sea salt, optional

Pepper, coarsely ground, optional

Prepare the quinoa according to package directions.

In a large mixing bowl, chop the cucumbers and avocados and add to the mint.

In a small mixing bowl, whisk together the oil, lemon juice, balsamic vinegar, and honey. Pour over the cucumbers, avocados, and mint. Combine gently.

Plate 4 plates with 2 cups mixed greens and ¾ cup cooked quinoa. Top with the cucumber, avocado, and mint mixture. Season with salt and coarsely ground pepper to taste (if using).

Per serving: 475 calories, 31 g total fat (5 g saturated), 0 mg cholesterol, 44 mg sodium, 780 mg potassium, 46 g carbohydrates (9 g sugar), 14 g fiber, 10 g protein

TIP: If you're not a fan of mint, try using Italian parsley or basil instead.

DINNER

Curried Mustard Greens with Lentils and Eggs

Detoxifying, anti-inflammatory, antimicrobial, cholesterol-lowering, and belly-fat-fighting (11 grams of fiber!) activity abounds in this supercharged, supergreen dish.

MAKES 4 SERVINGS

2 cups black (or any color) lentils

2 tablespoons extra-virgin olive oil

1 medium onion

3 garlic cloves

2 tablespoons minced fresh ginger

$\frac{1}{4}$ cup organic tomato paste

2 tablespoons curry powder

1 teaspoon crushed red-pepper flakes

6 cups mustard greens

2 tablespoons water

$\frac{1}{2}$ cup low-sodium vegetable broth

4 eggs

Sea salt, optional

Pepper, optional

Prepare the lentils according to package directions.

Heat the oil in an extra-large sauté pan or wok over medium-high heat. Sauté the onion, garlic, and ginger for 2 to 3 minutes, until translucent.

Add the tomato paste, curry powder, and red-pepper flakes. Sauté for 1 to 2 minutes, or until the spices are fragrant. Add the mustard greens and water, stirring often, and sauté for 4 to 5 minutes, or until the mustard greens begin to wilt.

Add the broth and cooked lentils and sauté for 4 to 5 minutes, until the greens and lentils are heated through. Transfer to a covered serving dish.

Rinse the sauté pan, brush generously with oil, return to medium heat until the oil sizzles, and crack the eggs into the pan. When the white is solid, swiftly but gently flip with a spatula and allow 30 to 40 seconds for the white to set. Transfer the eggs to a serving dish atop the greens. Season with salt and pepper (if using).

Per serving: 263 calories, 13 g total fat (3 g saturated), 186 mg cholesterol, 256 mg sodium, 965 mg potassium, 24 g carbohydrates (3 g sugar), 11 g fiber, 17 g protein

TIP: Pacific, Trader Joe's, and Whole Foods all sell organic, gluten-free, low-sodium veggie broth.

Day 21 Mind-Body Detox

VISUALIZE A PEACEFUL PLACE

Meditation isn't the answer for everyone. For some people, visualization feels better. Rather than working to clear the mind by focusing on the breath or a mantra, visualization works by actively creating a rich inner tapestry of sensation—sights, sounds, smells, feelings—aimed at creating a relaxation response. There are many good guided visualization audio programs out there, but you can also create your own experience. I suggest imagining a time and place when you were surrounded by comfort in nature, completely at peace and feeling at home in the world. It may have been at the beach, in the desert, playing in a field, walking through a forest, or sitting by a mountain stream. Then use your mind to re-create and focus on the scene—noticing every little detail.

I like to use meditation based on a walk through the woods, which I offer here as an example. You might use this, if the woods also have a positive association for you; if not, use it as a guideline for creating your own visualization. (I work through this scene while listening to a recording of nature sounds, which help me feel immersed in the experience.)

A Walk in the Woods

You are strolling through a wooded glade
On a path covered with soft pine needles
Nearby, you hear the babbling of a clear mountain stream
All around you, you see dappled light shining through the trees
The air is warm, but crisp—it is early autumn
The trees around you are robed in glorious color
Regal red, deep orange, and clear, bright yellow
Hear the breeze rustle through the treetops
Listen as the birds and insects sing to each other
From the corner of your eye, you see them flit from branch to branch
There is a sense of magic in the air, as if fairies are at play nearby
As you inhale the clean, fragrant air, you feel it supercharging your body
The smell of pine, maple, and a distant fire soothe your mind
With every step, you feel more connected to this wood, to this place
You are safe in the arms of your own Mother Earth.

You Did It!

Congratulations on completing the entire Detox Prescription. There is absolutely no reason you can't keep on going with this plan for another week or two or three . . . or for the rest of your life. The 21-Day Clean and Lean Diet was designed to be doable for the long term.

You can get back to your real life and still stick with the principles we've outlined here: Eat a diet that is centered on vegetables, fruits, and whole grains; choose organics whenever you can; make the menu colorful, spicy, and broadly sourced; and keep animal proteins to a minimum (erring on the side of the highest quality and lowest fat).

If you want to return to eating a little more animal protein or maybe having a couple of drinks a week, or even a slice of birthday cake now and again, you can do that without spiraling out of control: Moderation is the key to maintaining your good health. If you overdo a bit, don't give up. Rather, just remember your long-term goal of feeling and looking your best, and pick up where you left off. You can return to the 3-Day Turbo Cleanse any time you need a "tune-up," then add in the rest of the 7-Day In-Depth Detox—doing it once or twice a year can really help you stay in touch with your commitment to living a clean lifestyle.

Now that the Detox Prescription is completed, you should definitely take time to retake both the Medical Symptom Questionnaire (page 35) and the Environmental Factors Questionnaire (page 42). You should now see wonderful improvements on both scales from the time you started the plan.

To review your progress, take out your journal. Look at what you wrote when you started this plan (see page 91) and what you wrote at every step along the way—at the end of the 3-Day Turbo Cleanse, at the end of the 7-Day In-Depth Detox, and last week, midway through the 21-Day Clean and Lean Diet. Where were you then? And where are you now?

You should see a serious arc of improvement. You've been through a lot, you've learned a lot, you've done a lot for yourself over the last 3 weeks. How do you feel about it? How is your energy level? Did you lose weight? Do you look better? Are you less anxious or depressed? Do you have less fatigue or fogginess? Are you now experiencing fewer headaches, or stomachaches, or allergy symptoms? Is your skin clear? Are you feeling less bloated? Is your digestion running well?

Take a minute to write down every one of your "wins"—the ways in which you are feeling better. Once you've done this, take inventory of your wishes. Is there room for improvement? Is there anything you're still struggling with in terms of pesky symptoms? If you haven't gotten all the results you wanted, don't panic. There is still more you can do.

Stick with the diet plan outlined in the 21-Day Clean and Lean Diet, and turn to Chapter 8 to go Beyond the Detox Prescription.

beyond the detox prescription

Once you've finished the Detox Prescription, you should be feeling remarkably better. If you'd like to get a read on just how much better, it's a good time to turn to page 35 and take the Medical Symptom Questionnaire again—if you didn't already do that. You should notice a significant improvement across the board from the first time you took the test.

It's completely possible, however, that you're still dealing with troubling symptoms in one or two areas. If so, you may need to take additional steps to detoxify your body and keep your health moving in a positive direction. That's what this chapter is all about: taking things to the next level. Nothing here is a substitute for any part of the plan in the preceding pages. But if you feel strongly that you want to continue with the detoxifying diet laid out in Chapter 7 *and* kick things up a notch by adding in smart supplements, more intensive lifestyle practices, and adjunctive therapies, you can do a lot—and possibly get incredible results.

I say "possibly" because it really all depends on what is going on with you. I don't hesitate to state outright that the Detox Prescription is helpful for nearly everyone, but neither do I claim that it's any kind of miracle cure. If you have an underlying condition, such as parasitic infection, Lyme disease, hormone imbalance, or chronic fatigue syndrome, you will need to seek the help of a qualified physician to address that problem directly. (See "Do You Need Further Testing" on page 32 for a more comprehensive list of conditions to talk to your doc about.) Chronic conditions such as heart disease and diabetes might well have improved over the course of the Detox Prescription, but it will take more work to reverse or eliminate them entirely. You cannot detox all your health problems away. I wish it were that simple; it is not.

What you *can* detox away is that general malaise—achiness, weight gain, mental fogginess, fatigue, mild depression—that sometimes keeps you from seeing what is really going on. Sometimes, when the fog lifts, it becomes clear what the true underlying complaint really is. That's a good thing for you—and a good thing for your physician, who can now help you in a more targeted way. Take the new energy you have derived from 3 weeks of eating healthy whole foods and use it to get yourself going on a healing plan, working with people who can truly help you. That's the most helpful next step you can take.

I am a firm believer in finding a practitioner who is versed in functional medicine—be it a medical doctor (MD), naturopath (ND), osteopath (DO), nurse practitioner (NP), or other licensed health care provider. Functional medicine doctors are trained to combine the best of Western medicine with nutritional therapy and the integrative approaches laid out in this chapter. They are the best resource for dealing with chronic conditions. If you don't already have access to such a person, you can find one near you using the excellent database of the Institute for Functional Medicine (functionalmedicine.org).

If there's no such health concern and you still want to go further—or if you're working in conjunction with a knowledgeable health care provider and want to do even more to increase your odds of healing—consider the following options. There are nine of them, and certainly you don't have to do all of them. They're not cumulative, and you don't get bonus points for heaping them on. Rather, read through this chapter and see what might apply to you, specifically. Then add them to your already cleaned-up diet and lifestyle.

1. Make Meditation a Priority

If you've gotten through all 21 days of the Detox Prescription diet but haven't settled into a regular meditation practice, make this your first priority. If you want to get more hard-core results, you will have to delve beyond the physical for them. The mind is the most powerful healing tool you have. Period. By actively working to release dysfunctional patterns of mental and emotional stress, we can finally free the body from the sympathetic nervous system's overdrive, and from the cascade of endogenous toxins (hormones, free radicals, etc.) associated with nonstop exposure to stress hormones. Of all the lifestyle changes you can make, the single most powerful is gaining control of your mind. This will improve your general state of well-being and help put an end to common complaints, such as headaches, IBS, musculoskeletal pain, and allergies. But to stop the madness, you have to stop the madness.

Theoretically, it shouldn't be hard to do. Your meditation practice doesn't have to be strict, New Agey, or religious in nature. Chapters 5, 6, and 7 are filled with Mind-Body Detox meditation techniques for you to try—if you skipped over these, go back and read them now. Walking meditation (page 195), mantra repetition (page 162), breathing techniques (pages 13 and 89), thought clearing (page 132), visualization (page 286), mindful eating (page 155), and candle gazing (page 248) are all good ways to focus attention, engage the calming parasympathetic nervous system, unwind stress, and begin to teach the mind how to be present in a peaceful, easy, less-toxic way. Each of these techniques is simple to grasp and do. Try them on for size; if you find one that seems to fit, do it every day. You don't have to do it for long to see results. Setting aside just 10 minutes can make a big difference (or in the case of the breathing exercises, just four or five rounds can do for a start).

If all else fails, try this simple exercise: Sit down, shut your eyes, focus on your breath, and count to 42. You don't have to do anything to change your breathing, just notice it. Keep your attention focused on it. Breathe in, breathe out—that's one. Breathe in again, breathe out again—that's two. If your mind wanders, just bring it back. Don't hurry, but don't slow things down either. Find a natural rhythm that feels good. If you lose your focus or find that your mind has wandered, no big deal. Start over again.

Stick with this exercise until you can make it through 42 breaths. It might feel uncomfortable at first, even difficult. Your mind will serve up its objections and distractions—that's what minds do. But in meditation, you learn that you don't have to react to these thoughts. They are just thoughts, which come and go, the good ones and bad ones. Behind those thoughts is the real you—a more solid, stable presence that can't be touched by stressful thinking.

If you like gadgetry and want to meditate the high-tech way, that's an equally valid path, by the way. There are plenty of Web sites, Blu-rays, podcasts, and apps dedicated to helping you transcend the merely technical difficulties of everyday living. My favorite is the app Headspace (getsomeheadspace.com), a progressive program of daily guided meditations, along with podcasts and some really clever support videos that explain the process.

2. Do an Elimination Diet

The next thing to do is get a handle on the foods that might be undermining your health without your even knowing it. The Detox Prescription is an excellent way to eliminate common trigger foods from your diet—it is completely free of wheat and gluten and all inflammatory red meats. The first 7 days are also free from dairy and eggs—which are limited throughout the entire 21 days. During this time, you may have seen a big change. If these were problematic foods for you when you started the plan, even if you didn't realize it before you started, you may have seen dramatic or even near-miraculous results while off them. (Hopefully, you saw our advice on page 183 in Chapter 7 to pay attention when you added each new food back to your diet, and noticed when and if you hit a trouble spot. If not, read on.)

There are two main types of reactions to food: allergies and sensitivities. **Food allergies** are just that—allergic reactions wherein the immune system identifies a food as a foreign invader and mounts an attack on it, unleashing the inflammatory cascade. Symptoms can be as subtle as an itchy tongue or throat, or as overt and life-threatening as anaphylactic shock, as can happen with peanut or shellfish allergies. If you experience severe and immediate symptoms after eating a particular food, this is an **IgE allergic reaction**—the kind of allergy that is in your face and relatively easy to diagnose. You eat a food, you react directly—it's pretty clear.

But there is another kind of food allergy, an **IgG allergic reaction**, wherein symptoms may be much less pronounced and can take 2 or 3 days to develop. With IgG reactions, it's much trickier to make the connections to particular foods—in part because so much time may have elapsed from the time you ate the food until a reaction is evident. Symptoms of this type of food allergy are often vague and insidious (and in some ways pretty close to that foggy malaise I just described): fatigue, allergies, headaches, joint pain, gastrointestinal distress, and rashes are common. Because these symptoms are associated with so many other issues—including general toxicity—it is impossible to say whether they definitely herald a food allergy.

Meanwhile, **food sensitivities** aren't allergies at all. Rather, they have to do with the body's hyperreactivity to certain components of foods. The allergic response is not involved, and yet food sensitivities can cause very real physical problems for the body—including damage to the walls of the small intestine, setting the body up for leaky gut syndrome, a condition in which proteins and toxins can pass through the intestinal lining when they shouldn't. Two common and highly problematic sensitivities are dairy and gluten intolerance—the latter of which can actually lead to toxic consequences for the brain, as recorded in multiple studies published in neurological journals. Food sensitivities can be serious.

You can take medical tests that will show you when you are reacting to a food as an allergen. Besides the classic skin tests, which are less accurate for foods than for inhaled allergens, there are blood tests—chief among them the whole-blood ALCAT test available through Cell Science Systems, IgE and IgG antibody testing available through Genova Diagnostics or Metametrix Clinical Labs, or the ELISA/ACT available through ELISA/ACT Biotechnologies. Few food sensitivities can be tested at all (dairy and gluten being notable exceptions).

If you suspect a food sensitivity, or if it's not clear whether you're experiencing an allergy or a sensitivity (wheat and dairy can cause both types of reactions, for instance)—you can diagnose it yourself by testing within the laboratory of your own body using an elimination diet (See "Food Elimination Strategies," page 296) followed by a food challenge. An elimination diet will reveal both allergies and sensitivities.

You can't eliminate everything, of course—even though it's true that even the most mild-mannered foods can pose big problems for some people. What you can do is look at the categories with the most risk of food allergy.

Eliminate these all at once if you want, or do them one group at a time to check for results. Please note that you'll need to be off the food *for at least 3 weeks* to know for sure.

COMMON FOOD TRIGGERS

Anyone who is experiencing symptoms that they would describe as frequent, chronic, or daily should seriously consider whether the foods they eat frequently or daily may be contributing to the problem. Along with wheat, dairy, and eggs, here are a few other common culprits.

• **SOY FOODS:** These include soybeans, milks, tofu, and many processed health foods. Read labels carefully.

• **NUTS:** Peanuts, macadamias, pecans, walnuts, almonds, cashews, pistachios, Brazil nuts. Nut allergies can be quite severe—as with the peanut allergy epidemic we are seeing among children.

• **FISH AND SHELLFISH:** Especially shrimp.

• **CORN:** Corn is one of the "big eight" food triggers, along with soy, wheat, peanuts, tree nuts, dairy, shellfish, and eggs. It's a tough one to uncover, because unfortunately corn is everywhere—as a whole grain, as corn syrup (which is ubiquitous as high-fructose corn syrup), and as cornstarch. You will have to read labels like crazy to eliminate this one, but it can be life changing if you discover a problem and are able to address it.

Certain food groups that share a chemical constituent are often overlooked. These can be very important triggers of inflammation and physical disease and should be considered if you are suffering from headaches (especially migraines), allergies and asthma, skin rashes, joint pain, or digestive complaints.

• **NIGHTSHADE VEGETABLES:** This category of vegetables—which includes tomatoes, potatoes, eggplants, tomatillos, and both sweet and hot peppers—contains a naturally occurring class of toxic alkaloids (primarily solanine and chaonine). Nightshades may be a problem for anyone experiencing joint pain or digestive symptoms. (Interestingly, tobacco is also a nightshade and contains the alkaloid nicotine. Vegetables also contain nicotine, but not as much as tobacco!)

• **HISTAMINES:** Histamines are produced by the natural breakdown of the amino acid histidine in the food aging process. Foods that are fermented, aged, or stale may have high histamine content. Common suspects include processed or cured meats, cheese, canned fish, chocolate, vinegar, alcohol, some nuts, and common condiments like ketchup, mustard, and soy sauce. Histamines are a common trigger for migraine headaches.

• **TYRAMINES:** Tyramines are produced by the natural breakdown of the amino acid tyrosine in the food aging process. As with histamines, foods that are fermented, aged, or stale may have high tyramine content. Cheese, wine, nuts, seeds, and pickled vegetables may be particularly problematic. Tyramines are also a common trigger for migraine headaches.

• **SULFITES:** Sulfites are a group of sulfur compounds commonly added to enhance or preserve packaged or processed food. They may be present in dried fruits, nuts, trail mix, baked goods, wine, beer, and many condiments. Read labels carefully—if you see "sulf," stay away. Sulfites are a common trigger for respiratory and skin dysfunctions.

• **SALICYLATES:** Salicylates are naturally occurring compounds found in many vegetables, fruits, nuts/seeds, and herbs and spices. Basically, they are a kind of natural pesticide and as such are concentrated in higher amounts in the skin and peels of vegetables and fruits. (Salicylates can also be found in preservatives, perfumes, and medications, including aspirin.) To eliminate this, remove all rinds and peels from your produce and cut out dried fruits, oranges, grapes, plums, pineapples, and tangerines. Salicylates are a common trigger for respiratory and skin dysfunctions.

• **YEAST:** Many people feel much better when they cut out foods that are leavened, flavored, or fermented with yeast. This includes solid baked (baker's yeast) and liquid (brewer's yeast), as well as other nutritional yeasts, but excludes baked goods leavened with baking soda (e.g., Irish soda bread, biscuits, and pancakes, though these are not exactly health foods). Sourdough made with naturally occurring yeast and lactobacillus bacteria also contains some potentially irritating yeast species. On ingredient labels, look for "autolyzed" or "hydrolyzed" yeasts. The main yeast-containing culprits include breads, alcohol (especially wine and beer), vinegar (and anything containing vinegar such as ketchup and mustard), soy sauce, pickles, cheese, some dried fruits and mushrooms (which may have natural yeasts on their surface), the probiotic saccharomyces, and even some gravies, broths, and canned soups. Fermented foods can cause general symptoms such as fatigue, headache, joint and muscle aches, irritable bowel, and rashes.

Food Elimination Strategies

An elimination diet is a straightforward process: Decide what food, or group of foods, you want to test, then eliminate it entirely from your diet for 3 or 4 weeks. This might take a little research and label reading. In some cases, you might have to be proactive and ask about the source and treatment of your food—for instance, whether dried fruits from a health food store bin were treated with sulfites or not.

• While you are eliminating, start keeping a food and symptom diary. This is a good habit in general, and it will give you a place to record both what you ate and how it made you feel. Record any symptoms and cravings you're experiencing, too. Write down what time you ate or drank, and what you ate or drank. Record the time symptoms occur, and watch for trends. Does your mouth itch every time you eat an eggplant? (You might be sensitive to nightshades.) Do you start itching or even break out in hives whenever you drink chamomile tea? (It's in the ragweed family.) This exercise will help you identify your triggers and link them to reactions, and it will give you a baseline to look back on when you reintroduce the food.

• Once the elimination period has passed, you want to reintroduce one food at a time to your diet in a fairly intensive way—you are trying to provoke a response you can notice, after all. (Or not—hopefully, the latter.)

• Choose the food you want to test and eat it frequently over the course of 2 days. If you're testing nuts, have peanut butter on rice cakes for breakfast, walnut milk for lunch, a handful of almonds for a snack, and maybe a cashew curry for dinner. Then keep an eye on your responses for the next 1 to 2 days. Watch head to toe for any kind of negative reaction—for headaches, allergies or stuffy sinuses, scratchy throat, heartburn, wheezing, GI complaints, diarrhea and/or constipation, skin rashes, fatigue, increased depression, confusion, or anxiety. All of these might be caused by, or exacerbated by, food allergies or sensitivities. Take copious notes.

• If by the end of the third day you have logged no response, the food is probably okay for you. If you have noticed a small response but you're not sure or wonder if it could be coincidental, wait a few more days, then reintroduce the food. It should be clear whether or not it causes a reaction. Refer to your diary to compare notes.

• If you find you are having a reaction, you also have a cure: elimination. The best way to treat a food allergy or sensitivity is with avoidance. This used to be the only way. However, over the last few years, allergists have pioneered a technique sublingual desensitization, in which the specialist gives you minute—but ever-increasing—doses of the food you are reactive to, and over time, allergies and sensitivities decrease. Talk to your doctor about whether it's an option for you.

3. Add Integrative Therapies

The next step, in my opinion, is to consider integrating some helpful holistic and mind-body therapies—once considered alternative and now part of the standard integrative armamentarium. These are invaluable in terms of healing and can be a great way to relieve or eliminate problematic symptoms—or even get to the root cause of the symptoms, as is always preferable.

Many integrative therapies work, too, as a path for relaxation and self-discovery and are therefore invaluable for anyone seeking to live a less-toxic lifestyle. I am not discounting their very real therapeutic effects—however, in each of these instances, practitioners consider the body on an energetic as well as a mechanical/physical level. When you work with them, you may be introduced to new ways of thinking about your life and your self, and you will probably learn new ways to engage your mind and body. These are good things, in almost every case. (If you have a practitioner you don't like, or who is not taking the time to explain what he or she is doing, it can work against you—exercise your right to leave treatment at any moment.)

You might have to do a little exploration to find what is right for you; you may want to try something entirely new (and not listed here) based on what's available in your area and who is doing it. So long as your primary care provider agrees, or you're not experiencing debilitating symptoms, it's fine . . . as long as you feel good about it, it makes you feel good, and you can afford it. A few of my favorite alternative therapies include:

HOLISTIC THERAPIES

TRADITIONAL CHINESE MEDICINE (TCM) AND AYURVEDA: These are two prominent examples of ancient healing modalities—from China and India. They are, in fact, entire medical systems, with branches including herbalism, massage, diet therapy, exercise, and bodily manipulation. Whereas Western medicine tends to focus on problem solving around a set of symptoms, both TCM and Ayurveda create a diagnosis based on your own constitutional body type, as well as the energy patterns prevailing in your life.

In TCM, this energy is called chi, and it is moved powerfully through the practice of acupuncture, the placing of thin needles along the energy channels (meridians) of the body. I have found in my practice of it for the last 25 years—and studies have now confirmed—that acupuncture is incredibly helpful in dealing with any kind of musculoskeletal pain, from lower-back pain to carpal tunnel syndrome. It's also effective for IBS, headaches, and reducing addictions—to name a few from a very long list.

Ayurveda focuses more on striking a balance in the vital energies of the body, called *doshas*—*vata*, which is airy creative energy, *pitta*, which is fiery focused energy, and *kapha*, which is earthy stable energy. Whereas TCM uses needles to manipulate the body, Ayurveda uses massage therapy to move energy—to stimulate, calm, or pacify as needed. (FYI: Ayurveda also focuses intensively on detox—in fact, some Ayurveda centers offer something called *panchakarma*, which might involve diet, supplements, enemas, and other purgative therapies.)

Both of these systems have vast herbal traditions, largely focused on healing and bitter herbs—which are among the most powerful healing tools on the planet. Both also prescribe individualized diet, exercise, and meditation regimens designed to promote perfect harmony of mind and body. Keep an open mind. You can learn a lot and leave with some life-changing tools. Find a practitioner of TCM and/or acupuncture at the National Certification Commission for Acupuncture and Oriental Medicine (nccaom. org); find a practitioner of Ayurveda at the National Ayurvedic Medical Association (ayurvedanama.org). Many states have formal licensure for acupuncturists, but not for practitioners of Ayurveda: *caveat emptor.*

HOMEOPATHY: Based on the principle of "like cures like," homeopathy works by using a minuscule dose of a substance that would in larger doses aggravate or even cause the symptoms it is treating. Simplistically, it works like a vaccination to help the body to overcome a problem. It's a controversial idea, but one that's been around since the 1800s, when it was crystallized by the German physician Samuel Hahnemann, who was reacting to the harsh medical treatments of his day, including bloodletting and deliberate poisoning with mercury and arsenic. (Fascinating trivia: He was a contemporary of Edward Jenner, an English scientist who was at the same time experimenting with less-dilute live substances from cow infections to vaccinate against human disease—cowpox vs. smallpox.)

Over the last 2 decades, dozens of published articles have shown homeopathy's effectiveness (when compared with placebo). Now, such remedies as arnica (for bruises), chamomilla (for teething babies), and nux vomica (for nausea and hangovers) have become so popular and widely accepted that you can find them in any pharmacy. (Other examples you might have heard of include the formulas Oscillococcinum for flu, Sabadil for allergies, and Calms Forte for general tension—or topical Topricin or Traumeel for musculoskeletal injuries.) Certainly, these remedies can be quite effective, and they are rarely, if ever, harmful—certainly never in the way their pharmaceutical counterparts can be. But in my opinion, and personal experience, homeopathy is at its best when you work with a qualified practitioner to find your own constitutional remedy. That means that rather than treating simple symptoms as they pop up, you are treating the person behind those symptoms (actually the vital force, the homeopathic equivalent of chi). It will take time for a practitioner to find that remedy, and he or she will ask you hundreds of questions to attempt to "peel back the onion" of symptom complexes to find what lies at the core. The right remedy can be powerfully supportive—to both a detox process and to a life in general. To find a qualified homeopathic practitioner, visit the Web site for the National Center for Homeopathy (nationalcenterforhomeopathy.org).

BOTANICAL MEDICINE: All world cultures have incredibly deep herbal healing traditions. And today, you can access many of them, such as Native American, Hawaiian, Amazonian, Japanese, and Central/South American, through seasoned practitioners. Herbs are food, but they can also be used as serious medicine, with potential for interaction, toxicity, and even very serious side effects. Our Western mind-set encourages us to go reaching for them as miracle cures, and too often we extrapolate from encouraging studies in unhelpful ways. One of my favorite examples is ginkgo. Ginkgo has been shown to improve memory—*on people slipping into early senility*. For these people, ginkgo's ability to act as an antioxidant and thin the blood can help improve circulation going to the brain cells. What it *cannot* do, despite the marketing efforts of so many companies to tell you that it can, is help an 18-year-old studying for a final exam—or even a 60-year-old who is having a harder time remembering formerly easy things (names, numbers, etc.). For these people, there are many other, better options . . . as any herbalist would know. Many modern practitioners are trained to integrate herbs from many cultures. Finding those practitioners can be tricky, however—licensing and professional training requirements for "herbalists" are loose, to say the least. Your best bet may be to find a naturopath or doctor of Oriental medicine (OMD) who is credentialed in herbs, or an osteopath, integrative physician, or nurse practitioner who specializes in botanical medicine. If you are on medication or at medical risk for any reason, do not explore botanical medicine without the supervision of your doctor or pharmacist—herb-drug interactions can be just as problematic as drug-drug interactions.

MIND-BODY THERAPIES

HYPNOSIS: Hypnosis can be an especially useful tool for exploring the kind of anxiety that stems from stress, social isolation, or long-term depression. Working with a qualified practitioner, you can both explore your own consciousness for clues about how and why you feel the way you do, gain new insights that will help you live more skillfully in the world, and develop skills to help you cope with any dysfunctional or self-undermining behaviors. Hypnosis can also be used to reduce pain, as with headaches, and symptoms related to gastrointestinal issues, or allergies. It has even been used successfully to reduce the need for surgical anesthesia. I'm a big fan of self-hypnosis techniques that help you help yourself on a subconscious (as well as a conscious) level in maintaining your commitment to a healthy lifestyle or avoiding unhealthy behaviors. It can be a powerful way to release toxic habits or thoughts. Visit the Web site for the American Society of Clinical Hypnosis to find a qualified practitioner near you (asch.net).

BIOFEEDBACK: Biofeedback aims to take the mind-body link and make it tangible, using a variety of instruments to let you see how your thoughts and your breath can create very real changes in your physical responses. This technique is especially good for conditions arising from a chronic state of overdrive of the sympathetic nervous system (that is to say, the nonstop adrenaline state), and I often recommend it for overworkers and stressed-out caregivers. It's also a very good form of meditation for those who need to "see" immediate results. You can work with a professional trained to provide biofeedback therapy (psychologists often offer this service), or make a small investment in home equipment that lets you do it for yourself, such as the emWave system from the Institute of HeartMath (heartmath.org), the Iom Active Feedback hardware from Wild Divine (wilddivine.com), and RespeRate (resperate.com), a device approved by the FDA for use in lowering blood pressure.

GUIDED IMAGERY: Here, you use the power of imagination to lead your mind to a place of healing. Guided imagery exercises can reduce stress and relieve symptoms, such as headaches or asthma. Imagery is particularly powerful in helping to relieve back pain and is, in fact, the driving therapy behind the phenomenally successful book *Healing Back Pain* by John Sarno. The psychotherapist Belleruth Naparstek, LISW, has been a pioneer in using guided imagery in treating depression, insomnia, anxiety, PTSD, IBD and IBS, fertility problems, and pain syndromes, and offers many programs via her Web site, belleruthnaparstek.com.

BODY WORK: Peruse the menu at any day spa and you might think all you need to do to detox is surrender $90 and an hour of your time—most offer an array of facials, ionic footbaths, herbal body wraps, showers, scrubs, and massage claiming to cleanse and purify the body. Unfortunately, there's not much science to support those claims. They may feel good and be utterly relaxing (and so support detoxification of the mind), but they won't do much to release physical toxins from the body.

The single exception is lymphatic drainage massage. There are good studies to show that this technique—which has been used since Greek and Roman times to improve health—really can improve lymphatic flow. And since we know that the lymphatic system's main function is to remove toxins, debris, and excess fluids from the body, it just makes sense that lymphatic drainage massage would help in detoxification—even though there's no gold-standard study to explicitly prove that it does.

4. Pump Up the Probiotics

Twenty years ago, nobody was talking about the importance of maintaining healthy intestinal flora. But microbiologists have increasingly established just how important to human health friendly bacteria can be. We know now that microorganisms help break down food in the gut and are critical in the digestion (and even production) of some nutrients, including vitamin B_{12}. Recent studies have shown that they are also very important in strengthening our immune system—60 percent of which resides in the gut, communicating actively with the rest of the body. Of course, microorganisms can be hazardous, too—some species work to steal nutrition rather than contribute, and undo the products of phase II detoxification coming out of the liver. Others wreak outright havoc: Consider the handiwork of headline makers E. coli and salmonella.

We all play host to the good and the bad, and plenty of it—at least 1,000 different species that comprise 90 percent of our bodies' total DNA. The balance between human and bacterial cells is what microbiologists call the *microbiome*, and it has been radically transformed in recent years by changes in agricultural practices and in the chemical landscape. Scientists are only beginning to scratch the surface in the field, though they speculate that these microbiome changes may be behind some of our modern health epidemics, including the rise in food allergies, auto-immune disorders, diabetes, obesity, digestive complaints like irritable bowel syndrome (IBS) and the more destructive inflammatory bowel disease (IBD), and heart disease.

Taking a *probiotic* supplement lets you tip the balance a bit by introducing more of the friendly guys into your digestive tract. Keeping the flora friendly will help shore up the walls of the small intestine so that more toxins are kept out of the system overall (see more on this in Chapter 9), and the workload on the liver is kept to a minimum.

Prebiotics are carefully selected, carbohydrate food–based substances such as beta-glucan or inulin that fuel the growth of friendly bacteria colonies and can inhibit the growth of more pathological ones. These are also found in natural foods such as Jerusalem artichokes, chicory, burdock, leeks, onions, and garlic (and yes, they work when you eat them). Prebiotics will also minimize inflammation and support good nutrient assimilation— and therefore boost overall health. Taking them is just a good idea in general, especially if you're still having symptoms of toxicity: many probiotic supplements are already fortified with prebiotics.

You can take probiotics in capsule or liquid form (most are freeze-dried, but there are some—such as Bio-K—that are liquid yogurts with living cultures). Look for a supplement that contains members of both the lacto-bacillus and bifidobacterium families (or combine two supplements, such as Culturelle and Align, to get both). Choose one that offers between 5 billion and 20 billion live bacteria per dose, and take it once or twice daily. If you are suffering from IBS or IBD, you might choose a higher-dose supplement, such as VSL#3, which has 250 billion live bacteria per dose (though you should only go this high if you are working with a doctor). Here are a few brands I like and trust, along with what you get from them:

- VSL#3 (medical therapeutic grade)
- Metagenics (UltraFlora and others)
- Bio-K (yogurt with 50 billion live bacteria per container; comes in dairy, soy, and rice versions)
- Pharmax (many varieties)
- Culturelle (lactobacillus GG)
- Align (*Bifidobacterium infantis*)
- Florastor (beneficial yeast *saccharomyces*)
- Jarrow Formulas (many varieties and quite affordable)
- Klaire Labs (many varieties)

5. Consider Using Medical Foods

Some physicians use medical foods—nutritionally engineered meal-replacement powders designed to improve particular conditions—as the basis for their entire detox plan. And although, as I've said before, I believe that a whole-foods, fruit- and vegetable-dense diet (such as the one you just completed) is unequivocally the best way to cleanse your body, there are times when I do turn to these medical foods. Many have been formulated by nutritional biochemists to provide nutrients for specific health challenges. If you find yourself with remaining difficulties after the 21-Day Clean and Lean Diet, you might want to consult with a functional/integrative medicine specialist to see if one or more of these will be helpful additions for you.

Functional medical foods are designed to be complete meal replacements, to provide the body with a low-carb, medium-fiber, low-fat (with added "good fats"), relatively high-protein mix of nutrition that delivers all the vitamins and minerals needed to heal and detoxify (typically, each serving contains about a third of the recommended daily amount). These foods also include many targeted phytonutrients and nutraceuticals designed to address particular problems.

Generally speaking, you can use two scoops of medical food powders as a base for a smoothie, or mix with water, juice, or even nut milk. The following are some of the best products available.

- *Detoxification* support medical foods: These are low-allergy formulas, made without gluten, dairy, soy, egg, corn, and yeast and fortified with vitamins and minerals. They may contain some combination of detox-specific ingredients such as milk thistle, dandelion, artichoke, curcumin, NAC, and glutathione. Examples include Designs for Health *Paleo Cleanse*, Metagenics *UltraClear*, Thorne *MediClear*, and Xymogen *OptiCleanse*.

- *Gastrointestinal* support medical foods: These formulas are tremendously helpful for leaky gut syndrome, a condition in which the lining of the small intestine has been damaged (see page 334 for more information). They are also useful for people who are experiencing a more temporary bowel dysfunction after a round of antibiotics, food poisoning, or a bout with a virus. They may contain such gut-fortifying ingredients as glutamine, quercetin, aloe vera, licorice, slippery elm bark, marshmallow root, fibers, gums, probiotics, and prebiotics. Examples include Designs for Health GI Revive, Metagenics UltraClear Sustain, and Xymogen OptiCleanse GHI.

- *Anti-inflammatory* medical foods: These are for those suffering from inflammatory conditions, such as colitis or arthritis. They may contain ingredients such as specific amino acids, high-dose antioxidants, green tea, ginger, turmeric, holy basil, NAC, fish oil, sulfur compounds, and glutathione. Examples include Metagenics UltraInflamX and Thorne MediClear Plus.

- *Low glycemic index* medical foods: These are designed for diabetics to help lower blood sugar and improve the body's sensitivity to insulin. They can also help stabilize blood sugar for those with hypoglycemia. They may contain ingredients such as chromium and vanadium, cinnamon, gymnema, fenugreek, glucomannan, chlorogenic acid, fiber, gums, and pectin. Examples include Metagenics UltraGlycemX and Xymogen OptiGlycemX.

- *Fiber supplements:* For people who need additional fiber besides what they can get in food, the Fiber Boosters discussed on page 104 are excellent. There are also combination (soluble and insoluble) powdered forms that can be added to shakes or taken alone. Examples are Metagenics' Meta Fiber, Renew Life Organic Clear Fiber, Garden of Life Raw Fiber, and Thorne MediBulk.

Simple Meal Replacements

Sometimes having a simple, clean protein powder on hand makes it easy to keep yourself well fed. Occasionally I use meal replacement powders and bars to supplement my own diet when I don't have time to stop for lunch or when I need to boost my stamina so I can make it until dinner. And it happens.

Most medical foods companies make a basic product that doesn't "do" much more than replace a meal—but they do a good job of it, using whole foods and providing a good, balanced blend of protein, carbohydrates, and fats with added fiber, vitamins, minerals, food concentrates, culinary spices, herbs, and sometimes probiotics. They're not quite the same as a good meal—but they're quick and easy, and they certainly make good snacks.

Why didn't I tell you about them sooner? Because, as I explained, whole foods are superior—and I believe everyone should understand how to prepare for themselves (and their families) a balanced diet that's low in toxins and high in nutrition. The 21 days of detox should include a releasing of your reliance on unnatural, manufactured foods (at least for a little while). But these are certainly okay to use and can stand in for any meal during days 8 through 21 and beyond.

One of my favorites is the Ultimate Meal (theultimatelife.net), a powder made completely from raw, whole foods—though it is best when blended with a bit of fruit, as suggested by the manufacturer. If that's too much effort, or if you have food allergies or intolerances, another excellent powder mix is Metagenics UltraMeal (metagenics.com). It comes in whey, rice, and soy formulas with a dozen different flavors—and it comes in bars, too. My favorite liquid is Orgain (orgain.com), a pre-mixed organic drink that tastes so (slightly) sweet and delicious (flavors include mocha, chocolate, vanilla bean, and strawberries and cream) that you'd never know you were getting kale, beets, spinach, carrots, and tomatoes with every sip.

If grab-and-go bars are more your style, you'll have to settle for snack status (it's hard to get everything you need for a meal in a bar), but there are a few good choices: Paleobars by Designs for Health (designsforhealth.com), ImmunoBar by Xymogen (xymogen.com), SoLo bars (solo-gi.com), Raw Revolution (rawrev.com), and Keen-Wah Decadence bars (yogaearth.com). Note that these are prepared foods and many do contain some sugar—not ideal for frequent use but okay in a pinch.

6. Sweat Things Out

Saunas have been used for thousands of years to promote health by practically every major world civilization (Roman, Greek, Russian, Scandinavian, Turkish, Mayan, Inuit, and Native American) and are highly valued for their rejuvenating effects. Now we know that that rejuvenation comes partly from the offloading of toxins through the sweat (as well as improving circulation and relaxation . . . both of which help in detoxification!).

Scientists have long understood that the skin is a major organ of detoxification and that such chemicals and metals as mercury, PCBs, dioxins, and drugs (including cocaine, heroin, and antibiotics) can be efficiently released from the body via the sweat and oil glands.

What's less well understood is whether raising core body temperature, as saunas do, actually helps release deposits of these chemical and metal invaders from their long-term storage in the fat cells of the body. The best thinking at the moment is that yes, they can—and that infrared saunas might be particularly effective in this area, as they warm the core body temperature before the skin, sweating you from the inside out, so to speak (as opposed to conventional saunas, which do the opposite . . . though they are still efficient). There is some evidence that PCB concentrations in fat cells are reduced after using a sauna. The jury is still out on that one, though I believe the practice is not only not harmful, but for most, an incredibly enjoyable and energizing experience and therefore one that's very much worth exploring.

However, note that while saunas can lower blood pressure, for some, the dry heat can raise blood pressure, so those struggling with hypertension or serious kidney disease should not do saunas without checking in with their doctors first. The same rule applies to anyone with internal metallic implants, on blood pressure medication, on multiple medications, with serious illness, or who is pregnant. Start by getting in the sauna for 10 to 15 minutes at a time, and work up to 20-minute sessions. The maximum session should be 30 minutes a day.

Don't forget the other way to raise your core body temperature and get your sweat on: good, old-fashioned exercise. Sweating once a day for 20 minutes would be ideal if you're combining it with the heart-healthy benefits of aerobic exercise; four or five times per week will do, if you can't swing a daily sweat.

7. Explore Enzymes

Enzymes have long been an overlooked secret to helping our bodies heal. Every plant contains naturally occurring enzymes that help us digest the plant's nutrients, making them more readily available to the body. These enzymes help in improving digestion, aid in absorption, reduce inflammation, and in the case of fiber, help the intestines better eliminate toxins. (I think there are untold other ways they help the body's unimaginably complex machinery operate better, too, as enzymes facilitate nearly every process in the human body.) Nature designed things so that we would get plenty of these from our food—they are literally all around us!

Trouble is, too often, these plant enzymes are lost in our diet because our food is so often processed, not so fresh (picked long ago and far away), or cooked—the slightest bit of heat, over 140°F, destroys them. The Detox Prescription is high in natural plant enzymes because it is full of juices and fresh greens (in the form of salad). But for some, adding an enzyme supplement can improve the results of their detox.

How is this done? You can take enzymes with food to help with digestion in a very straightforward way. Or you can take them between meals so that they are absorbed into the bloodstream—and this is when they can really do some amazing things. Perhaps most relevant here: They can reduce inflammation directly in the liver. They can also improve circulation, promote healing of tissue throughout the body, help with glycation (simply put, the body's processing of sugars on a molecular level), and boost kidney function. Here's a brief guide to choosing the enzyme/supplement that best meets your needs:

- **IF YOU HAVE TROUBLE DIGESTING BEANS:** An enzyme called *alpha galactosidase* will help digest undigestible starches in beans that cause gas/bloating/cramping. Beano is a readily available product you can find in any pharmacy, as well as Bean Assist by Enzymedica.

- **IF YOU ARE LACTOSE INTOLERANT:** You can take the enzyme *lactase* to help break down the lactose in dairy products. Good products include Identify Dairy by Enzyme Science, Lacto by Enzymedica, and Lactaid.

- **IF YOU ARE GLUTEN INTOLERANT:** Gluten-digesting enzymes *DPP IV* can help digest trace amounts of gluten for individuals who dine out and are exposed to gluten contamination, which can cause local and systemic inflammation. Products I like include GlutenEase 2X by Enzymedica and Identify Gluten by Enzyme Science.

• **IF YOUR DIGESTION IS SLUGGISH:** Most good general enzyme formulas include *proteases* to help with protein digestion, *amylase* for carbohydrate digestion, and *lipases* for fats. These will maximize digestion when taken with meals and absorption of critical nutrients when taken between meals. Some excellent formulas are ATPro Digest Gold by Enzymedica, Vital-Zymes Complete by Klaire Labs, Similase by Integrative Therapeutics, and Critical Digestion by Enzyme Science.

• **IF YOU HAVE INFLAMMATION-RELATED DISORDERS:** For any kind of inflammation disorder—arthritis, headaches, IBS—proteolytic enzymes can be powerful medicine. Taken between meals, they can help reduce systemic inflammation and promote absorption and are an excellent choice for anyone who feels he or she may need a bit of liver repair, as they help all bodily tissues (including organs). An excellent product in this category is Wobenzym N, which contains a proprietary mix of pancreatin, papain, bromelain, papain, trypsin, and chymotrypsin. A recent powerful addition to the repertoire of anti-inflammatory enzymes is serratiopeptidase, found in Enzymedica's Serra Gold. There is ongoing research on using enzymes to break up common chemicals in food that produce (nonallergic) reactions. Some of these include the biogenic amines histamine and tyramine. (Hist-DAO by Xymogen is one of the new enzyme products.)

8. Supplement Your Diet Smartly

Did you skip ahead to this section? I put it last for a reason. Too often, my patients want to bypass the hard work of doing a detox diet, thinking that taking just a supplement or two will do the work for them. That's in sync with our general Western mind-set—that we should be able to just pop a pill that will make everything better. Unfortunately, it doesn't work that way. Supplements are just that, *supplements* to a healthy lifestyle and whole-foods diet. They can help add a few key nutrients here and there, maybe give the body a little push in the right direction in a few critical places. Sometimes they can help a lot. But they can't do the work for you, and they can never replace clean living and eating. Enough said?

There's a lot to consider when you're choosing a supplement. Quality is always a serious consideration (see "Choosing the Best Supplements," page 314) with anything you put in your mouth—taking something that's ineffective or, worse, toxic is worse than taking nothing at all. Also, what's right for one person isn't always right for another. When I make recommendations to a patient, it is always within a highly personal context that takes under consideration their health status, habits, and unique constellation of symptoms. It is very difficult to make meaningful general recommendations—particularly in the realm of herbs, which really are at their best when treated as medicine, and prescribed as such by a professional who understands their wide range of systemic biochemical effects. This is especially important when pharmaceuticals are also being used, as context is everything—and contraindications are entirely possible.

Still, food-based supplements are a good way to pump up the power of certain types of nutrition we know are helpful to the detox process. They are a way to add nutrients to the diet when you can't or won't eat a certain kind of food because you don't like the flavor or texture (say, turmeric or seaweed), or don't have the time or resources to deal with juicing or cooking whole foods (as with green powders). In some cases, they are a way to add elements of nutrition that you simply wouldn't naturally eat, even though you could (as with milk thistle). Capsules, powders, and liquid extracts make these foods more readily available.

Here is what you can use to "supplement" your detoxification efforts with food-based nutrients. Take one or two of these based on your needs. For example, if you just can't stomach broccoli and kale, a green powder is a good choice. If you're also highly stressed, consider adding a green tea extract for its calming L-theanine. If you have arthritis, the anti-inflammatory power of turmeric or garlic will support your joints as well as your liver. Read through the entire list and choose the supplements that make the most sense for your situation. Or if you really want to power up your detox, you can put them all together (see Dr. Merrell's Detox Super Shooter, page 311):

• **Green superfood powders:** Don't have enough time in the day to get kale, broccoli, romaine, Brussels sprouts, and spinach? Green powders can deliver all that, plus a host of other green foods—including seaweeds and grasses. These are dehydrated whole foods. Not as good as a whole thing, in that you're missing out on all the fiber and super-fresh enzymes. But a pretty close second. . . . There are many good products out there, but my favorite is NutriCology ProGreens (nutricology.com), which contains probiotics, as well as a good dose of thistles (see below). Add one scoop daily to juices, nut milks, and smoothies.

• **Red superfood powders:** If you're not getting your daily quota of raspberries, cranberries, cherries, tomatoes, and red cabbage, red powders can deliver a lot of that goodness, plus what you'd find in a host of other red foods—including tropical superfruits like camu camu. Good blends will veer into the yellow and blue ends of the spectrum, too. As with green powders, they're not quite as good as real foods, but close. Add one scoop daily to juices, nut milks, and smoothies.

• **Chlorella or spirulina:** Western diets don't feature much seaweed. It's too bad, since these foods do everything other green foods do . . . plus a little more. Because they are living cellular organisms, they contain an abundance of nutrients, including protein, as well as iodine, increasingly lacking in the American diet as we continue to gravitate toward noniodized sea salts. But to the point of this book in particular, they have been shown to directly chelate heavy metals (lead, mercury, arsenic, cadmium). If you know you are borderline to high in heavy metals, you should be taking a daily seaweed supplement (don't guess, get tested; see page 35). Cilantro supplements can work, too. Use three 500- or 600-milligram capsules twice daily.

• **Turmeric:** Study after study shows that turmeric—notably its chief constituent, curcumin—has incredible antioxidant, anti-inflammatory, and detoxifying powers. Brain health, heart health, endocrine health, and even cellular health (yes, the stuff has anticancer power) are all improved by curcumin. It has been shown to support both phase I and phase II detoxification, and there's some evidence to show that it may help to directly chelate arsenic. You can certainly cook with more turmeric—it's delicious and contains curcumin within a context of other phytonutrients, which may boost effectiveness in ways we don't yet understand. Find a supplement that contains the form called Meriva; these are made by a number of companies. Take one 500-milligram capsule twice daily.

• **Thistles:** Dandelion leaf, artichoke, blessed thistle, and all other members of the thistle family are *cholagogues*, meaning that they promote the

The Ultimate "Drink to Your Health"

In my opinion, if you're going to add anything to the Detox Prescription, you simply can't do better than this mix. Add it into any smoothie or juice recipe, or use a shaker cup to mix it with 12 ounces of filtered water or organic pineapple juice (you'll benefit from that fruit's natural enzymes, including the powerful anti-inflammatory protease enzyme bromelain) to make a stand-alone drink. I've called for my favorite brand names here to make shopping easiest. You can make substitutions (as noted below). One caveat—if you are substituting another greens powder, you'll have to take an extra probiotic supplement to equal what's in ProGreens.

Dr. Merrell's Detox Super Shooter

1 scoop of Nutricology ProGreens*

1 serving Trace Minerals Research Red Pak**

1 dropperful Herb Pharm liquid green tea extract

1 dropperful Herb Pharm liquid turmeric extract (or contents of Meriva capsule)

1 dropperful Herb Pharm liquid milk thistle extract

1 ounce organic pomegranate or black cherry juice

Optional: 1 capsule New Chapter Garlic Force, pierced and squeezed into drink

(or 1 capsule quercetin if garlic is a problem)

12 ounces filtered water or organic pineapple juice

*Other green superfood powder blends: GOL Perfect Food Super Green powder, Sun Warrior Ormus Supergreens, Barlean's Organic Greens, Davinci Spectra Greens, Invite Greens Hx, Amazing Grass Green SuperFood All Natural, and Vibrant Health Field of Greens. Individual superfood greens (not blended greens) can be found in the Rainbow Superfoods Boosters on page 103.

**Other red superfood powder blends: Garden of Life Fruits of Life powder, Invite Reds Hx. Individual superfood red powders (not blended reds) can be found in the Rainbow Superfoods Boosters on page 103.

*/**Powder blends containing both greens and reds include: Metagenics Phytoganix, Source Naturals Life Greens and Berries, AmazingGrass Green SuperFood Berry Drink Powder, and New Chapter Berry Greens.

production and flow of bile. From a detox perspective, milk thistle is a substance so powerfully liver enhancing that it has been found to medically prevent poisoning from the deadly amanita mushroom. Take one 500-milligram capsule twice daily.

• **Green tea extract:** Nature's premier antioxidant supports phase I and phase II detox, with a nice relaxing bonus: L-theanine, which crosses the blood-brain barrier to promote the work of calming neurotransmitters. The L-theanine offsets green tea's natural caffeine, but sensitive people may want to opt for a decaffeinated supplement. Buy this in a tincture form, and take one dropperful once or twice daily.

• **Garlic:** This antioxidant, anti-inflammatory substance helps with phase II detox (in particular, sulfation) and may help to directly chelate lead, mercury, cadmium, and arsenic. In Ayurveda, garlic is considered *rasayana*, or universal medicine. It may affect digestion—deodorized garlic works for most, but not for all. (If not you, consider one of its bioflavonoids, quercetin, as a good substitute—see page 326 for more information.) Take 500 milligrams twice daily.

9. Troubleshoot Your Symptoms

So you've talked to your doctor, you've done a bunch of tests, and you've ruled things out. You don't have diabetes, or heart disease, or a thyroid problem, or a kidney or liver or lung or autoimmune issue. In fact, from a physical perspective, it's all systems go!

But you're still feeling less than well. There may be no disease, per se, but there is still discomfort in the physical body. What's going on?

It could be that you are still in the process of detoxifying. There are symptoms that both herald the need to detox and crop up as a result of your efforts as your body processes and releases toxins stored in the fat tissue. Are they chickens or eggs? We may never be absolutely sure.

Headaches, skin rashes, allergies and asthma, GERD and IBS, and joint pain are just such complaints. They may come and go and be maddeningly hard for even you to pin down (let alone anyone who's trying to help you). These can, of course, be associated with serious illness. But they can also arise with no discernible underlying cause that Western medicine can identify, so they lump them into a category they call "functional disorders," meaning there may be a problem, but there's no "proof" of disease. They may also be classified as psychosomatic and dismissed—or worse, treated in a way that really isn't that helpful. (Antidepressants aren't for everyone.)

Assuming you've done your homework and talked with your doctor, we'll offer a little troubleshooting for these pesky symptoms. If you're sure there's no disease at the root of them, integrative approaches are the logical next step for your self-care explorations. Used in conjunction with a detoxification diet and the techniques laid out earlier in this chapter—meditation and acupuncture help everything, for example—these supplements and strategies can alleviate or even eliminate the problems. Talk to your doctor—hopefully an integrative or functional one!—about how best to use them in the context of your own treatment plan.

Gastritis/GERD

- **DGL (DEGLYCYRRHIZINATED LICORICE):** has been shown to heal the stomach lining
- **DIGESTIVE ENZYMES:** reduce digestive work in the stomach and duodenum
- **MASTIC GUM:** binds to the lining of the stomach to help protect it
- **ZINC CARNOSINE:** helps inflamed stomach lining heal
- **HEAD ELEVATION:** sleeping with the head elevated prevents gastric juices from trickling up the esophagus

IBS

- **ALOE:** soothing to the stomach and intestinal lining
- **BITTERS (ANGOSTURA, SWEDISH):** stimulate digestion in stomach and duodenum
- **ENTERIC-COATED PEPPERMINT OIL:** helps to relax the small intestine (only when enteric coated; otherwise, irritates the stomach)
- **ENZYMES:** help to break down food more efficiently
- **MAGNESIUM CITRATE:** promotes better bowel movement and is especially useful for constipation
- **PREBIOTICS (INULIN, BETA GLUCAN, FOS):** support the growth of beneficial

(continued on page 316)

Choosing the Best Supplements

In the world of supplement shopping, it is caveat emptor—let the buyer beware. And beware you should, as there isn't much regulation of the production of vitamins, minerals, and herbs in this country, even though it's a $20 billion–plus industry. That's because the Dietary Supplement Health and Education Act of 1994 defined supplements as food, not drugs, meaning they are free from regulation by the FDA (unless they make claims that they act like drugs, in which case the FDA can act, though it rarely does because it lacks manpower and funding). Therefore, it is mostly up to the *honesty of the company* to give you what they say is in their product—and to do their own extensive, exacting, and expensive quality-control testing. Especially when the product is expensive to make or hard to get, there is an incentive to cheat.

Since supplements can have biological consequences for every cell of your body, it's critical that they be high quality—especially when they are plant derived (as with herbs) with hundreds of active substances (even when standardized for only one). Here are just a few of the things that need to be considered before you swallow any supplement. These things can compromise quality and effectiveness:

- poor soil and weather conditions

- cross-species contamination

- use of chemical fertilizers and pesticides

- heavy metal contamination

- extraction method (alcohol versus water)

- unregulated fillers

- lack of dose standardization

It's a lot to think about. But you can shortcut all of the above provisos by knowing that some companies *do* have exacting quality control—often equal to any pharmaceutical products. There is even a label for this: cGMP, current good manufacturing practices, which means that dietary supplements voluntarily comply with manufacturing guidelines to ensure consistency with regard to identity, purity, strength, and composition.

Let me make things easy for you. The following is a list I've compiled of the best and most reliable companies I know; they have a proven track record of the highest quality control in the industry. If you can find a generic product that is half the price of the brand name, you are often getting what you are paying for. Pick the most reliable brands you can afford—these brand names are worth the investment.

FOR NUTRACEUTICALS (VITAMINS AND MINERALS) AND BOTANICALS (HERBS):

- Complementary Prescriptions
- Design for Health
- Douglas Labs
- Enzymatic Therapy
- Integrative Therapeutics
- Metagenics
- Phytopharmica (only herbs)
- Pure Encapsulations
- Rainbow Light
- Thorne
- Vital Nutrients
- Xymogen

FOR HERBAL TINCTURES:

- Gaia herbs
- Herb Pharm
- Quantum herbs

FOR HOMEOPATHIC REMEDIES:

- BHI-HEEL
- Boiron
- Standard Homeopathics

FOR OMEGA-3 FATTY ACIDS:

- Barlean's (vegan)
- Nordic Naturals
- Nutramins (algae, non-fish-based DHA)
- Pharmax (British)
- Udo's (vegan)
- Vital Nutrients

IBS (cont.)

bacteria and inhibit the growth of more harmful bacteria (can cause gas)

- **PROBIOTICS:** higher doses of lactobacillus and bifidobacterium can reset levels of friendly intestinal flora

- **SMALL, FREQUENT MEALS:** eliminates burdens to system

Chronic allergies and respiratory congestion

- **BROMELAIN:** mucolytic enzyme that can reduce inflammation and act as a preventive

- **BUTTERBUR:** reduces inflammation in the nasal passages

- **ESSENTIAL OIL SUCH AS YOUNG LIVING THIEVES:** combined with steam inhalation, these act as expectorants and decongestants (they're also germicidal)

- **NAC:** (N-acetyl-cysteine) helps break up mucus

- **NAZANOL BY METAGENICS:** a nondrying, nonstimulating decongestant

- **NETTLES:** natural herbal antihistamine

- **QUERCETIN:** reduces inflammation that leads to allergies and sinusitis

Asthma

- **BUTTERBUR:** decreases inflammation and spasming

- **EPA:** helps reduce inflammation that triggers bronchial spasming

- **GINKGO BILOBA:** also helps reduce bronchial spasming

- **MAGNESIUM:** helps relax muscles in lungs; IV drips can stop acute attacks

- **KUNDALINI YOGA:** a type of yoga that uses breath-based techniques that serve as asthma prevention

Eczema/psoriasis/chronic dermatitis

- **EPA:** reduces topical inflammation (as well as inflammation in general)

- **GLA:** curbs inflammation—evening primrose oil, which contains GLA, is a good choice for eczema

- **OATMEAL BATHS:** very soothing for skin and mind

- **TURMERIC:** the active ingredient, curcumin, is a powerful anti-inflammatory
- **DIET:** it's critical to do an elimination diet, especially a gluten-free trial, for psoriasis
- **MEDITATION:** skin conditions are highly influenced by emotions—one study showed mindfulness meditation dramatically reduced psoriasis

Headaches (general and migraine)

- **BUTTERBUR:** decreases inflammation and spasming; endorsed by the American Headache Society for migraine prevention
- **FEVERFEW:** evidence supports use as a preventive (contains salicylates)
- **MAGNESIUM:** deficiencies have proven to increase migraines, and magnesium is proven to help prevent them
- **RIBOFLAVIN:** a B vitamin that has been shown in some studies to prevent headaches
- **BIOFEEDBACK:** a powerful treatment that triggers the relaxation response
- **CRANIOSACRAL THERAPY:** a wonderful, gentle soft-touch massage technique focused on the head and neck

Joint and musculoskeletal pain

- **BOSWELLIA:** Ayurvedic herb (frankincense) reduces joint inflammation
- **CAPSAICIN TOPICAL:** depletes substance P in nerves, which causes pain; good for diffuse muscular pain (as with fibromyalgia)
- **ENZYMES:** proteolytic enzymes such as Wobenzym N and Enzymedica's Serra Gold have been shown to survive intact absorbed from the intestinal tract when taken in between meals and have good efficacy in relieving joint pain
- **GINGER:** also an anti-inflammatory
- **GLUCOSAMINE AND CHONDROITIN:** studies show these cartilage building blocks help repair damaged cartilage
- **MSM:** (methylsulfonylmethane) helps make all connective tissues more supple, both inside and outside of joints
- **OMEGA-3 FATTY ACIDS:** (e.g., flax or fish oil) has been shown in numerous studies to reduce inflammation that causes these conditions

- **RHUS TOX:** oral homeopathic remedy for chronic sprains
- **SAMe:** (S-adenosyl-methionine) reduces inflammation within joins in arthritis
- **TOPRICIN TOPICAL:** effectively reduces joint and general musculoskeletal inflammation and pain
- **TURMERIC:** excellent general anti-inflammatory
- **MAGNETS (APPLIED TO POINT OF PAIN):** studies support use in relieving discomfort; Nikken is a reliable supplier

What Next?

If you've tried everything and you're still hungry for more—whether you feel you need it because you're experiencing symptoms or you just want to know how good you can feel—you can take your detox to still another level. You'll need to bone up on some basic science to do it.

Don't worry, though. I'll make it simple. In the next chapter, I'll explain in more detail exactly how the detox process works, as well as exactly what things you're doing to help and hurt that process. In so doing I will hopefully shed some light on the unique set of challenges to your body—and the next logical step you can take to up your detox game if needed. A few more supplements can be useful in the effort to detox, powerful and targeted nutraceuticals that directly feed phase I and especially phase II. I highly recommend them—if you understand which one or two you really need and can take them appropriately. In Chapter 9, we can figure that out together.

If you're ready to dig deeper, let's get into the Science of Detox.

the science of detox

I n a very real sense, you are a detoxification machine. Nearly every cell in your body has the power to detoxify, 24/7, 365. That's a good thing, as you are under constant attack from without and within.

From the dawn of time, man has encountered toxins in our air, water, and food. Moreover, toxins have always been natural internal byproducts of metabolism and the stress response. As we experiment with food and fire, we encounter occasional poisons and noxious gases. As we burn energy internally, we produce free radicals; as we respond to the environment around us, we metabolize hormones, neurotransmitters, and countless other intrinsic chemicals that the body has to clear. Bacteria in our intestines can produce endotoxins. To be alive is to be constantly in equilibrium with a toxic state. To thrive is to detoxify effectively and efficiently.

Nowadays, of course, the toxic inputs have become amplified. We're no longer dealing with an occasional poisonous mushroom or saber-toothed tiger encounter. Today, the body faces an unprecedented array of exogenous, or external, chemical stressors in our food, air, and water—many of them purposely engineered into our diet and medicine. We've already talked about what they are and where they come from (see page 8). We've talked about what you can do about it on the most practical level—the Detox Prescription—and by now you may even have done it. We have even gone beyond that to explore integrative approaches to the deepest levels of detox.

But if you're curious to learn even more, read on: Here we explore in depth how the body operates on a physiological level to protect itself in the face of a toxic threat. My hope is that by understanding the machinery better, you'll be a better mechanic—and as a better mechanic, able to keep yourself clean, cared for, highly tuned, and running well at all times.

Hell on the Cells

The common perception about detoxification is that it all happens in the liver. Not true. Detox happens within the body's cells, all over, all the time. You can literally detox from the top of your head to the tips of your toes. Heart, kidney, ovary, testicle, brain, lung, skin, intestines—these are all organs of detoxification. The liver is merely a specialist (being loaded with cells that are highly prepared for the task).

Every cell in the body is surrounded by a permeable layer of proteins and lipids that respond to sugars, nutrients, and natural hormones, all of which act like keys to open locks on the cell wall to let them in or to relay messages to receptors for internal messengers to transmit throughout the cell. Often, modern toxins—especially pesticides and herbicides—mimic these natural substances, effectively picking the locks that protect the cells or turning them on from the outside with a fake ID. (This is a big part of endocrine disruption—many toxins mimic hormones such as estrogen so closely that cells can't tell the difference.)

When and if toxins, having settled on the cell's surface, breach the protective membrane, they have a lot of options. The toxins can remain in the soup of the cell (the cytosol), latching on to whatever molecules they are best at poisoning. These might be messenger molecules (such as kinase enzymes) coming from the inner cell membrane on their way to the nucleus or mitochondria, or they might be components of the Krebs cycle—the critical process that, with the help of a factory's worth of supportive nutrients such as iron, copper, selenium, molybdenum, and B vitamins, prepares oxygen, water, and sugar to be converted into energy (ATP) inside the mitochondria. This interference inhibits the cell's ability to create energy.

Toxins can also proceed directly into the mitochondria—the cell's tiny energy factories, and the relatively unprotected mitochondrial DNA is very susceptible to damage. When the body is overwhelmed with toxins and/or nutrition is inadequate to mop up the damage (antioxidants such as vitamins E and C and the body's own glutathione can help quench free radicals), the energy that can move from the mitochondria to the cell is greatly reduced. Eventually, the mitochondria are barely able to function at all—meaning there is less energy available to support life, literally.

Toxins have a harder time penetrating the nucleus, which enjoys far more protection than any other part of the cell. But when you keep adding to the army of toxic warriors, you can expect that eventually their spear-chucking and cannon blasts will be successful. Once inside, they encounter the epigene—the shield that surrounds the chromosome, acting as both protector and external control center of our DNA. The epigene determines to a large extent which of our genetic tendencies are expressed and which stay suppressed: *It is the software to our genetic hardware.* It receives information from the environment and is remarkably responsive to the world around it. But it has to deal with both positive and negative messages—and you don't get more negative than a toxic poison trying to shut you down with both misinformation and direct damage. This damage short-circuits some of the critical control mechanisms that tell our DNA what to do.

The nuclear chromosomes' genes are well protected—tightly wound in their famous double helix, which is enfolded on itself and wrapped in a layer of histones and other protectors. It's the ultimate inner sanctum—the computer room that exists in a nearly hermetically sealed environment. But once a threshold number of toxins have arrived to overwhelm the epigene's defense mechanisms—toxins can make it into the DNA and latch on to specific nucleic acids within our genes. They can actually rewrite our genetic code, changing the sequences by which our nucleic acids manifest. The tiniest change in one sequence of the genes' nucleic acids can make a huge difference. It can result in aberrant messages being sent from the nucleus into the rest of the cell—turning off some defenses, instructing other organelles within the cell to make dysfunctional molecules to deliver to the rest of the body, increasing inflammation, and even allowing cancerous genes to dominate.

However, this cascade of events doesn't have to be inevitable. You can protect your DNA and every part of the magnificent machine. By taking in enough nutrient-dense foods, you can fuel the intracellular detoxification processes that can disarm the bad guys before they get a chance to do any damage to the cells. And better still, you can switch to a clean, plant-based diet that does not introduce toxins in the first place.

The Detox Defense

When it comes to detox, the best offense is a good defense. The single best way to avoid becoming toxic is to avoid toxins, period. Beyond that, the most proactive thing you can do is to get yourself ready by eating as many organic, whole, nutrient-dense fruits and vegetables as you can so that the processes of detoxification are fully available and well supported whenever and wherever they are needed. If you're eating according to the Detox Prescription, you are already getting exactly what you need—and avoiding what you don't want inside you. If not, you'll want to amp up the produce, with its heavy artillery of vitamins, minerals, phytonutrients, and fiber.

There are just two phases of detoxification, as we've described already: phase I, which identifies the toxins and readies them for chelation, or binding, and phase II, which chelates or binds the toxins to neutralize them so that they can be safely eliminated from the body. You might think of phase I as "modification" and phase II as "conjugation" (followed, of course, by what some people describe as the third phase, "elimination"). Here's how the system works in more detail:

PHASE I: **MODIFICATION**

When the cell recognizes something to be harmful, its first reaction is to call on one of the phase I enzymes to alter it. These enzymes are called cytochromes, and there are hundreds of variations of them in each cell. Though it may seem counterintuitive, the job of phase I is not only to identify potentially toxic molecules but to destabilize them through oxidative chemical processes to create new, highly unstable molecules, called "toxic intermediaries."

These are free radicals, created by the body on purpose. Why? These toxic intermediaries are then available to be chelated by (or bound up with) one of the phase II conjugators waiting to do exactly this job. The binding renders the toxic molecule harmless and water-soluble, so that it may exit the body via the kidneys or colon. (By the way, that's another pretty good reason not to get dehydrated—you want to help this process along.)

However, the body can encounter problems when the detoxification pathways become stressed. First, there's a lot of competition for phase I enzymes. The body can make these pretty easily from basic proteins and vitamins found in cruciferous vegetables and protein-rich foods, but nearly 50 percent of the drugs we take compete for just one kind of phase I enzyme. The body's hormones, too, must go through the processes of detoxification and compete with all the pharmaceuticals and other chemicals. If we overload this pathway, or do something to undermine these enzymes' ability to work properly (such as drink grapefruit juice, oddly enough, which can inhibit phase I enzyme production by as much as 30 percent), the detox mechanism becomes deficient, allowing the offending chemicals to accumulate in the body—not just medications, but also hormones, drugs, pesticides, herbicides, and any other substance that might also need to be processed by the same phase I enzyme. Another type of phase I enzyme not only detoxes caffeine but is also needed to process pesticides, tobacco carcinogens, and polyaromatic amines (a toxic by-product of charbroiled beef). If some of these pathways are overloaded, the toxins will quickly begin degrading the function of the cellular machinery.

An even worse-case scenario, though, is when phase I takes place just fine and the toxic intermediaries (or free radicals) are created . . . but can't find the phase II conjugators (or chelators) they need to neutralize them. These unmoored toxic intermediaries *will* grab on to something, anything—chemically speaking, they must. Because they are free radicals, they can and will do a lot of damage, some of which we have discussed: disrupting the mitochondria's ability to create energy, short-circuiting the cell's enzymatic and genetic mechanisms to produce molecules needed to sustain it, interrupting the epigene's role in helping to direct our genetic functions, and even directly damaging our genes' DNA. The toxic intermediaries are often actually more toxic than the toxins themselves. The moral of the story: Phase I detox without phase II is complete disaster. Read on.

PHASE II: **CONJUGATION**

Here's the best reason I know why you should never go on a water fast, and why you should always do a cleanse that supplies plenty of micromolecules (vitamins, minerals, and phytonutrients) and macromolecules (protein, good fats, and carbohydrates)—all of which are abundant in the Detox Prescription. Phase II of the detoxification process is all about having the right nutrition at the right time. (*Note:* The 3-Day Turbo Cleanse is lower in proteins by design, to rest the gut and deliver a blast of needed micronutrients to the body quickly and efficiently through the intestines.)

As described above, the conjugators, or chelators, are the substances needed to bind with the toxic intermediaries in phase II processes. There are about a hundred of these, but the most important include:

Methylation

Sulfation

Glucuronidation

Acetylation

Glutathione conjugation

Amino acid conjugation

Particular toxic inputs will create stressors for each one of these systems, while different foods will support them, as you might have noticed in the notes that precede each recipe in this book. Garlic and onions provide the building blocks for sulfation, for example; broccoli, kale, and other cruciferous vegetables support glucuronidation. Strawberries, citrus fruits, and salmon fuel methylation. Berries of all types support acetylation. Beans support amino acid conjugation. Green tea, olive oil, and aromatic spices support glutathione conjugation. And that's just scratching the surface. (The chart on page 327, "Stressors and Supporters," is more in-depth.)

The molecules in these foods do more than provide nutrition to bind with toxins, by the way—they also help make red blood cells. They are involved in the production of neurotransmitters. They can even work to repair damage to the DNA. So providing your body with abundant nutrition has far-reaching consequences.

If you are, say, doing a water fast, your body simply won't have what it needs—especially if it was nutrient depleted when you started. There will be a dumping of toxins into phase I, but not enough nutrition to chelate them in phase II. The body will end up marinating in highly toxic intermediaries or free radicals—compounding the problem that you may have been trying to correct with a fast. You will be worse off than when you started.

Here is a graphic that illustrates this process.

Phases of Detoxification

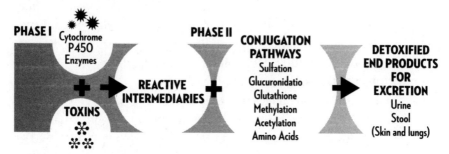

You can also support some of these phase II pathways with targeted supplements called nutraceuticals. There are six, in particular, that I like and that have been shown to be safe and effective: NAC, MSM, SAMe, calcium D-glucarate, quercetin, and curcumin. Being concentrated, nutraceuticals can be more powerful in their actions (and often more expensive) for a specific purpose than whole foods. But they lack the panoply of supportive nutrients that are in the whole food. This trade-off is worth it when the specific nutraceutical ingredient is desired for a specific biochemical purpose. (The FDA does not technically allow for the prescription of these nutrient-only substances, which are not regulated as drugs.) They are best used under the advice of a qualified physician who knows and understands your own health history—especially if you are ill or have had trouble getting the results you want from your detox (or pharmaceutical) efforts or are on medications. I recommend finding someone qualified to practice integrative, functional medicine (visit functionalmedicine.org). But in the interest of sharing the best information, here is what they do:

NAC: N-acetyl cysteine is, hands-down, my favorite supplement for detoxification, because it supports phase II sulfation, as well as amino acid and glutathione conjugation. (It is used in ERs to counteract Tylenol poisoning, which depletes the body of glutathione, even fatally.) It also has kidney-protective and immune-boosting properties and is converted by the body into glutathione, which is sometimes called "the master antioxidant." Usually 500 milligrams twice daily, or as recommended by your physician.

MSM: Methylsulfylmethane is an organosulfur that supports phase II sulfation and glutathione conjugation. It is also widely used to help reduce many kinds of musculoskeletal inflammation (joint, muscle, tendon). Usually taken as 500 milligrams once or twice daily.

SAMe: S-adenosyl-L-methionine strongly supports phase II methylation and glutathione. Besides helping the liver detox, it has some other wide-ranging benefits—these include reducing arthritis, repairing DNA damage, and increasing production of mood-uplifting neurotransmitters. Recommendation is typically 200 to 400 milligrams twice a day to start.

CALCIUM D-GLUCARATE: Naturally found in fruits and vegetables, calcium D-glucarate prevents compounds that have already been phase II–conjugated by glucuronidation from being *de*conjugated and reentering circulation. Notably, it helps clear estrogens from the body—making it a supportive choice for women. Glucaric acid protects DNA by preventing toxins from binding; 500 milligrams two or three times daily is typical.

CURCUMIN: Curcumin, the most active extracted ingredient of turmeric, is a more powerful nutraceutical that supports both phase I and phase II detoxification. Studies have demonstrated that curcumin can also chelate heavy metals directly, has powerful anti-inflammatory effects, may protect against cancer, and may prevent some of the damage that leads to neurodegenerative diseases such as Alzheimer's. The most reliable products are those that contain patented Meriva curcumin. Take 500 milligrams once or twice daily.

QUERCETIN: Quercetin is a flavonoid (naturally found in oranges and onions) that supports both phases of detoxification and is particularly supportive to glucuronidation. It is used by allergy sufferers, as it inhibits the inflammatory cascade; 500 milligrams two or three times daily.

Do they all sound good to you? They all *are* good, for some people, at some times. However, food is still your best medicine. You can spend a lot of money buying supplements. The smart money is on the supplements you truly need—and the best way to know that is to get a professional who is skilled in nutrition and in detoxification science to assess you and make personal recommendations. This should be—and is slowly becoming—the standard of care in this country. However, until that is universally true, I advise you to get proactive in researching your own health care team. Find a provider who knows functional and integrative medicine. Also, find a pharmacist who knows supplements (part of a growing field called pharmacognosy). Learn all you can and remember the smart supplement shoppers' mantra: *caveat emptor.*

Stressors and Supporters

Food is the only source of fuel for both phases of detox—and is especially important for phase II detoxification. Without enough phase II nutrition available in the cells, you stand no chance of winning the war on toxins.

Here is a beginner's list of some of what we know about which particular toxins—from drugs and environmental sources, as well as internal processes—are processed by which phase II detox pathways, and which foods then serve to fuel those pathways. I call them "stressors" and "supporters" of the system. I offer you this detailed information in the hopes that you might use it to fine-tune your diet.

PATHWAY: GLUCURONIDATION

Stressors	Supporters
Acetaminophen	Almond
Amphetamines	Apple
Benzodiazepines	Broccoli
Bisphenol A	Carrot
Estrogen	Chile pepper
NSAIDs	Cocoa
Opiates	Cranberries
Phenobarbital	Halibut
Propranolol	Pumpkin
Salicylates	Sweet potato
Steroid hormones	Turmeric
Tobacco smoke	
Tricyclic antidepressants	

PATHWAY: AMINO ACID CONJUGATION

Stressors	Supporters
Acids	Beans
Antihistamines	Legumes
Salicylates	

(continued)

Stressors and Supporters—*Continued*

PATHWAY: SULFATION

Stressors

Acetaminophen
Adrenaline
Alcohol
Cholesterol
Estrogens
Food additives (flavors and dyes)
Heterocyclic amines
Methyldopa
Minoxidil
Neurotransmitters(incl serotonin)
Phenylephrine
Steroid hormones
Tamoxifen
Thyroid hormone

Supporters

Almond
Brazil nuts
Egg
Leek
Onion
Potato
Scallops
Spinach

PATHWAY: METHYLATION

Stressors

ACE inhibitors
Arsenic
Adrenaline
Dopamine
Estrogens
Histamine
Lead
Mercury
Opiates

Supporters

Banana
Beans
Beets
Broccoli
Brussels sprouts
Cabbage
Cauliflower
Egg
Legumes
Potato
Soy foods
Spinach
Sweet potato

PATHWAY: GLUTATHIONE CONJUGATION

Stressors

Acetaminophen
Alcohol
Chemotherapies (many)
Chlorobenzene
Endotoxins
Heavy metals
Herbicides/insecticides
Industrial solvents
Naphthalene
Penicillin
Petroleum products
Prostaglandins
Styrene
Tetracycline

Supporters

Apples
Artichoke hearts
Asparagus
Cruciferous vegetables
Egg
Green tea
Oats
Pomegranate
Red peppers
Sprouted lentils
Turmeric
Yogurt

PATHWAY: ACETYLATION

Stressors

Aniline (dyes)
Benzodiazepines
Caffeine
Car exhaust fumes
Heterocyclic amines
Histamine
Serotonin
Sulfa antibiotics
Tobacco smoke

Supporters

Berries
Bok choy
Broccoli
Brussels sprouts
Cabbage
Cauliflower
Garlic
Grapes
Kale
Onions
Soy foods

Tune Up the Digestive Symphony

The liver plays a starring role in the detoxification process. Not all of the toxins we're exposed to come from food, but most do, and the digestive tract is designed so that everything we put in our mouths runs through the liver for a chance at detoxification. (The other portals of entry—lungs, skin, and mucous membranes—allow substances to pass through cells via diffusion and enter directly into the circulatory system, where they sidestep a first pass through the liver.) However, its work doesn't take place in a vacuum—the liver's detoxifying dance is interwoven into the full digestive, assimilative, and eliminative systems of the gastrointestinal system.

These interdependent systems need each other to be functioning well to provide the body with a sense of harmony. Think of them as one highly tuned orchestra. The liver plays a key part, but if it's not working from the same score as the stomach, small intestine, colon, kidneys, gallbladder, pancreas, and even the tongue, then it really doesn't matter how well you tune it up. You'll still be experiencing major, screechy, unpleasant health discord.

So the liver is no soloist. It *must* work in tune with every other digestive organ to optimally process toxins. I feel strongly that if you understand the score, you can be a good conductor. So read on for more on the wonderful, orchestral work that is you.

BEFORE THE BITE

Everything starts with the mere thought of eating. This is when you have the power to make a decision that will either be toxic (a burger with chips and beer?) or healing (Wild Arctic Char and Roasted Radicchio and a Hot Tomato Juice?) for your body. As soon as you think about food, your body starts to generate salivary enzymes and digestive hormones. The digestive process begins with the *mere thought* of a good meal.

The next step in the process is pure aromatherapy. Unlike all the other nerves in your body, which have multiple checkpoints that slow messages down, the smell receptors in your nose are hardwired straight to the brain—no filter. You smell the food, you feel hungry (or react to foods in some prepatterned—both positive and occasionally negative—ways). A cascade of digestive enzymes and hormones is unleashed—not just in the mouth, but throughout the body. The appetite-stimulating hormone ghrelin is released in the stomach (and in the brain—also heightening your sense of smell). Your body recognizes that dinner is coming and in its infinite intelligence is getting itself ready to receive the food—not just to enjoy the experience, but to use it for all it's worth. Don't bypass this crucial step of digestion—stop, look, and smell before you dig in.

CHEW, CHEW, CHEW

When you do, take the time to chew. First and most obviously, this is where a lot of the sensory enjoyment of food happens. The tongue is a sensitive organ made to help us understand and savor our food, its textures and flavors, leading us to feel satisfied. Whereas if you wolf down your food, you may hardly even realize you've eaten.

But even more important, chewing kick-starts the chemical and physical processes of digestion. The teeth grind and pulverize the food—a critical step, as food should never leave the mouth in anything chunkier than a gruel consistency. The jaw provides brute force that will be hard for the body to make up for later—use it now, especially if you're eating food that is tough or chunky or fibrous (as with broccoli and other cruciferous vegetables, as well as animal foods, if you are eating those). A good 20 or 30 times makes sense—maybe 12 if you're in a hurry or the food is soft. But three or five bites won't cut it, and could wreak havoc later . . . as you will see.

As you chew, the salivary glands release key enzymes to help break down the food into even smaller chunks. Chewing your food, obviously, exposes them to these enzymes longer, allowing them time to do their work. It's also a good reason to chew everything, even if you don't think you need to—I even advise patients to chew their juices, smoothies, and nut milks, as I did during the 3-Day Turbo Cleanse. If there is nutrition in it, the act of chewing will help your body unlock that nutrition. It is worth the extra 10 seconds of work—you might even be surprised to find that during the process of chewing these kinds of liquids, you discover a new world of flavors in them. You'll slow down in general, allowing more time for your body to register that it is full. Moreover, chewing triggers the release of the hormone CCK (cholecystokinin) in the stomach, which signals ahead to the pancreas and gallbladder to get busy doing their work: Dinner is coming!

DOWN THE HATCH

Once the food is pulverized, nice and moist (another key role of saliva), and ready to go, you swallow—it's down the esophagus and into the stomach. This is a one-way ride, unless something is wrong and you have a condition like GERD (or gastroesophageal reflux, see page 313) and the esophageal sphincter relaxes too much, allowing food and acid to make an unwanted and unpleasant return.

The stomach works as an agitator to literally grind the food it takes in— it is composed of smooth muscle, built to churn. This mechanical action isn't as efficient or as effective as what the mouth can do, but so long as food is present, its muscular action is trying to break it down. Bigger hunks of food mean extra churning.

There's help for this churning, of course. The stomach has lots of chemical allies, chief among them hydrochloric acid, or HCl. If you made it through seventh-grade chemistry class, you might remember this one: It's pretty brutal stuff, eats through (almost) anything, and can be problematic if you spill it where it's not supposed to go (like onto your jeans or into the esophagus). In the stomach, if everything is going according to plan, the HCl is working to break food down into its tiniest particles and is killing any microorganisms that might have hitched a ride in on the food.

HCl levels naturally decline as you age, unfortunately, leaving a little more work for the rest of the system to handle. If you suffer from GERD or gastric ulcers, a painful defect in the stomach lining, you may be prescribed acid-suppressing medications such as proton-pump inhibitors (Zegerid, Nexium, Prilosec) or histamine-2-receptor antagonists (Zantac, Axid, Tagamet). If you take them, your symptoms will be relieved, but HCl levels will be suppressed, "paying forward" a heavier load for the rest of the digestive system to handle (for better alternatives, see my suggestions on page 313) and reducing absorption of nutrients that need acid to prepare them for absorption (e.g., calcium).

Meanwhile, the stomach lining is busy, too. It's producing the enzymes pepsin, which begins to cleave apart protein molecules, and gastrin, which stimulates the secretion of more HCl. It's making mucin, which creates the mucous layer that protects the stomach lining from all that corrosive HCl. And it's triggering the release of the hormone leptin, which reduces appetite and acts as an antagonist to the appetite-promoting hormone ghrelin.

ASSIMILATION ASSIGNATION

If all has gone well and the stomach has done its job, it moves the food in a (hopefully) gruel-like pulp called chyme through the valve at the bottom of the stomach (the pyloric valve) into the duodenum. The duodenum is the first part (about 12 inches) of the small intestine, a small organ unto itself, with an incredibly important job.

As chyme moves into the duodenum, the pancreas and gallbladder come into play—and digestion begins to overlap with assimilation.

Most people think of the pancreas as the organ that produces insulin to handle our blood sugar, but that endocrine function is only half its job. Its other function, called exocrine, is producing the chemicals the duodenum needs to function properly. Perhaps first and foremost, the pancreas releases sodium bicarbonate (or bicarb), which neutralizes stomach acid. In the alkaline environment of the duodenum, the pancreas's enzymes can then take over. Along with bicarb, the pancreas releases into the duodenum a host of enzymes, primary among which are amylase, which further breaks down carbohydrates; lipase, which breaks down fats; and trypsin, which breaks down proteins. Meanwhile, the gallbladder also squirts some bile, an alkaline greenish-brown fluid produced by the liver, into the duodenum to assist in the breakdown of fats (and it also carries some detoxified fat-soluble substances from the liver for elimination out the intestines).

Whereas HCl acted as a machete to crudely hack apart hunks of food in the stomach, enzymes in the duodenum are more like scalpels, reducing food to its molecular components so that it can be absorbed in the small intestine. Vitamins, minerals, phytonutrients, amino acids, carbohydrates, fatty acids . . . all are released from the food and readied to be soaked in and used by the body.

Hopefully, you've chewed well and your stomach has had a chance to do its job perfectly; if not, the duodenum will take up the slack. Here's the rub: If larger chunks of food have gotten through, more enzymes and bile will be needed to process that food. That means more stress on the pancreas and ultimately the liver, which will kick up bile production and send it in via the gallbladder. Unfortunately, these two organs have other important jobs to do, namely regulating insulin (pancreas) and detoxifying the body (liver). Can you see how stressing the system day after day with unchewed, unprocessed, undigested food might result in some unpleasant side effects?

Once food moves out of the duodenum and into the rest of the 20 feet of small intestine, coaxed along via peristaltic waves (rhythmic contractions of the smooth muscles), the heavy work of digestion should have been done, and assimilation gets going. The design and function of the small intestine (let's call it SI) is truly marvelous—you cannot help but be amazed at how magnificently the body has been designed in harmony with the natural world, and how, even amidst our best efforts to undermine it, it keeps on chugging to serve us!

To maximize the absorption area of the SI, it is lined with hundreds of thousands of small projections called *villi*, which also make a few more enzymes to further facilitate sugar breakdown. Here is where the most usable nutrition gets passed into the blood vessels through tightly packed cells (epithelial tissue) that line the villi, and what is not useful gets pushed on through the system and into the large intestine for disposal.

The cells that line these villi are first of all guardians—they try to keep out anything harmful. In that way, they are the body's first line of detoxification. Each of them has thousands of tiny channels that open and close to let in only selective nutrients that have been properly prepared. Between each cell, there is a tight junction that is meant to prevent leakage of anything into the body—specifically into the interstitial space behind the cells. This interstitial space is a soupy area where nutrients (including oxygen) come from the arterial capillaries to supply the cells. This is a heavy exchange zone, as processed toxins and other waste and debris (including CO_2) are moved into the lymphatics (which eliminate fats and heavier molecules) and venous capillaries, for elimination from the body.

If the small intestine is damaged (by drugs, toxins, or free radicals) or diseased (as with celiac disease, infection, or inflammatory conditions such as Crohn's disease), it can develop "leaky gut syndrome," in which the normally tight junctions between the small intestine cells essentially have holes punched in them, allowing material to flow freely into this interstitial space and be circulated within the body—often creating big problems. This is a problem in celiac disease, when the gluten molecules enter into this space and are circulated—even as far away as the brain. It's often hard to know for sure if you have leaky gut, though if you have food allergies or sensitivities, such as lactose intolerance, it's likely that you do. If so, the treatment is to eliminate from your diet and lifestyle all things that might cause further trauma—such as food allergens, charbroiled beef, food additives, toxic plasticizers (to name but a few of hundreds)—and allow the gut to heal itself. That's exactly what we're doing with the Detox Prescription.

THE LIVER SPOT

Everything—and that means *everything*—that passes into the interstitial space from the small intestinal cells is absorbed into the portal vein. This is a big vein whose only purpose is to carry all absorbed things into the liver, which as you recall is the body's main organ of detoxification. We've already said that the liver creates bile to help digest fats. It also produces many other molecules that are critical to maintaining human health, including clotting factors, most of the cholesterol your body needs to maintain cell membranes, and steroid hormones (among other things). It also serves as a storage area, most notably for iron and vitamin B_{12}, but also for fat. (Too much fat gums up the works; fatty liver disease is a scourge associated with obesity in Western culture. Science is now beginning to show how our overconsumption of fructose is linked to fatty liver.)

Unless the liver is overloaded, toxins will get processed here. If proper nutrition has been provided, phase I begins—and within a nanosecond a toxic intermediary (those free radicals!) is created and bound by a phase II conjugator (see page 322 to review the process). It's been several pages in the reading, but it's less than the blink of an eye in the happening.

OUT YOU GO

Once detoxified, there are a number of elimination routes out of the body for toxins. Most bound toxins, once safely conjugated, are rendered water-soluble and released by the cell into the interstitial fluid. They make their way into the hepatic vein, up to the heart where they are are pumped out, and eventually are excreted from the body via the kidneys. (Yet another good reason to keep up your water intake!) Some fat-soluble bound toxins (processed estrogens are a good example) are put by the liver into bile to be released into the intestines.

There are two other eliminative organs: lungs and skin.

The lungs only eliminate gases (mostly CO_2)—along with whatever the lungs' mucosal lining has been able to trap and move out. But every bit of tar you have ever smoked is still in the interstitial spaces, depleting the lungs' oxygen-absorbing capacity—and, if enough of it is there, causing emphysema and cancer. (Any toxic gases you have inhaled have already either damaged the lung tissue directly or been absorbed into the circulation to wreak havoc elsewhere.)

The skin can release toxins via sweat and oil glands. Research on saunas has demonstrated their ability to excrete myriad toxins (including illicit drugs, toxic chemicals, and even antibiotics). The more you sweat, the more toxins are released. So try to sweat every day (see page 306).

All the substances that made it through the small intestine now need to be eliminated out the large intestine (aka colon). The colon has only a small role in active detoxification, by the cells lining its interior and by some of the bacteria. It functions mainly to package waste for removal. For this, the more fiber (and water) you have taken in, the better. Some of the fiber, besides soaking up water to give bulk for better bowel movements, has absorbed toxins from the small intestine for elimination. In the colon, friendly bacteria (probiotics) also play a role by trying to keep the more pathological bacteria at bay—thus reducing the amount of bacterial endotoxins released into the body from the colon.

I want to say a word here about methods used for "colon detoxification," aka colonics. Colonics mainly remove stool. That makes some people feel good temporarily—primarily because they may lose as much as 5 pounds of waste matter. (This will come back anyway over the next few days.) But it does no more "detoxification" than simple waste management—the popular but misguided theory that coffee shot through the colonic will go to the liver and enhance bile flow, resulting in better detoxification, has never been proven. The action for detoxification happens earlier in the process—in the small intestine and liver. And for this you need to feed the system from above, not below.

Repair the Future

There's really good news for anyone willing to put in the time and effort to do the Detox Prescription. By eliminating toxic exposures, introducing a few key mind-body practices to help you manage stress effectively, exercising/sweating regularly, resting sufficiently, and eating a nutrient-dense, plant-based diet that will fuel phase I detox and feed phase II, you can not only detox in the present but in the future, too. The nutrients that feed detox feed everything else that happens in the body—including DNA repair. You can quite literally eat—and act—your way to a brighter future.

The growing field of epigenetics is showing how our choices today impact how our genes are interpreted tomorrow, and next month . . . and next year. Now we understand that our genes do not write our story—indeed, we write it ourselves with our lifestyle choices. It is estimated that we can affect a minimum of 70 percent of disease through our environmental and health choices that influence the epigene, and only 30 percent (some say as little as 10 percent) is manifest destiny from our genes. Yes, we are hardwired in a particular way, but our bodies are like the world's most sophisticated computers—and we are all software engineers. We write our own code when we choose to exercise (or not), when we sleep (or not), when we connect with others (or not), when we relax (or not), when we eat nourishing foods (or not), when we breathe (or not). Every decision you make about your health will affect your health—will you decide for the good or not?

One other thing to consider: Changes we make to the epigene are inherited by our progeny. So we not only make ourselves better by cleaning up our lifestyle, but we pass it on to future generations—often trumping genetic predispositions, such as hypertension and high blood pressure, diabetes, arthritis, etc. That's right. You can not only experience better health but leave a legacy for your children—and your children's children. Or not.

I think it wise to choose to live in a way that minimizes your exposure to toxins and maximizes your chances of experiencing optimal health and energy right now. Do it for yourself. Do it for your health and energy, and for your very DNA. Do it for your legacy.

You can. That's why I wrote *The Detox Prescription*. I've drawn on all of my experience to outline a way of living and eating that can be, for many people, absolutely transformative. I think that once you experience the benefits, you won't be able to imagine living any other way.

Acknowledgments

I t sounds like a cliché, but at this point in my career and life, I realize increasingly that every encounter I have with a patient—as well as with friends, family, and colleagues—provides a moment for learning, reflection, and growth. This book is the culmination of what I have learned from dozens of masters and hundreds of "teaching assistants." I have a few people especially to thank for helping this book come to fruition.

First and foremost, I want to thank my editor at Rodale, Alex Postman. Every author should be so lucky to have such a wise, helpful, and supportive editor holding their hand every step of the way, ever since our very first meeting about the book over breakfast at Le Pain Quotidian 2 years ago.

My coauthors have been wonderful. Mary Beth Augustine's knowledge base of nutritional science is vast and deep. She kept peppering us with extraordinary new studies on the power of food to change our lives while creating more than 100 wonderful recipes to make the science real (and delicious). Hillari Dowdle made the writing process so smooth: She has an awe-inspiring ability to take my medical-speak and organize and transform it into engaging prose. I am also indebted to her for her knowledgeable input on the yoga, meditation, and stress-busting strategies.

Dean Ornish has been a mentor, colleague, and friend for years. I thank him for all he has given me personally, as well as having had not only the brilliance to carry out groundbreaking studies published in major journals, but also the perseverance for more than 16 years with Medicare and insurance companies to make his life-extending and disease-reversing program reimbursable as a model for optimal health (www.pmri.org).

The Environmental Working Group (www.ewg.org), headed by Ken Cook, has become a beacon of truth, showing us the evidence we desperately need to know to help counter the ever-increasing pollution of our planet.

The Institute of Functional Medicine (www.functionalmedicine.org) and its brilliant physician leaders and teachers has been an invaluable resource for clinicians wanting to take back their medical education and make it practical for their patients—using the leading edge of health science to transform health practices. Mark Hyman, Laurie Hoffman, and David Jones are treasures for their commitment to this cause. Jeff Bland, PhD, is the IFM's founder and is the current president of his new foundation, Preventive Lifestyle Medicine Institute. He is the dean of this field and has had a profound influence on my life and practice.

I thank my deeply committed colleagues at the Continuum Center for Health and Healing of Beth Israel Medical Center (www.healthandhealingny.org) for their inspired collaboration.

I'm also very grateful to the whole Rodale team, including Nancy Bailey, Chris Rhoads, Aly Mostel, and Brent Gallenberger, for their hard work and energetic support throughout the book-writing process.

And most specially, I thank my patients, for working with and inspiring me all these years.

I wouldn't be able to do what I do without the incredible loving collaboration with my wife, Kathy—health science writer par excellence, coauthor of our last book, *The Source* (*Power Up* in paperback), primary author of our Web site www.iwellville.com, and loving mother of our two wonderful daughters.

A Note on Resources

There's an enormous amount of emerging science on the subject of detoxification—too much, in fact, to list in these pages. To learn more about the research underpinning *The Detox Prescription* and to browse additional resources, see www.woodsonmerrell.com.

Index

Underscored page references indicate boxed text. **Boldface** references indicate illustrations.

Acetaminophen, 40, 327, 328
Acid-suppressing medications, 40–41, 332
Acorn squash
  Baked Acorn Squash with Apples and
    Walnuts, 225
Acupuncture, 81, 297–98
Adenosine triphosphate (ATP), 136
Adrenaline, toxic effects of, 7
Afternoon Snack 1, in 3-Day Turbo Cleanse
  Carotenoid Smoothie, 122
  Pineapple Sizzle Juice, 130
  Sunburst Juice, 114
Afternoon Snack 2, in 3-Day Turbo Cleanse
  Bravocado! Smoothie, 123
  Crucifer Crusader, 131
  Limetastic! Juice, 115
Agave nectar and syrup, 198
Agriculture
  chemicals in, 30, 60, 67 (see also Pesticides)
  preserving diversity in, 66
Air, toxins in, 7, 48–49
Alcohol, 20, 85, 287
Allergies
  chronic, treatments for, 316
  food (see Food allergies and sensitivities)
Almond butter
  Almond Butter Banana-Raspberry Tortilla,
    150
Almonds
  Raw Almond Milk, 112, 123
American diet, health hazards from, xv, 16
Apples
  Baked Acorn Squash with Apples and
    Walnuts, 225
  Cranberry Supreme Juice, 113
  Get-Up-and-Go Juice, 119
  Limetastic! Juice, 115
  Nutty Baked Apples, 188
  organic, 95
  Polenta with Apple Compote, 218
  Polenta with Granny Smith Apple Compote,
    164–65
  Twice-Baked Fruit-and-Nut-Stuffed Sweet
    Potatoes, 275

Arctic char
  Wild Arctic Char and Roasted Radicchio,
    201
Arsenic toxicity, 34
Asthma treatments, 316
Atrazine, 8
Augustine, Mary Beth, xvii, 11, 72, 109, 135,
    138, 144, 178, 198, 238, 239
Avocados
  Bravocado! Smoothie, 123
  Chickpea and Arugula-Stuffed Avocado,
    213
  "Creamy" Avocado-Broccoli Soup, 233–34
  Green Gazpacho with Chive-Cayenne Oil
    and Tortilla Toasts, 276–77
  Green Goodness Smoothie, 111
  Moo-Less Avocado-Chocolate Mousse, 183,
    189
  Poached Egg–Avocado Tortilla, 257
  Red Quinoa–Avocado Salad, 284
Ayurveda, 297, 298

Bacteria
  good vs. bad, 56, 134, 302
  in probiotics, 179, 302, 336
Bananas
  Almond Butter Banana-Raspberry Tortilla,
    150
  Buckwheat-Banana-Walnut Cereal, 232
Beano, 141, 147, 307
Beans
  guide to, 146–48
  Mediterranean Kidney Beans, 161
  Middle Eastern White Beans, 154
  in 7-Day In-Depth Detox, 138–40
  Southwestern Black-Bean Mash, 169
  Spicy White Bean and Spinach Soup, 222
  Stuffed Black Bean–Cabbage Rolls, 205–6
  Three-Bean Kale Sauté with Brown Rice,
    174–75
  Tomato and Kidney Bean Soup with Maple-
    Sesame Oranges, 253–54
  Tuna Niçoise and White Bean Salad, 270
Beef, 58, 59

Beets
    Just Beet It Juice, 121
    Roasted Root Vegetables, 220–21
Berries. *See also* Blueberries; Cranberries;
        Raspberries
    Coconut Yogurt, Berry, and Hemp Heart
        Parfait, 157
Beverages. *See also specific beverages*
    for hydration, 90
Biofeedback, 300
Bison, 58
Bisphenol A. *See* BPA
Blackburn, Elizabeth, xiv, 53
Bland, Jeffrey, 339
Blenders, 73, 78
Blood pressure caution, in 3-Day Turbo
        Cleanse, 97
Blood sugar
    Detox Prescription lowering, xviii, 97
    foods raising, 82
    foods stabilizing, 100, 104, 304
Blueberries
    Black Rice Porridge with Blueberries and
        Toasted Walnuts, 283
    Chia Seed Porridge with Blueberries, 243
Blueprint Cleanse, 72
Blue Zones, 57
Body work, 301
Boosters, for 3-Day Turbo Cleanse recipes,
        102–6
Botanical medicine, 299–300
Bowels, as detoxification organ, 4
BPA, 3, 6, 8, 30, 49, 61, 75
BPA-free containers, 75, 77
Breakfasts
    for blood sugar stability, 82
    3-Day Turbo Cleanse
        Get-Up-and-Go Juice, 119
        Green Goodness Smoothie, 111
        Kale-icious! Smoothie, 127
    7-Day In-Depth Detox
        Almond Butter Banana-Raspberry
            Tortilla, 150
        Coconut Yogurt, Berry, and Hemp Heart
            Parfait, 157
        Polenta with Granny Smith Apple
            Compote, 164–65
        Savory Green Tea–Buckwheat Cereal,
            172
    21-Day Clean and Lean Diet
        Baked Acorn Squash with Apples and
            Walnuts, 225
        Black Rice Porridge with Blueberries and
            Toasted Walnuts, 283
        Buckwheat-Banana-Walnut Cereal, 232
        Chia Seed Porridge with Blueberries, 243
        Kick-Butt Coconut Oatmeal, 191
        Orange-Pecan-Millet Cereal, 269
        Parsnip and Pear Puree, 197

    Poached Egg–Avocado Tortilla, 257
    Polenta with Apple Compote, 218
    Pumpkin-Oat Pancakes, 250
    Tofu-Veggie Scramble with Gluten-Free
        Toast, 263
    Twice-Baked Fruit-and-Nut-Stuffed
        Sweet Potatoes, 275
    Vanilla Cashew Cream, 219
    Vanilla Quinoa with Raspberry Compote,
        204
    Zucchini and Sweet Potato Frittata,
        211–12
Breathing techniques
    for Day 1 of Turbo Cleanse, 117
    meditative, xiv, 12, 13, 15, 291–92
    for stress reduction, 89, 91
    for thought clearing, 132
Broccoli
    "Creamy" Avocado-Broccoli Soup, 233–34
    Crucifer Crusader, 131
    Peanut Satay Tofu Stir-Fry with Broccoli,
        214–15
Brown rice syrup, 198
Brussels sprouts
    Roasted Brussels Sprouts and Hazelnuts
        with Miso Soup, 264–65
Buckwheat
    Buckwheat-Banana-Walnut Cereal, 232
    Savory Green Tea–Buckwheat Cereal, 172
    Tahini-Buckwheat Tabbouleh, 153
Burdock root tea, 141
Burger
    Chickpea Burger with Tahini Dressing and
        Red Cabbage Slaw, 278–79
Butter, reducing consumption of, 86
Butterbur, for migraine prevention, 12
Butternut squash
    Curry Butternut Squash Soup with
        Cayenne-Roasted Butternut Squash
        Seeds, 151–52

Cabbage
    Chickpea Burger with Tahini Dressing and
        Red Cabbage Slaw, 278–79
    Red Cabbage Slaw, 280
    Stuffed Black Bean–Cabbage Rolls, 205–6
Caffeine, 84, 99
Calcium D-glucarate, for detoxification
        support, 326
Cancer
    chemotherapy for, 41, 96
    contributors to, 6, 8, 9, 30, 322, 336
    preventing, xiii–xiv, 53, 62, 66, 85, 103,
        104, 105, 106, 141, 147, 178, 310, 326
Carrots
    Carrot-Rhubarb Soup, 173
    Just Beet It Juice, 121
    Roasted Root Vegetables, 220–21
    Sunburst Juice, 114

Cashews
    Lentil-Cashew–Stuffed Peppers, 158–59
    Raw Cashew Milk, 120, 131
    Red Pepper–Cashew Endive with Grape
        Salad, 192
    Vanilla Cashew Cream, 219
Cauliflower
    Cauliflower "Rice," 246–47
Celery
    Get-Up-and-Go Juice, 119
Celiac disease, 26, 27, 32, 83, 334
Cells, effect of toxins on, 320–22
Cereals
    Buckwheat-Banana-Walnut Cereal, 232
    Orange-Pecan-Millet Cereal, 269
    Savory Green Tea–Buckwheat Cereal, 172
Champion Juicer, 74
Cheese, 55, 86
Chemicals. See also Toxins
    prevalence of, 30–31
    toxic effects of, 3–4
Chemotherapy, 41, 96
Cherries
    Kale, Pecan, and Dried Cherry Salad with
        Rosemary Quinoa, 251–52
Chewing
    juices and smoothies, 99, 137
    in mindful eating, 155
    for optimal digestion, 135, 137, 331
Chia seeds
    Chia Seed Porridge with Blueberries, 243
Chickpeas
    Chickpea and Arugula-Stuffed Avocado,
        213
    Chickpea Burger with Tahini Dressing and
        Red Cabbage Slaw, 278–79
Chicory root tea, 141
Chive-cayenne oil
    Green Gazpacho with Chive-Cayenne Oil
        and Tortilla Toasts, 276–77
Chlorella, 310
Chocolate
    dark, 143, 175
    Moo-Less Avocado-Chocolate Mousse, 183,
        189
    Rawsome Chocolate Truffles, 183, 186–87
Chronic diseases, xii, 100, 290
Clean Fifteen produce, 61, 63
Cleaning products. See Household cleaning
    products
Coconut milk
    Bravocado Smothie, 123
    Kick-Butt Coconut Oatmeal, 191
Coconut sweeteners, 198
Coffee
    teas replacing, 140–41
    weaning from, 84–85
Colon, in detoxification, 336
Colonics, 336

Complementary healing practices, xii–xiii
Conjugation phase of detoxification, 324–26
    stressors and supporters of, 327–29
Convenience foods, as toxic trigger, 17. See
    also Processed foods
Cooked foods, benefits of, 136
Cookware, avoiding toxins from, 74–75
Corticosteroids, 41
Cortisol, 7
Cranberries
    Cranberry Supreme Juice, 113
Cravings, sugar, 82
Crohn's disease. See Inflammatory bowel
    disease
Crostini
    Spinach-Tofu Soup with Gluten-Free Garlic
        Crostini, 271–72
Cucumbers
    Get-Up-and-Go Juice, 119
    Green Gazpacho with Chive-Cayenne Oil
        and Tortilla Toasts, 276–77
    Green Goodness Smoothie, 111
    Limetastic! Juice, 115
Curcumin, for detoxification support, 326
Curry powder
    Curried Lentils with Sweet Potato and
        Chard, 193–94
    Curried Mustard Greens with Lentils and
        Eggs, 285
    Curry Butternut Squash Soup with
        Cayenne-Roasted Butternut Squash
        Seeds, 151–52

Dairy products
    nonfat vs. full-fat, 55–56
    reducing consumption of, 86
    sensitivity to, 55
    toxins in, 6
Dandelion root tea, 140–41
Davis, William, 27
DDT, 3, 6, 9, 80
Dehydration, avoiding, 90
Desserts
    fruit as, 143, 183
    in 21-Day Clean and Lean Diet, 182–83,
        186
    Just Peachy, 187
    Moo-Less Avocado-Chocolate Mousse,
        183, 189
    Nutty Baked Apples, 188
    Rawsome Chocolate Truffles, 183, 186–
        87
Detox boosters, 106
Detoxification
    in cells, 320
    digestive system for, 330–35, 336
    effective, outcomes of, 4
    food-based, 30
    future repair from, 336–37

ineffective methods of, 4–5
lungs for, 335–36
overloaded mechanisms of, 4
phases of, 5, **325**
    conjugation, 324–26, <u>328</u>, <u>329</u>
    modification, 322–23
skin for, 336
steps toward, 49–58 (see also Detox
    Prescription program)
sweating for, <u>202</u>, 306, 336
Detox Prescription program
food preparation for, 93–97
foods in, xi, 8, 70
options for moving beyond, 290
    elimination diet, 292–96
    enzymes, 307–8
    integrative therapies, 297–301
    medical foods, 303–4
    meditation, 291–92
    probiotics, 301–3
    supplements, 308–12, <u>314–15</u>
    sweating, 306
    troubleshooting symptoms, 312–13, 316–18
overview of, xvi–xviii, 9–10
phases of (see 3-Day Turbo Cleanse; 7-Day
    In-Depth Detox; 21-Day Clean and
    Lean Diet)
planning and preparation for, 71
    of body, 78–86
    in kitchen, 72–79
    of mind, 87–93
principles of
    clean eating, 67–68
    dietary diversity, 61–62, <u>64–65</u>, 66
    doable diets, 68–69
    organic foods, 59–61
results from, xvi, 71–72
setbacks in, <u>148</u>
symptoms after completion of, 289, 290
Detox-retox cycle, 79–80
Detox teas, morning, <u>140–41</u>
Dietary diversity, 61–62, <u>64–65</u>, 66
Diets
    detoxification, 50
    ineffective, 21, 69–70
    for slow weight loss, 68–69
Digestion
    enzymes helping, 307, 308
    process of, 135
    for detoxification, 330–35, 336
Digital devices, logging off, <u>255</u>
Dinners
    3-Day Turbo Cleanse
        Raw Almond Milk, 123
        Raw Cashew Milk, 131
        Raw Walnut Milk, 116
    7-Day In-Depth Detox
        Mediterranean Kidney Beans, 161
        Middle Eastern White Beans, 154

Roasted Lemon-Garlic Artichokes, 160
Rosemary Celeriac and Root Vegetables,
    168
Southwestern Black-Bean Mash, 169
Tahini-Buckwheat Tabbouleh, 153
Three-Bean Kale Sauté with Brown Rice,
    174–75
21-Day Clean and Lean Diet
    Black Bean and Spinach Tortilla, 235
    Broiled Wild Salmon, 245
    Caramelized Sea Scallops with Bok Choy,
        228–29
    Cauliflower "Rice," 246–47
    Chickpea Burger with Tahini Dressing
        and Red Cabbage Slaw, 278–79
    Curried Lentils with Sweet Potato and
        Chard, 193–94
    Curried Mustard Greens with Lentils and
        Eggs, 285
    Peanut Satay Tofu Stir-Fry with Broccoli,
        214–15
    Quinoa with Asian Mushrooms and
        Black Truffle Oil, 266
    Red Cabbage Slaw, 280
    Roasted Spaghetti Squash and Tomatoes,
        259–60
    Rosemary-Portobello Mushrooms, 207
    Spicy White Bean and Spinach Soup, 222
    Spinach-Tofu Soup with Gluten-Free
        Garlic Crostini, 271–72
    Tahini Green Beans, 208
    Tomato and Kidney Bean Soup with
        Maple-Sesame Oranges, 253–54
    Wild Arctic Char and Roasted Radicchio,
        201
Dioxins, 3, <u>8</u>, 306
Dirty Dozen produce, 61, <u>63</u>, 94
Disease, taxonomy of, xiii
Dressings, 142–43, 144
    Chickpea Burger with Tahini Dressing and
        Red Cabbage Slaw, 278–79
    Citrus Zinger Detox Dressing, 144, 145
    Honey-Mustard Detox Dressing, 144, 146
    Lemon-Tahini Dressing, 144, 145
    Sesame-Ginger Detox Dressing, 144, 147
Dr. Merrell's Detox Super Shooter, <u>311</u>

Eating out or on the move, <u>238–39</u>
Eggplant
    Roasted Veggie and Hummus Romaine
        Wraps, 258
Eggs
    Curried Mustard Greens with Lentils and
        Eggs, 285
    health benefits from, 56–57, 180
    Poached Egg–Avocado Tortilla, 257
    reducing consumption of, 86
    Zucchini and Sweet Potato Frittata, 211–12
Elimination diet, 11–12, 292–96, 316

EMFs (electromagnetic fields), 9, 43, 255
Energy, from raw foods, 136
Energy boosters, 103
Environmental Defense Fund, 57, 181, 239
Environmental Factors Questionnaire, 31,
    39–42, 42–47, 133, 176, 237, 287
Environmental Working Group, 30, 61, 63,
    338
Enzymes, 307–8, 317
Epigenetics, xiv, 53, 337
Essential fatty acid boosters, 102, 105
Essential fatty acids, 56, 99. See also Omega-3
    fatty acids
Exercise, xiv, 91, 92, 182
    sweating from, 202, 306

Fat, body
    inflammation from, 7
    rapid weight loss and, 68–69
Fiber, for removing toxins, 140–41, 336
Fiber boosters, 104–5
Fish
    Broiled Wild Salmon, 245
    guide to choosing, 181
    health benefits from, 57, 180
    safety of, 57, 180, 181
    Tuna Niçoise and White Bean Salad, 270
    Wild Arctic Char and Roasted Radicchio,
        201
Food allergies and sensitivities, 26, 27, 183,
    292–93, 296
    common triggers of, 294–95
Free radicals, 5, 15, 88, 144, 291, 319, 321,
    323, 325
Frittata
    Zucchini and Sweet Potato Frittata, 211–12
Fruits. See also specific fruits
    for dessert, 143, 183
    Dirty Dozen and Clean Fifteen, 61, 63, 94
    organic, 59–61 (see also Organic foods,
        produce)
    sugar in, 100
    toxins in, 6
    Twice-Baked Fruit-and-Nut-Stuffed Sweet
        Potatoes, 275

Gallbladder, in digestive process, 333
Game meats, 58–59
Garlic
    "Creamy" Garlic Soup with Spinach, 226–
        27
    Roasted Lemon-Garlic Artichokes, 160
    Spinach-Tofu Soup with Gluten-Free Garlic
        Crostini, 271–72
    as supplement, 312
Gastritis treatments, 313
Gazpacho
    Green Gazpacho with Chive-Cayenne Oil
        and Tortilla Toasts, 276–77

Genes, effect of toxins on, 321–22
Genuis, Stephen, xiii, xv
GERD, 26, 27, 83, 312, 313, 332
Ginkgo, 299
Gluten intolerance, 293, 307–8
Gluten sensitivity, 27
Grains, as wheat alternative, 178, 179
Grapes
    Red Pepper–Cashew Endive with Grape
        Salad, 192
Green beans
    Tahini Green Beans, 208
Greenhouse gas emissions, 67
Greens, salad, 142, 144
Green superfood powders, 309–10
Green tea, 84
    Savory Green Tea–Buckwheat Cereal, 172
Green tea extract, 312
Guided imagery, 300–301

Headaches
    caffeine, 84
    from food allergies, 28
    migraine, case history about, 10–13
    treatments for, 317
Health care costs, xii
Heart attacks, morning, 132
Heart disease
    contributors to, 6, 16, 24, 27, 74, 92, 94,
        182, 186, 302
    eggs and, 56, 180
    preventing, xiii, 85, 91, 147
    reversing, 53, 290
Heavy metal testing, 30, 34
Hemp
    Coconut Yogurt, Berry, and Hemp Heart
        Parfait, 157
    Raw Hemp Milk, 128
Herbal medicine, 298, 299–300
Holistic therapies, 297–300
Home environment, detoxifying, 49–50
Homeopathy, 298–99
Honey
    Honey-Mustard Detox Dressing, 144, 146
    as sweetener, 198–99
Household cleaning products
    chemicals to avoid in, 75
    ecofriendly, 75–76
    as toxic, 7, 25, 49
Hummus
    Hummus and Veggie Rainbow Tortilla,
        200
    Roasted Veggie and Hummus Romaine
        Wraps, 258
Hydration guidelines, 90
Hyman, Mark, 68, 339

IBD. See Inflammatory bowel disease
IBS. See Irritable bowel syndrome

Inflammatory bowel disease (IBD), 30, 32,
    96–97, 301, 302, 304, 334
Insomnia, yoga pose after, 267
Institute for Functional Medicine, 31, 33, 33,
    290
Integrative/functional medicine practitioners,
    31, 33, 38, 47, 290
Integrative therapies, 297–301
Irritable bowel syndrome (IBS), 26, 27, 28, 83,
    291, 298, 301, 302, 308, 312, 313, 316

Joint pain, treating, 317–18
Journaling, 91–93, 133, 176, 237, 261, 287–88
Juice delivery services, 72
Juicers, 72, 73–74, 79
Juices, 3-Day Turbo Cleanse, 99–100, 101
    boosters for, 102–6
    chewing, 99, 137
    Cranberry Supreme Juice, 113
    Get-Up-and-Go Juice, 119
    Hot Tomato! Juice, 129
    Just Beet It Juice, 121
    Limetastic! Juice, 115
    Pineapple Sizzle Juice, 130
    Sunburst Juice, 114
Juicing
    DIY, 72
        equipment for, 72–74
        raw food benefits from, 136

Kale
    Kale, Pecan, and Dried Cherry Salad with
        Rosemary Quinoa, 251–52
    Kale-icious! Smoothie, 127
    Three-Bean Kale Sauté with Brown Rice,
        174–75
Kidneys, as detoxification organ, 4
Kitchen equipment, 72–74, 76–77, 78–79

L

Lactose intolerance, 6, 307
Lamb, 59
Large intestine, in detoxification, 336
Lead toxicity, 34
Leaky gut syndrome, 293, 304, 334
Lemons
    Citrus Zinger Detox Dressing, 144, 145
    juicing and zesting, 77
    Lemon-Tahini Dressing, 144, 145
    Roasted Lemon-Garlic Artichokes, 160
Lentils, 142–43
    Curried Lentils with Sweet Potato and
        Chard, 193–94
    Curried Mustard Greens with Lentils and
        Eggs, 285
    Lentil-Cashew–Stuffed Peppers, 158–59
    Lentil-Walnut Pâté, 244
Lifestyle changes, professional help with, 47
Lifestyle medicine, xii–xiii, 33

Limes
    Limetastic! Juice, 115
Liver
    alcohol as toxic to, 85
    as detoxification organ, 4, 320, 330, 333,
        335
    in digestive process, 333, 335
Lunches
    3-Day Turbo Cleanse
        Cranberry Supreme Juice, 113
        Hot Tomato! Juice, 129
        Just Beet It Juice, 121
    7-Day In-Depth Detox
        Carrot-Rhubarb Soup, 173
        Curry Butternut Squash Soup with
            Cayenne-Roasted Butternut Squash
            Seeds, 151–52
        Lentil-Cashew–Stuffed Peppers, 158–59
        Savory Mushroom Soup, 166–67
    21-Day Clean and Lean Diet
        Chickpea and Arugula-Stuffed Avocado,
            213
        "Creamy" Avocado-Broccoli Soup,
            233–34
        "Creamy" Garlic Soup with Spinach,
            226–27
        Green Gazpacho with Chive-Cayenne Oil
            and Tortilla Toasts, 276–77
        Hummus and Veggie Rainbow Tortilla,
            200
        Kale, Pecan, and Dried Cherry Salad with
            Rosemary Quinoa, 251
        Lentil-Walnut Pâté, 244
        Red Pepper–Cashew Endive with Grape
            Salad, 192
        Red Quinoa–Avocado Salad, 284
        Roasted Brussels Sprouts and Hazelnuts
            with Miso Soup, 264–65
        Roasted Root Vegetables, 220–21
        Roasted Veggie and Hummus Romaine
            Wraps, 258
        Stuffed Black Bean–Cabbage Rolls,
            205–6
        Tuna Niçoise and White Bean Salad, 270
Lungs, for detoxification, 335–36
Lymphatic drainage massage, 301

Magnesium, for migraine prevention, 12
Maple syrup, 199
    Tomato and Kidney Bean Soup with Maple-
        Sesame Oranges, 253–54
Massage, 223
    lymphatic drainage, 301
Master Cleanse detox, 4, 5, 70
Meal replacements, 305
Meats
    best choices of, 58–59
    consequences of producing, 67
    factory-farmed, 68

Meats *(cont.)*
  problems with, 58
  reducing consumption of, 85–86
  toxins in, 6
Medical foods, 303–4
Medical Symptom Questionnaire, 31, 33, 35,
  35–38, 133, 176, 237, 287, 289
Medications. *See* Pharmaceuticals
Meditation techniques
  breathing (*see* Breathing techniques,
    meditative)
  candle gazing before sleep, 248
  health benefits of, xiv, 12, 13
  mantra repetition, 291
  mindful eating, 155
  regular practice of, 291–92
  thought clearing, 132
  visualization vs., 286
  walking, 195
Mercury toxicity, 34, 181
Metabolic syndrome, xv
Microbiome, 56, 302
Midmorning snacks
  in 3-Day Turbo Cleanse
    Raw Almond Milk, 112
    Raw Cashew Milk, 120
    Raw Hemp Milk, 128
  in 21-Day Clean and Lean Diet, 180, 182
Migraine headaches, case history about,
    10–13. *See also* Headaches
Milk, reducing consumption of, 86
Milks, nut. *See* Nut milks
Milk thistle, 312
Mind-body therapies, 300–301
Mindful eating, 155
Miso soup
  Roasted Brussels Sprouts and Hazelnuts
    with Miso Soup, 264–65
Modification phase of detoxification, 322–23
Molasses, 199
Morning detox teas, 140–41
Mousse
  Moo-Less Avocado-Chocolate Mousse, 183,
    189
MSM, for detoxification support, 326
Muscle loss, from rapid weight loss, 68
Musculoskeletal pain, treating, 317–18
Mushrooms
  Quinoa with Asian Mushrooms and Black
    Truffle Oil, 266
  Rosemary-Portobello Mushrooms, 207
  Savory Mushroom Soup, 166–67
Mustard greens
  Curried Mustard Greens with Lentils and
    Eggs, 285

NAC (N-acetyl cysteine), for detoxification,
    325
Naparstek, Belleruth, 301

Nonstick cookware, avoiding toxins from,
    74–75
Nut butters. *See* Almond butter;
    Peanut butter
Nut milks
  in 7-Day In-Depth Detox, 138, 144
  in 3-Day Turbo Cleanse, 99, 100
  boosters for, 102–6
  Raw Almond Milk, 112, 123
  Raw Cashew Milk, 120, 131
  Raw Hemp Milk, 128
  Raw Walnut Milk, 116
Nutraceuticals, for detoxification support,
    325–26
Nutrition, for detoxification, xv, xvi, xvii, 4,
    5, 8, 38, 52, 53–54, 99
Nutritional deficiency, xiii–xiv, 3, 32, 33
Nuts. *See also* Almonds; Cashews; Hazelnuts;
    Pecans; Walnuts
  allergies to, 294
  Nutty Baked Apples, 188
  Twice-Baked Fruit-and-Nut-Stuffed Sweet
    Potatoes, 275

Oats
  Kick-Butt Coconut Oatmeal, 191
  Pumpkin-Oat Pancakes, 250
Obesity, toxic effects of, 7
Omega-3 fatty acids, 56, 57, 180, 181
Onions
  Roasted Veggie and Hummus Romaine
    Wraps, 258
Oranges
  Citrus Zinger Detox Dressing, 144, 145
  Orange-Pecan-Millet Cereal, 269
  Tomato and Kidney Bean Soup with Maple-
    Sesame Oranges, 253–54
Organic foods, 14, 15, 18, 19, 22, 68, 70, 86,
    96, 287
  dairy, 56, 182
  Dirty Doezen/Clean 15, 61, 63
  effect on genetics, 53–54
  eggs, 56, 86, 180
  juices, 72, 182, 311
  produce, xvi, 6, 53, 59–61, 62, 63, 66,
    94–95, 96, 97, 138, 186, 322
  protein powders, 102
Ornish, Dean, xiv, 53
Over-the-counter medications, reducing use
    of, 40–41
Overweight
  case history about, 16–18
  toxic effects of, 7
Overwork, as migraine trigger, 15
Ovolactopescovegetarian (OLPV), 55

Pancakes
  Pumpkin-Oat Pancakes, 250
Pancreas, in digestive process, 333

Papayas
  Sunburst Juice, 114
Parabens, 9
Parasympathetic nervous system, 13
Parsnips
  Parsnip and Pear Puree, 197
  Roasted Root Vegetables, 220–21
  Rosemary Celeriac and Root Vegetables,
    168
Pâté
  Lentil-Walnut Pâté, 244
Patients
  common symptoms of, 1–2
  individuality of, xi–xii
  toxicity of, 3
PBDE, 9
PCBs, 8, 21, 57, 84, 179, 181, 306
Peaches
  Just Peachy, 187
Peanut butter
  Peanut Satay Tofu Stir-Fry with Broccoli,
    214–15
Pears
  Bravocado! Smoothie, 123
  Parsnip and Pear Puree, 197
Pecans
  Kale, Pecan, and Dried Cherry Salad with
    Rosemary Quinoa, 251–52
  Nutty Baked Apples, 188
  Orange-Pecan-Millet Cereal, 269
  Twice-Baked Fruit-and-Nut-Stuffed Sweet
    Potatoes, 275
Peppers, bell
  Lentil-Cashew–Stuffed Peppers, 158–59
  Red Pepper–Cashew Endive with Grape
    Salad, 192
  Roasted Veggie and Hummus Romaine
    Wraps, 258
  Tofu-Veggie Scramble with Gluten-Free
    Toast, 263
Perchlorate, 9
Perfluorooctanoic acid. See PFOA
Pesticides
  effects of, xv, 21, 60, 67, 69, 320
  in environment, 49
  in foods, 6, 17, 39, 42, 49, 54, 57, 60, 61,
    63, 95, 295
  medications and, 40
  organic foods for avoiding, 14
  phase I detox and, 323
  removal of, 96, 136
  in supplements, 314
  types of, 8, 9
PFOA, 6, 8, 74–75
Pharmaceuticals
  alternatives to, xiii
  overreliance on, xi, 2
  reducing use of, 40–41
  as toxic, 7, 20

Phthalates, 7, 8, 49, 327
Phytonutrients
  in rainbow of foods, 62, 66
  in 7-Day In-Depth Detox, 138
  in 3-Day Turbo Cleanse, 100, 136
Pineapple
  Pineapple Sizzle Juice, 130
Plastic containers, avoiding, 18, 75
Plastics, as toxic, 6, 39
Polenta
  Polenta with Apple Compote, 218
  Polenta with Granny Smith Apple Compote,
    164–65
Pork, 59
Porridges
  Black Rice Porridge with Blueberries and
    Toasted Walnuts, 283
  Chia Seed Porridge with Blueberries, 243
Poultry, choosing, 58
Prebiotics, 302, 313, 316
Probiotics, 56, 301–3, 316
Processed foods
  eliminating, 81–82
  encouragement to eat, xv
  harmful effects of, 54
  overreliance on, 2
Prostate cancer, vegan diet and, 53
Protein
  calculating need for, 182
  eating more, 287
  in 7-Day In-Depth Detox, 138
Protein powders, 102
Psoriasis. See Skin conditions
Psychological dysfunction, disease from, xiii
Pumpkin
  Pumpkin-Oat Pancakes, 250
Pushups, 230

Quercetin, for detoxification support, 326
Questionnaires, for assessing toxicity,
    31–32
  Environmental Factors Questionnaire, 31,
    39–42, 42–47, 133, 176, 237, 287
  Medical Symptom Questionnaire, 31, 33,
    35, 35–38, 133, 176, 237, 287, 289
Quinoa
  Kale, Pecan, and Dried Cherry Salad with
    Rosemary Quinoa, 251–52
  Quinoa with Asian Mushrooms and Black
    Truffle Oil, 266
  Red Quinoa–Avocado Salad, 284
  Vanilla Quinoa with Raspberry Compote,
    204
  as wheat alternative, 28

Radiation, 41
Rainbow of foods, 61–62, 64–65, 66, 138,
    178
Rainbow superfood boosters, 103–4

Raspberries
  Almond Butter Banana-Raspberry Tortilla,
    150
  Vanilla Quinoa with Raspberry Compote,
    204
Raw cane sugar, 199
Raw foods, benefits of, 136
Recreational drugs, as toxic trigger, 19, 20
Red superfood powders, 310
Retox, 80, 178
Rheumatoid arthritis, xvi–xvii, 51, 53
Rhubarb
  Carrot-Rhubarb Soup, 173
Rice. See Black rice; Brown Rice
Rosemary
  Kale, Pecan, and Dried Cherry Salad with
    Rosemary Quinoa, 251–52
  Rosemary Celeriac and Root Vegetables,
    168
  Rosemary-Portobello Mushrooms, 207

Salad dressings. See Dressings
Salads
  in 7-Day In-Depth Detox, 141–42
  in 21-Day Clean and Lean Diet
    Kale, Pecan, and Dried Cherry Salad with
      Rosemary Quinoa, 251–52
    Red Pepper–Cashew Endive with Grape
      Salad, 192
    Red Quinoa–Avocado Salad, 284
    Tuna Niçoise and White Bean Salad, 270
Salmon, 181
  Broiled Wild Salmon, 245
SAMe, for detoxification support, 326
Sauce
  Peanut Satay Sauce, 215
Saunas, for detoxification, 202, 306, 336
Scallops
  Caramelized Sea Scallops with Bok Choy,
    228–29
Sensitive Superstar case history, 25–28
Sesame oil
  Sesame-Ginger Detox Dressing, 144, 147
Sesame seeds
  Tomato and Kidney Bean Soup with Maple-
    Sesame Oranges, 253–54
Setbacks, managing, 148
7-Day In-Depth Detox, xvi
  advance meal preparation for, 133, 155,
    159, 170
  assessing completion of, 176
  menus, 137
    Day 4, 149–54
    Day 5, 156–61
    Day 6, 163–69
    Day 7, 171–75
  Mind-Body Detoxes for, 155, 162, 170, 175
  overview of, 53–54
  results from, xvi, 135

  setbacks in, 148
  snacks in, 139
  for "tune-ups," 287
  types of food in, 135, 136–44, 136
Shellfish
  Caramelized Sea Scallops with Bok Choy,
    228–29
Shopping
  for foods, 72, 93, 94–95, 96–97
  for supplements, 314–15
Shopping lists, for 3-Day Turbo Cleanse,
    107–8
Skin, as organ of detoxification, 336
Skin conditions, treating, 316–17
Slaw
  Chickpea Burger with Tahini Dressing and
    Red Cabbage Slaw, 278–79
  Red Cabbage Slaw, 280
Sleep
  caffeine preventing, 84
  importance of, xiv
  improving, 15, 87–88
  inadequate, yoga pose after, 267
  lack of, case history about, 13–15
  meditative technique before, 248
Small intestine, role of, 334
Smoking, as toxic, 7, 20
Smoking cessation, 80–81
Smoothies
  equipment for making, 73
  3-Day Turbo Cleanse, 99, 100
    boosters for, 102–6
    Bravocado! Smoothie, 123
    Carotenoid Smoothie, 122
    chewing, 99, 137
    Green Goodness Smoothie, 111
    Kale-icious! Smoothie, 127
    options for making, 101
Snacks. See also Afternoon Snack 1, in 3-Day
    Turbo Cleanse; Afternoon Snack 2, in
    3-Day Turbo Cleanse; Midmorning
    snacks
  in 7-Day In-Depth Detox, 139
  in 21-Day Clean and Lean Diet, 182
Soups
  7-Day In-Depth Detox, 144
    Carrot-Rhubarb Soup, 173
    Curry Butternut Squash Soup with
      Cayenne-Roasted Butternut Squash
      Seeds, 151–52
    Savory Mushroom Soup, 166–67
  21-Day Clean and Lean Diet
    "Creamy" Avocado-Broccoli Soup,
      233–34
    "Creamy" Garlic Soup with Spinach,
      226–27
    Roasted Brussels Sprouts and Hazelnuts
      with Miso Soup, 264–65
    Spicy White Bean and Spinach Soup, 222

Spinach-Tofu Soup with Gluten-Free
    Garlic Crostini, 271–72
Tomato and Kidney Bean Soup with
    Maple-Sesame Oranges, 253–54
Spaghetti squash
    Roasted Spaghetti Squash and Tomatoes,
    259–60
Spinach
    Black Bean and Spinach Tortilla, 235
    "Creamy" Garlic Soup with Spinach,
    226–27
    Crucifer Crusader, 131
    Green Goodness Smoothie, 111
    Spicy White Bean and Spinach Soup, 222
    Spinach-Tofu Soup with Gluten-Free Garlic
    Crostini, 271–72
Spirulina, 310
Stir-fry
    Peanut Satay Tofu Stir-Fry with Broccoli,
    214–15
Stomach, in digestive process, 332, 333
Storage, food, 93–94
Stress, toxic effects of, 7, 87, 89
Stress hormones, 7, 89
Stress-reduction techniques, 89, 91. See also
    Meditation techniques
Stretching, 91, 92
Sugar
    alternatives to, 198–99
    toxic effects of, 6, 182, 186
Sugary foods, eliminating, 81–82
Sun Salutation yoga series, 124–25
Supplements, 308–12, 314–15
Support groups, 95
Sweating, for detoxification, 202, 306, 336
Sweeteners
    natural, 198–99
    nonfood, 236
Sweet potatoes
    Carotenoid Smoothie, 122
    Curried Lentils with Sweet Potato and
    Chard, 193–94
    Roasted Root Vegetables, 220–21
    Rosemary Celeriac and Root Vegetables,
    168
    Twice-Baked Fruit-and-Nut-Stuffed Sweet
    Potatoes, 275
    Zucchini and Sweet Potato Frittata, 211–12
Sympathetic nervous system, 13
Symptom troubleshooting, 312–13, 316–18

T

Tabbouleh
    Tahini-Buckwheat Tabbouleh, 153
Tahini
    Chickpea Burger with Tahini Dressing and
    Red Cabbage Slaw, 278–79
    Lemon-Tahini Dressing, 144, 145
    Tahini-Buckwheat Tabbouleh, 153

Tahini Green Beans, 208
Taxonomy of disease, xiii
Teas
    after-dinner, 143
    morning detox, 140–41
Telomeres, lengthening, 53
Tests, for evaluating toxicity, 29–30, 32–34
Thickeners, 106
Thistles, 310, 312
3-Day Turbo Cleanse
    assessing completion of, 133
    boosters for, 102–6
    case histories about, 14, 15, 16–17, 19, 21,
    27
    caution with, 96–97
    menus, 109
        Day 1, 110–16
        Day 2, 118–23
        Day 3, 126–31
    Mind-Body Detoxes for, 117, 124–25, 132
    origin of, xvi–xvii
    overview of, 51–52, 98–101
    results from, xvii, 52, 134, 136
    self-discipline for, 10, 98–99
    setbacks in, 148
    shopping lists for, 107–8
    for "tune-ups," 287
Tofu
    Peanut Satay Tofu Stir-Fry with Broccoli,
    214–15
    Spinach-Tofu Soup with Gluten-Free Garlic
    Crostini, 271–72
    Tofu-Veggie Scramble with Gluten-Free
    Toast, 263
Tomatoes
    Hot Tomato! Juice, 129
    Roasted Spaghetti Squash and Tomatoes,
    259–60
    Tofu-Veggie Scramble with Gluten-Free
    Toast, 263
    Tomato and Kidney Bean Soup with Maple-
    Sesame Oranges, 253–54
Tortillas
    Almond Butter Banana-Raspberry Tortilla,
    150
    Black Bean and Spinach Tortilla, 235
    Green Gazpacho with Chive-Cayenne Oil
    and Tortilla Toasts, 276–77
    Hummus and Veggie Rainbow Tortilla,
    200
    Poached Egg–Avocado Tortilla, 257
Toxicity
    assessing (see Questionnaires, for assessing
    toxicity)
    from chemicals, 3–4
    diagnoses related to, 3
    prevalence of, 30–31
    preventing disease from, xiii–xiv
    testing for, 29–30, 32–34

Toxic triggers
  bad habits, 19–20
  convenience foods, 17
  household cleaners, 25
  lack of sleep, 15
  overwork, 13
  travel, 22
  wheat, 27
Toxins
  effect on cells, 320–22
  in foods, 49, 60, 66, 180, 181, 330
  journaling about, 91–93
  in kitchen, 74–75
  prevalence of, 3–4, 48–49, 319–20
  primary sources of, 6–7, 8–9
  from rapid weight loss, 68–69
  released by Detox Prescription, xvi, xvii, 5,
      100, 140, 179, 312
  from smoking, 80, 81
  from stress, 89, 291
Traditional Chinese Medicine, 297–98
Travel, as toxic trigger, 22
Triclosan, 9
Truffles
  Rawsome Chocolate Truffles, 183, 186–87
Tuna
  Tuna Niçoise and White Bean Salad, 270
Turmeric, 310, 317, 318
21-Day Clean and Lean Diet
  advance meal preparation for, 176, 194,
      202, 207, 216, 223, 229, 236, 248,
      254, 260, 267, 273, 281
  assessing completion of, 237, 287–88
  characteristics of, 178–80
  foods added to, 138, 139, 180–83, 186–89
  menus, 184–85, 240–41
    Day 8, 190–94
    Day 9, 196–97, 200–201
    Day 10, 203–8
    Day 11, 210–15
    Day 12, 217–22
    Day 13, 224–29
    Day 14, 231–35
    Day 15, 242–47
    Day 16, 249–54
    Day 17, 256–60
    Day 18, 262–66
    Day 19, 268–72
    Day 20, 274–80
    Day 21, 282–85
  Mind-Body Detoxes for, 195, 202, 209,
      216, 223, 230, 236, 248, 255, 261,
      267, 273, 281, 286
  overview of, 54–58
  results from, xviii, 27
  setbacks in, 148
  transitioning to, 177–78

Ulcerative colitis. See Inflammatory bowel
  disease

Vegan diet. See also 7-Day In-Depth Detox
  beans in, 138
  health benefits of, 53–54
  resistance to, 54–55
  rotating carnivorous foods with, 57–58
Vegetables. See also specific vegetables
  Dirty Dozen and Clean Fifteen, 61, 63
  Hummus and Veggie Rainbow Tortilla, 200
  organic, 59–61 (see also Organic foods,
      produce)
  Roasted Root Vegetables, 220–21
  Roasted Veggie and Hummus Romaine
      Wraps, 258
  Tofu-Veggie Scramble with Gluten-Free
      Toast, 263
  toxins in, 6

Walking, 91, 216, 230
Walking buddy, 95
Walnuts
  Baked Acorn Squash with Apples and
      Walnuts, 225
  Black Rice Porridge with Blueberries and
      Toasted Walnuts, 283
  Buckwheat-Banana-Walnut Cereal, 232
  Lentil-Walnut Pâté, 244
  Nutty Baked Apples, 188
  Raw Walnut Milk, 116
Water
  drinking, 90
  toxins in, 7, 49
Weight, excess
  case history about, 16–18
  toxic effects of, 7
Weight gain, case histories about, 14–15, 18
Weight loss
  rapid, negative effects of, 68–69
  slow, benefits of, 69
  from 3-Day Turbo Cleanse, 21
  from 21-Day Clean and Lean Diet, 179
Wheat
  eliminating, 27–28, 83–84, 178–79
  as toxic trigger, 27
Wheat Belly, 27
Wheat sensitivity, 26–27, 83

Yacon syrup and powder, 199
Yoga poses
  Legs-Up-the-Wall, 267
  Sun Salutation, 124–25
  Warrior Flow, 209
Yogurt
  Coconut Yogurt, Berry, and Hemp Heart
      Parfait, 157
  health benefits of, 56

Zucchini
  Zucchini and Sweet Potato Frittata,
      211–12